Adrenal Disorders

100 Cases from the Adrenal Clinic

William F. Young, Jr., MD, MSc
Professor of Medicine
Tyson Family Endocrinology Clinical Professor
Division of Endocrinology, Diabetes, Metabolism, and Nutrition
Mayo Clinic
Rochester, MN, USA

Irina Bancos, MD
Associate Professor of Medicine
Division of Endocrinology, Diabetes, Metabolism, and Nutrition
Department of Laboratory Medicine and Pathology
Mayo Clinic
Rochester, MN, USA

ELSEVIER

Elsevier

1600 John F. Kennedy Blvd.
Ste 1600
Philadelphia, PA 19103-2899

Adrenal Disorders: 100 Cases from the Adrenal Clinic　　　　　　　ISBN: 9780323792851

Content Strategist: Humayra R. Khan
Senior Content Development Specialist: Malvika Shah
Publishing Services Manager: Shereen Jameel
Senior Project Manager: Kamatchi Madhavan
Design Direction: Amy Buxton

Printed in India
Last digit is the print number:　9　8　7　6　5　4　3　2

We dedicate this book to our patients. Adrenal gland disorders can present with some of the most challenging signs and symptoms across all fields of medicine. Many of our patients made long journeys in the health system before it was determined that they had an adrenal gland disorder. Individual perseverance and resiliency are documented in every page of this book. Our patients volunteered to have their stories shared herein and proceeds from this book will be devoted to adrenal-based research at the Mayo Clinic.

WILLIAM F. YOUNG, Jr., MD, MSc
IRINA BANCOS, MD

Preface

Why write a book of individual case reports in the era of evidence-based medicine and randomized controlled trials? Single case reports are passé: nothing to be learned there, right? Well, no. In the pages of this book, we impart valuable insights and clinical nuances you will not find in large case series or clinical trials. Many adrenal gland disorders are rare and not amenable to the rigors of advanced scientific trials. In addition, many of our best teaching moments have been based on the care of a single patient with a challenging clinical scenario. We have relied on decades of personal experience in managing rare and complex adrenal disorders, and with these 100 case scenarios we share our lessons learned.

William F. Young, Jr., MD, MSc

Irina Bancos, MD

Acknowledgments

The patients documented in these pages were not evaluated and managed by the authors alone. Successful care for patients with complex adrenal gland disorders can be accomplished only with a multidisciplinary team. Our team for these 100 patients included endocrine surgeons (Benzon M. Dy, MD; David R. Farley, MD; Trenton R. Foster, MD; Clive S. Grant, MD; Melanie L. Lyden, MD; Travis J. McKenzie, MD; Geoffrey B. Thompson; Jon van Heerden, MD); hepatobiliary and pancreas surgeons (Michael L. Kendrick, MD; David M. Nagorney, MD); pituitary neurosurgeons (John L. D. Atkinson, MD; Jamie J. Van Gompel, MD; Fredric B. Meyer, MD); cardiothoracic surgeons (Peter C. Pairolero, MD; Hartzell V. Schaff, MD; K. Robert Shen, MD); an otolaryngology–head and neck surgeon (Jan L. Kasperbauer, MD); vascular surgeon (Thomas C. Bower, MD); obstetricians and gynecologic surgeons (Norman P. Davies, MBBS, MD; Carl H. Rose, MD; C. Robert Stanhope, MD); interventional radiologists (James C. Andrews, MD; Thomas D. Atwell, MD; Patrick W. Eiken, MD; Anthony W. Stanson, MD); neuroradiologists (Harry Cloft, MD, PhD; David F. Kallmes, MD; Jonathan M. Morris, MD); endocrine pathologists (J. Aidan Carney, MD, PhD; Lori A. Erickson, MD; Ricardo V. Lloyd, MD, PhD; Michael Rivera, MD); medical oncologists (Keith C. Bible, MD, PhD; Ashish V. Chintakuntlawar, MBBS, PhD; Ronald L. Richardson, MD; Steven I. Robinson, MBBS; Mabel Ryder, MD); and endocrine laboratorians (Alicia Algeciras-Schimnich, PhD; Stefan K. Grebe, MD, PhD; Ravinder J. Singh, PhD).

In our Division of Endocrinology, Diabetes, Metabolism, and Nutrition at Mayo Clinic Rochester, we have special interest groups that we refer to as "core groups." Our Pituitary-Gonad-Adrenal Core Group membership over the decades during which we cared for the patients documented in these pages includes Charles F. Abboud, MB, BCh; Paul C. Carpenter, MD; Alice Y. Chang, MD; Caroline Davidge-Pitts, MB, BCh; Dana Erickson, MD; Neena Natt, MD; Todd B. Nippoldt, MD; Robert C. Northcutt, MD; Raymond V. Randall, MD; Robert M. Salassa, MD; and Richard E. Weeks, MD. Our approach to case management has been a group effort with our colleagues based on clinical practice experiences through which we learn not only from our patients but also from each other.

William F. Young, Jr., MD, MSc

Irina Bancos, MD

About the Authors

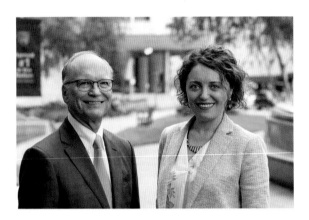

William F. Young, Jr, MD, MSc, is Professor of Medicine at Mayo Clinic College of Medicine, Mayo Clinic, Rochester, Minnesota, USA. He holds the Tyson Family Endocrinology Clinical Professorship in Honor of Vahab Fatourechi, MD. He received his bachelor degree and his medical degree from Michigan State University and his master of science degree from the University of Minnesota. Dr. Young trained in internal medicine at William Beaumont Hospital in Royal Oak, Michigan, and completed a fellowship in endocrinology and metabolism at Mayo Clinic in Rochester, Minnesota. He has been a member of the staff at Mayo Clinic since 1984. Dr. Young is the recipient of multiple education and leadership awards, he is a past president of the Endocrine Society, and past chair of the Division of Endocrinology at Mayo Clinic. Dr. Young's clinical research focuses on primary aldosteronism and pheochromocytoma. He has published more than 350 articles on endocrine hypertension and adrenal and pituitary disorders. Dr. Young has been the invited speaker for more than 30 named lectureships, delivered more than 650 presentations at national and international meetings, and he has been an invited visiting professor for more than 150 medical institutions.

Irina Bancos, MD, is Associate Professor of Medicine at Mayo Clinic College of Medicine, Mayo Clinic, Rochester, Minnesota, USA. She also serves as the associate program director for the clinical endocrinology training program. Dr. Bancos received her medical degree from the Iuliu Hatieganu Medical University in Cluj-Napoca, Romania. She completed her internal medicine residency at Danbury Hospital in Connecticut, USA and fellowship in endocrinology and metabolism at Mayo Clinic in Rochester, Minnesota. In addition, Dr. Bancos completed a 2-year adrenal research fellowship (Mayo Foundation Scholarship) at the University of Birmingham, UK. In 2015 she returned to Mayo Clinic, where her clinical and research interests include adrenal and pituitary tumors, pheochromocytoma/paraganglioma, primary aldosteronism, adrenal insufficiency, congenital adrenal hyperplasia, Cushing syndrome, and mechanisms of steroid regulation of health and disease. Between 2015 and 2018, Dr. Bancos was the principal investigator and leader of the Transform the Adrenal Practice team at Mayo Clinic. Dr. Bancos has been a recipient of several awards, including Teacher of the Year awards, Laureate award in Endocrinology, and the ENSAT award for research in adrenal adenomas. Dr. Bancos has published more than 140 scientific articles and currently holds several grants studying the impact of steroids on health.

Contents

Incidentally Discovered Adrenal Mass

Adrenal Incidentaloma

Adrenal incidentaloma is an adrenal mass discovered incidentally on cross-sectional abdominal imaging performed for indications other than suspected adrenal mass. Over the preceding two decades, the incidence rate of adrenal tumors increased 10-fold, most likely as a result of the widespread use of computed tomography (CT) imaging.[1] In a prospective study of adults undergoing abdominal CT imaging, the prevalence of adrenal tumors was 7%.[2] Adrenal tumors are rare in childhood and young adults and are usually diagnosed in the sixth decade.[1] The etiology of adrenal tumors can be broadly separated into five categories: (1) adrenocortical adenomas (85%), (2) other benign adrenal masses (4%–6%), (3) pheochromocytomas (1%–3%), (4) adrenocortical carcinomas (<1%–3%), and (5) other malignant adrenal masses (3%–8%)[1] (Table A.1). In any patient with an adrenal mass, workup needs to determine whether the adrenal mass is malignant and whether it is hormonally active.

Diagnosis of Malignant Adrenal Mass

Tumor size, tumor growth, history of extraadrenal malignancy, and imaging characteristics are helpful in diagnosing adrenal malignancy[3–6] (see Table A.1).

TUMOR SIZE AND TUMOR GROWTH

Adrenal tumors >4 cm in diameter represent 17% of adrenal tumors seen in the tertiary endocrine center.[7] The proportions of malignant adrenal tumors and pheochromocytomas is high in large adrenal tumors, representing 31% and 22%, respectively.[7] Accelerated tumor growth (>20% in 3–6 months) is suggestive of a malignant adrenal mass, while no or minimal tumor growth suggests a benign adrenal mass. Pheochromocytomas usually grow slowly, <1 cm per year. As reported in a systematic review of 2023 patients with adrenocortical adenomas, 2.5% of adenomas may demonstrate a growth >1 cm over 3–5 years, depending on when in relation to its natural history the tumor is first discovered.[8] However, the risk of malignant transformation was 0%.[8]

IMAGING CHARACTERISTICS

Hounsfield unit (HU) measurement of adrenal mass on unenhanced CT is an important diagnostic step that may distinguish benign adrenal mass from malignancy or pheochromocytoma. Adrenocortical adenomas can be lipid rich (with unenhanced CT attenuation <10 HU) in approximately 60% of cases, demonstrate an unenhanced CT attenuation between 10 and 20 HU in approximately 20%–25% of cases, and >20 HU (lipid poor) in 15%–20% of cases.[1,7] Adrenocortical carcinomas (ACCs), other malignant adrenal tumors (sarcomas, metastases), and pheochromocytomas usually demonstrate an unenhanced CT attenuation of >20–30 HU, and infrequently 10–20 HU (approximately 2%–5%).[1,4–7,9–11] Thus a homogeneous adrenal mass with an unenhanced CT attenuation of <10 HU excludes malignant adrenal tumors and pheochromocytomas, and imaging follow-up in these cases is not needed in most cases. Lipid-poor adrenal masses should either be resected or followed closely with serial imaging.[1,2]

TABLE A.1 Presentation of Adrenal Tumors	Benign Adrenal Mass	Malignant Adrenal Mass	Pheochromocytoma
Prevalence (population)	90%	9%	1%
Prevalence (endocrine clinic)	80%–85%	5%–10%	5%–10%
Mode of discovery	Most: incidental	Incidental: 40% Nonincidental (cancer staging, hormone excess, abdominal pain, B symptoms[1]): 60%	Incidental: 60% Hormone excess: 30% Genetic screening: 10%
Tumor size	Usually <4 cm	Adrenal cortical carcinoma: usually >6 cm Other malignancy: Variable	Usually >4 cm, variable (smaller when genetic screening and preclinical)
Tumor laterality	15%–20% bilateral	Adrenal cortical carcinoma <0.1% bilateral Other malignancy: 20%–40% bilateral	5%–10% bilateral (if genetic predisposition, e.g., VHL, MEN2, NF1.)
Unenhanced computed tomography attenuation, HU	HU <10: 50%–60% HU 10–20: 20%–30% HU >20: 10%–20%	HU>20 (usually >30 HU)	HU>20 (usually >30 HU)
Magnetic resonance imaging	Chemical shift: present – 60–80% Chemical shift: absent – 20–40%	Chemical shift: absent	Chemical shift: absent
[1]FDG-18 positron emission tomography	FDG-18 uptake – usually absent	FDG-18 uptake – present	FDG-18 uptake – present
Tumor growth	Usually <1 cm in 1 year	Usually >1 cm in 3–6 months	Usually <1 cm in 1 year

[1]a B symptom is a common way to describe fever, weight loss, and other symptoms related to malignancy. *FDG-18*, F-18 fluorodeoxyglucose; *HU*, Hounsfield units; *MEN2*, multiple endocrine neoplasia type 2; *NF1*, neurofibromatosis type 1; *VHL*, von Hippel-Lindau.

Magnetic resonance imaging (MRI) chemical shift analysis is similar in accuracy to the unenhanced CT attenuation.[5] F-18 fluorodeoxyglucose (FDG) positron emission tomography (PET) can also be used in diagnosis of malignant adrenal tumors, with positive FDG uptake in the adrenal mass that is greater than the uptake in liver suggestive of malignancy. However, FDG PET demonstrates sensitivity and specificity of approximately 85%–90%, with both false-positive (functioning adrenal adenoma, pheochromocytoma) and false-negative (small metastasis) results.[5,10]

URINE STEROID PROFILING

Urine steroid profiling has been recently validated as an accurate diagnostic test for ACC.[9] It is most useful in larger adrenal tumors with indeterminate imaging characteristics for diagnostic purposes, and can avoid unnecessary biopsy or surgery.[12]

ADRENAL BIOPSY

Adrenal biopsy is a procedure that is rarely needed in the workup of adrenal masses.[13,14] It is reserved for patients with indeterminate adrenal masses (e.g., unenhanced CT attenuation >10 HU), after excluding pheochromocytoma, and in someone likely to have an adrenal metastasis.[10,13,14] Adrenal metastasis should be suspected in any patient with a history of extraadrenal malignancy who presents with an indeterminate adrenal mass. In a retrospective study of 579 patients with adrenal metastases, 59% were discovered during cancer staging imaging, 36% were incidentally discovered during workup performed for another reason,

TABLE A.2 Hormonal Workup in Patients With Adrenal Tumors			
Adrenal Hormone Excess	**Indication for Testing**	**First-Line Testing**	**Additional or Confirmatory Testing**
Adrenal hypercortisolism (overt or mild)	Anyone with adrenal mass	1-mg overnight dexamethasone suppression test (abnormal: >1.8 mcg/dL)	ACTH, DHEA-S, 24-hour urine cortisol Repeat 1-mg or perform 8-mg dexamethasone suppression test
Adrenal hyperaldosteronism	Anyone with hypertension or spontaneous hypokalemia	Morning PAC and PRA or PRC (abnormal: aldosterone >10 ng/dL and suppressed renin)	Unnecessary if spontaneous hypokalemia, PAC >20 ng/dL, and PRA <1.0 ng/mL per hour Oral sodium loading test or saline infusion test
Catecholamine excess	Anyone with indeterminate adrenal mass (HU>10)	Plasma or 24-hour urine fractionated metanephrines	Usually not needed unless interfering medications are suspected

ACTH, Corticotropin; *DHEA-S*, dehydroepiandrosterone sulfate; *HU*, Hounsfield units; *PAC*, plasma aldosterone concentration; *PRA*, plasma renin activity; *PRC*, plasma renin concentration.

and 5% were detected as a result of other symptoms.[11] Adrenal metastases originated from the lung (39%), genitourinary (28%), gastrointestinal (14%), and other (20%) organ systems.[11]

Adrenal biopsy is not accurate in distinguishing between adrenocortical carcinoma and adrenocortical adenoma and should not be used with that intent.[15–17] The nondiagnostic rate for adrenal biopsy is around 5%, and complication rate is 3%.[15–17]

Diagnosis of Adrenal Hormonal Excess

Every patient with adrenal mass needs a careful evaluation for adrenal hormonal excess. Assessment includes workup for autonomous cortisol secretion, workup for primary aldosteronism, and workup for catecholamine excess (Table A.2).

Later sections in this book will address primary aldosteronism, overt Cushing syndrome, and pheochromocytoma.

MILD AUTONOMOUS CORTISOL SECRETION

The most common hormonal abnormality diagnosed in patients with adrenal incidentalomas is mild autonomous cortisol secretion (MACS). MACS is defined as abnormal overnight 1-mg dexamethasone suppression test (DST >1.8 mcg/dL) and is detected in up to 50% of

patients with adrenal cortical adenomas.[2,13,14] Patients with MACS demonstrate a higher prevalence of cardiovascular risk factors (e.g., hypertension, diabetes mellitus type 2, obesity, dyslipidemia), cardiovascular events and mortality, osteopenia, osteoporosis, and fractures.[8,18,19] In a systematic review and metaanalysis of adrenalectomy versus conservative management in MACS, patients undergoing adrenalectomy experienced improvement in diabetes mellitus type 2 and hypertension.[20] However, studies included in this systematic review were of low to moderate quality and had heterogeneous definitions of both MACS and comorbidity improvement. Identifying patients most likely to experience improvement in long-term outcomes is challenging, and thus the decision of adrenalectomy needs to be individualized. The decision on adrenalectomy versus conservative managements needs to be individualized to patient age, comorbidities, tumor imaging phenotype, local surgical expertise, and patient preference.

REFERENCES

1. Ebbehoj A, Li D, Kaur RJ, et al. Epidemiology of adrenal tumours in Olmsted County, Minnesota, USA: a population-based cohort study. *Lancet Diabetes Endocrinol.* 2020;8(11):894–902.
2. Reimondo G, Castellano E, Grosso M, et al. Adrenal incidentalomas are tied to increased risk of diabetes:

findings from a prospective study. *J Clin Endocrinol Metab*. 2020;105(4).

3. Bancos I, Arlt W. Diagnosis of a malignant adrenal mass: the role of urinary steroid metabolite profiling. *Curr Opin Endocrinol Diabetes Obes*. 2017;24(3):200–207.

4. Canu L, Van Hemert JAW, Kerstens MN, et al. CT Characteristics of pheochromocytoma: relevance for the evaluation of adrenal incidentaloma. *J Clin Endocrinol Metab*. 2019;104(2):312–318.

5. Dinnes J, Bancos I, Ferrante di Ruffano L, et al. management of endocrine disease: imaging for the diagnosis of malignancy in incidentally discovered adrenal masses: a systematic review and meta-analysis. *Eur J Endocrinol*. 2016;175(2):R51–R64.

6. Gruber LM, Strajina V, Bancos I, et al. Not all adrenal incidentalomas require biochemical testing to exclude pheochromocytoma: Mayo Clinic experience and a meta-analysis. *Gland Surg*. 2020;9(2):362–371.

7. Iniguez-Ariza NM, Kohlenberg JD, Delivanis DA, et al. Clinical, biochemical, and radiological characteristics of a single-center retrospective cohort of 705 large adrenal tumors. *Mayo Clin Proc Innov Qual Outcomes*. 2018;2(1):30–39.

8. Elhassan YS, Alahdab F, Prete A, et al. Natural history of adrenal incidentalomas with and without mild autonomous cortisol excess: a systematic review and meta-analysis. *Ann Intern Med*. 2019;171(2):107–116.

9. Bancos I, Taylor AE, Chortis V, et al. Urine steroid metabolomics for the differential diagnosis of adrenal incidentalomas in the EURINE-ACT study: a prospective test validation study. *Lancet Diabetes Endocrinol*. 2020;8(9):773–781.

10. Delivanis DA, Bancos I, Atwell TD, et al. Diagnostic performance of unenhanced computed tomography and (18) F-fluorodeoxyglucose positron emission tomography in indeterminate adrenal tumours. *Clin Endocrinol (Oxf)*. 2018;88(1):30–36.

11. Mao JJ, Dages KN, Suresh M, Bancos I. Presentation, disease progression and outcomes of adrenal gland metastases. *Clin Endocrinol (Oxf)*. 2020;93(5):546–554.

12. Chortis V, Bancos I, Nijman T, et al. Urine steroid metabolomics as a novel tool for detection of recurrent adrenocortical carcinoma. *J Clin Endocrinol Metab*. 2020;105(3).

13. Fassnacht M, Arlt W, Bancos I, et al. Management of adrenal incidentalomas: European Society of Endocrinology Clinical Practice Guideline in collaboration with the European Network for the Study of Adrenal Tumors. *Eur J Endocrinol*. 2016;175(2):G1–G34.

14. Vaidya A, Hamrahian A, Bancos I, Fleseriu M, Ghayee HK. The evaluation of incidentally discovered adrenal masses. *Endocr Pract*. 2019;25(2):178–192.

15. Bancos I, Tamhane S, Shah M, et al. diagnosis of endocrine disease: the diagnostic performance of adrenal biopsy: a systematic review and meta-analysis. *European Journal of Endocrinology*. 2016;175(2):R65–R80.

16. Delivanis DA, Erickson D, Atwell TD, et al. Procedural and clinical outcomes of percutaneous adrenal biopsy in a high-risk population for adrenal malignancy. *Clin Endocrinol (Oxf)*. 2016;85(5):710–716.

17. Zhang CD, Delivanis DA, Eiken PW, Atwell TD, Bancos I. Adrenal biopsy: performance and use. *Minerva Endocrinol*. 2019;44(3):288–300.

18. Delivanis DA, Athimulam S, Bancos I. Modern management of mild autonomous cortisol secretion. *Clin Pharmacol Ther*. 2019;106(6):1209–1221.

19. Athimulam S, Bancos I. Evaluation of bone health in patients with adrenal tumors. *Curr Opin Endocrinol Diabetes Obes*. 2019;26(3):125–132.

20. Bancos I, Alahdab F, Crowley RK, et al. therapy of endocrine disease: improvement of cardiovascular risk factors after adrenalectomy in patients with adrenal tumors and subclinical Cushing's syndrome: a systematic review and meta-analysis. *Eur J Endocrinol*. 2016;175(6):R283–R295.

45-Year-Old Woman With an Incidentally Discovered Large Adrenal Mass

Adrenal tumors >4 cm in diameter represent 17% of adrenal tumors seen in the tertiary endocrine center. The proportion of malignant adrenal tumors and pheochromocytomas is high in large adrenal tumors, representing 31% and 22%, respectively. Hounsfield unit (HU) measurement of adrenal mass on unenhanced computed tomography (CT) is an important diagnostic step that may distinguish benign adrenal mass from malignancy or pheochromocytoma.

Case Report

The patient was a 45-year-old woman with history of nephrolithiasis who was incidentally discovered with a 4.9 cm left adrenal mass on abdominal CT scan performed for abdominal pain. Past medical history included migraines, fibromyalgia, and gastric bypass performed 10 years prior. At the time of presentation, her weight was normal and she did not have hypertension or diabetes mellitus type 2. She denied symptoms consistent with catecholamine excess or Cushing syndrome.

INVESTIGATIONS

On unenhanced CT the left adrenal mass was homogeneous and lipid rich, measuring 4.9 cm in the largest diameter and demonstrating a CT attenuation of –13 HU (Fig. 1.1). The right adrenal gland appeared normal. Prior imaging from 8 years ago was obtained for comparison and revealed a 3.7 cm adrenal mass (–14 HU) (Fig. 1.2).

The baseline laboratory test results are shown in Table 1.1. The serum corticotropin (ACTH) and dehydroepiandrosterone-sulfate (DHEA-S) concentrations were not low and cortisol suppressed normally with an overnight 1-mg dexamethasone suppression test (DST) (Table 1.1). Thus, the adrenal adenoma was not secreting cortisol autonomously.

Discussion

In a study of 705 patients with adrenal tumors >4 cm from Mayo Clinic published in 2018, 31% represented benign adrenal cortical adenoma.[1] None of pheochromocytomas (22%) and malignant adrenal tumors (31%) demonstrated unenhanced CT attenuation <10 HU, with the lowest attenuation in malignant tumors and pheochromocytomas being 14 HU and 18 HU, respectively.[1] As reported in a systematic review of 2023 patients with adenomas, 2.5% of adenomas may demonstrate a growth >1 cm depending on when in relation to its natural history the tumor is first discovered.[2]

Treatment

The patient was counseled that adrenal mass was a benign nonfunctioning adrenal adenoma. This was concluded based on imaging phenotype of the adrenal mass with low unenhanced CT attenuation, but also based on a low growth rate of only 1.2 cm over 8 years. The patient was advised that no further endocrine follow-up was necessary.

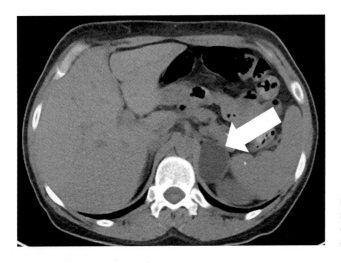

Fig. 1.1 Axial image from an unenhanced computed tomography (CT) scan showed a lipid-rich (−13 Hounsfield unit [HU]) 4.9 × 3.2 cm left adrenal nodule (*arrow*). The right adrenal gland appeared normal on all images.

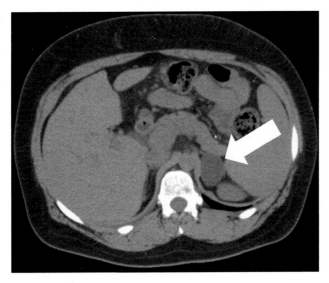

Fig. 1.2 Axial image from an unenhanced computed tomography (CT) scan performed 8 years earlier demonstrated a lipid-rich (−14 Hounsfield unit [HU]) 3.7 × 3.1 cm left adrenal nodule (*arrow*).

TABLE 1.1 Laboratory Tests		
Biochemical Test	**Result**	**Reference Range**
1-mg overnight DST, mcg/dL	1.1	<1.8
ACTH, pg/mL	28	7.2–63
DHEA-S, mcg/dL	178	18–284
Aldosterone, ng/dL	6.2	<21
Plasma renin activity, ng/mL per hour	3.2	2.9–10.8
Plasma metanephrine, nmol/L	0.22	<0.5
Plasma normetanephrine, nmol/L	0.7	<0.9
Urine free cortisol, mcg/24 h	21	3.5–45

ACTH, Corticotropin; *DHEA-S*, dehydroepiandrosterone-sulfate; *DST*, dexamethasone suppression test.

Key Points

- The risk of malignancy and pheochromocytoma is proportional to tumor size.
- In endocrine practice, 30% of adrenal tumors >4 cm in diameter are malignant and 22% are pheochromocytomas.
- Unenhanced CT attenuation <10 HU in a homogeneous adrenal mass excludes malignancy and pheochromocytoma.

REFERENCES

1. Iniguez-Ariza NM, Kohlenberg JD, Delivanis DA, et al. Clinical, biochemical, and radiological characteristics of a single-center retrospective cohort of 705 large adrenal tumors. *Mayo Clin Proc Innov Qual Outcomes*. 2018;2:30–39.
2. Elhassan YS, Alahdab F, Prete A, et al. Natural history of adrenal incidentalomas with and without mild autonomous cortisol excess: a systematic review and meta-analysis. *Ann Intern Med*. 2019;171:107–116.

Adrenal Mass in a Patient With a History of Extraadrenal Malignancy: The Role of Imaging

Adrenal metastasis should be suspected in any patient with a history of extraadrenal malignancy presenting with an indeterminate adrenal mass. Full hormonal workup and assessment of imaging characteristics are important even when the likelihood of adrenal metastasis is high.[1,2] Pheochromocytoma presents with similar indeterminate adrenal imaging, and, if mistaken for an adrenal metastasis, a biopsy can be inadvertently performed, resulting in potentially severe side effects.[3,4] Imaging characteristics of the adrenal mass can help exclude malignancy (as in lipid-rich tumors), and avoid additional testing, such as adrenal biopsy.[5,6] Finally, finding adrenal hormonal excess such as cortisol, androgen, or aldosterone excess can help diagnose an adrenocortical adenoma or carcinoma and exclude other etiologies of adrenal tumors that are incapable of steroid production.[4]

Case Report

The patient was a 66-year-old woman who was referred for evaluation of a newly found left 2.2 cm adrenal mass discovered on a contrast-enhanced computed tomography (CT) of the abdomen performed for breast cancer staging.

In addition to a recently diagnosed locally advanced left breast adenocarcinoma, the patient's past medical history was positive for hypertension and primary hypothyroidism. Her medications included levothyroxine and hydrochlorothiazide. At the time of evaluation, she had no symptoms to suggest adrenal hormonal excess and review of systems was negative. On physical examination, her body mass index (BMI) was 27.38 kg/m^2, blood pressure was 135/80 mmHg, and heart rate was 98 beats per minute.

INVESTIGATIONS

Baseline laboratory testing was obtained, and functioning pheochromocytoma and primary aldosteronism were excluded. However, the overnight dexamethasone suppression test was abnormal, and the patient was diagnosed with mild autonomous cortisol secretion (MACS) (Table 2.1). An unenhanced CT scan was obtained (Fig. 2.1) and demonstrated that the 2.2 × 2.0 × 1.8 cm left adrenal mass had an attenuation of –15 Hounsfield units (HU). A F-18 fluorodeoxyglucose (FDG) positron emission tomography (PET) scan was performed at the same time for breast cancer staging and revealed that the adrenal mass had FDG uptake of 5.3 maximum standard unit value (SUV_{max}) (Fig. 2.2).

TREATMENT AND FOLLOW-UP

The patient was advised that she had a lipid-rich adrenal adenoma with autonomous cortisol secretion. After consideration of management options, she elected conservative follow-up with periodic reevaluation for MACS-induced comorbidities.

Imaging Follow-Up

Although imaging was not recommended for follow-up of the adrenal mass, it was available because of follow-up of breast cancer for 8 years after the initial diagnosis. The adrenal mass was stable in size over 8 years of follow-up and demonstrated stable FDG uptake over the years.

TABLE 2.1 **Laboratory Tests**					
Biochemical Test	**Baseline**	**1 Year Later**	**2 Years Later**	**6 Years Later**	**Reference Range**
Post 1-mg DST serum cortisol, mcg/dL	2.6	3.1	2.5	2.9	<1.8
ACTH, pg/mL	30		54.2	21	10–60
DHEA-S, mcg/dL	34			51	15–157
Aldosterone, ng/dL	8.1				<21
Renin plasma activity, ng/mL per hour	1.3				<0.6–3
Plasma metanephrine, nmol/L	0.2				<0.5
Plasma normetanephrine, nmol/L	0.63				<0.9

ACTH, Corticotropin; *DHEA-S*, dehydroepiandrosterone-sulfate; *DST*, dexamethasone suppression test.

Biochemical Follow-Up

The patient had the 1-mg dexamethasone suppression test repeated several times over the years with little variability and consistent with MACS (Table 2.1).

Clinical Follow-Up

Bone mineral density was obtained at baseline and repeated 5 years later; it revealed no baseline osteoporosis or osteopenia and no significant decline of bone density over 5 years. At baseline the patient was tested for dyslipidemia and diabetes mellitus type 2, with normal results. At the time of last evaluation 6 years later, she developed prediabetes. Her BMI fluctuated between 22.4 and 27.6 kg/m^2, without an upward trend.

Discussion

Breast adenocarcinoma metastasis in the adrenal gland is infrequently seen, representing <2% of all adrenal metastases.[7] Adrenal metastasis should be suspected in any patient with a history of extraadrenal malignancy who presents with an indeterminate adrenal mass. Adrenal metastasis can be safely excluded if adrenal

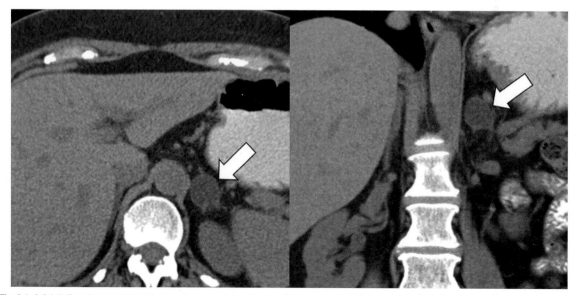

Fig. 2.1 Axial (*left*) and coronal (*right*) images from unenhanced computed tomography (CT) scan demonstrated a left adrenal mass (*arrows*) measuring 2.2 × 2.0 × 1.8 cm and with unenhanced CT attenuation of −16 Hounsfield units (HU).

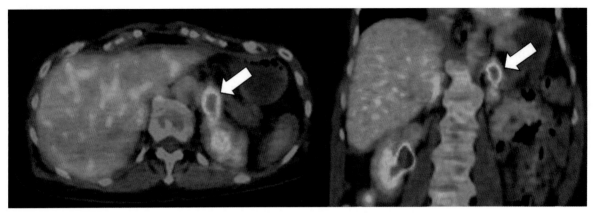

Fig. 2.2 Axial (*left*) and coronal (*right*) images from F-18 fluorodeoxyglucose (FDG) positron emission tomography (PET) scan demonstrated FDG uptake in the adrenal mass (*arrows*) measuring 5.3 maximum standard unit value (SUVmax), and no other foci of activity.

mass is lipid rich (i.e., unenhanced CT attenuation <10 HU), even if patient has a history of extraadrenal malignancy.[5,6,8] FDG PET scan is a valuable test for diagnosis of malignancy; however, both false-positive (functioning adrenal adenoma, pheochromocytoma) and false-negative (small metastasis) results occur.[5] In this case, FDG positivity was likely due to autonomous cortisol secretion from the adrenal adenoma.

The patient was diagnosed with MACS based on an abnormal dexamethasone suppression test.[1,2,9] She did have mild hypertension and eventually developed prediabetes. However, she did not have obesity, weight gain, osteoporosis, or other manifestations of MACS. As demonstrated in this case, MACS associated with a stable adrenal adenoma does not demonstrate worsening in cortisol autonomy and does not progress to overt Cushing syndrome.[10] However, comorbidities associated with MACS frequently do progress when compared to those in patients treated with adrenalectomy.[10,11] Patients with MACS also have a higher risk of cardiovascular events and mortality.[10,12] In this case, the patient decided against adrenalectomy because of mild manifestations of MACS and individual preference. In patients choosing conservative follow-up, yearly evaluation for and treatment of cardiovascular risk factors and bone health are recommended.[1,2]

Key Points

- Adrenal malignancy and pheochromocytoma can be excluded if the adrenal mass is homogeneous

  and demonstrates an unenhanced CT attenuation of <10 HU.
- FDG PET scan may be false positive in functioning adrenal adenomas.
- Patients with MACS due to unilateral adrenal adenoma do not develop overt Cushing syndrome, but are at higher risk for cardiovascular events, bone fragility, and mortality.
- Clinical monitoring and treatment of MACS-related comorbidities should be implemented in patients with MACS not treated with adrenalectomy.

REFERENCES

1. Fassnacht M, Arlt W, Bancos I, et al. Management of adrenal incidentalomas: European Society of Endocrinology Clinical Practice Guideline in collaboration with the European Network for the Study of Adrenal Tumors. *Eur J Endocrinol*. 2016;175(2):G1–G34.
2. Vaidya A, Hamrahian A, Bancos I, Fleseriu M, Ghayee HK. The evaluation of incidentally discovered adrenal masses. *Endocr Pract*. 2019;25(2):178–192.
3. Delivanis DA, Erickson D, Atwell TD, et al. Procedural and clinical outcomes of percutaneous adrenal biopsy in a high-risk population for adrenal malignancy. *Clin Endocrinol (Oxf)*. 2016;85(5):710–716.
4. Iniguez-Ariza NM, Kohlenberg JD, Delivanis DA, et al. Clinical, biochemical, and radiological characteristics of a single-center retrospective cohort of 705 large adrenal tumors. *Mayo Clin Proc Innov Qual Outcomes*. 2018;2(1):30–39.
5. Delivanis DA, Bancos I, Atwell TD, et al. Diagnostic performance of unenhanced computed tomography and (18) F-fluorodeoxyglucose positron emission tomography in indeterminate adrenal tumours. *Clin Endocrinol (Oxf)*. 2018;88(1):306.

6. Dinnes J, Bancos I, Ferrante di Ruffano L, et al. Management of endocrine disease: Imaging for the diagnosis of malignancy in incidentally discovered adrenal masses: a systematic review and meta-analysis. *Eur J Endocrinol*. 2016;175(2):R51–R64.

7. Mao JJ, Dages KN, Suresh M, Bancos I. Presentation, disease progression and outcomes of adrenal gland metastases. *Clin Endocrinol (Oxf)*. 2020;93(5):546–554.

8. Ebbehoj A, Li D, Kaur RJ, et al. Epidemiology of adrenal tumours in Olmsted County, Minnesota, USA: a population-based cohort study. *Lancet Diabetes Endocrinol*. 2020;8(11):894–902.

9. Delivanis DA, Athimulam S, Bancos I. Modern management of mild autonomous cortisol secretion. *Clin Pharmacol Ther*. 2019;106(6):1209–1221.

10. Elhassan YS, Alahdab F, Prete A, et al. Natural history of adrenal incidentalomas with and without mild autonomous cortisol excess: a systematic review and meta-analysis. *Ann Intern Med*. 2019;171(2):107–116.

11. Bancos I, Alahdab F, Crowley RK, et al. THERAPY OF ENDOCRINE DISEASE: Improvement of cardiovascular risk factors after adrenalectomy in patients with adrenal tumors and subclinical Cushing's syndrome: a systematic review and meta-analysis. *Eur J Endocrinol*. 2016;175(6):R283–R95.

12. Debono M, Bradburn M, Bull M, Harrison B, Ross RJ, Newell-Price J. Cortisol as a marker for increased mortality in patients with incidental adrenocortical adenomas. *J Clin Endocrinol Metab*. 2014;99(12):4462–4470.

13. Bancos I, Taylor AE, Chortis V, et al. Urine steroid metabolomics for the differential diagnosis of adrenal incidentalomas in the EURINE-ACT study: a prospective test validation study. *Lancet Diabetes Endocrinol*. 2020;8(9):773–781.

Incidentally Discovered Adrenal Mass in a Patient With a History of Extraadrenal Malignancy: The Role of Adrenal Biopsy

Adrenal metastasis should be suspected in any patient with history of extraadrenal malignancy presenting with an indeterminate adrenal mass. The most common extraadrenal malignancies that metastasize to adrenal gland include lung, renal, and gastrointestinal cancers, followed by melanoma, lymphoma, breast, and other cancers.[1] In this case, we illustrate the role of adrenal biopsy in the workup of adrenal mass and discuss the potential of adrenal insufficiency in these patients.

Case Report

The patient was a 77-year-old woman who was referred for evaluation of an incidentally discovered left adrenal mass on a renal ultrasound that was obtained for workup of hypertension and hyperkalemia. A subsequent computed tomography (CT) scan was obtained and demonstrated a heterogeneous left adrenal mass measuring $12.3 \times 8.3 \times 9.1$ cm (Fig. 3.1). No other lesions were seen.

The patient's past medical history was positive for renal cell carcinoma 12 years prior that was treated with right nephrectomy and right adrenalectomy. Periodic imaging was performed until 5 years prior and was negative for recurrence. At the time of evaluation, she had no symptoms to suggest adrenal hormonal excess and the review of systems was negative.

She had a history of hypertension, dyslipidemia, and type 2 diabetes mellitus. Her medications included amlodipine, losartan, metoprolol succinate, atorvastatin, and metformin. Her body mass index was 42.8 kg/m^2, and the physical examination was otherwise unrevealing.

INVESTIGATIONS

Baseline laboratory testing was obtained and excluded a functioning pheochromocytoma (Table 3.1). Initial testing also demonstrated possible primary adrenal insufficiency with elevated serum corticotropin (ACTH) concentration and low serum cortisol concentration. Follow-up cosyntropin stimulation testing was abnormal, with a peak serum cortisol concentration of 9 mcg/dL.

The patient was advised that she most likely had metastatic disease to the adrenal gland. A previous history of extraadrenal malignancy, a new diagnosis of an indeterminate adrenal mass, combined with the biochemical confirmation of primary adrenal insufficiency, supported the preliminary diagnosis of infiltrative metastatic disease in the setting of contralateral adrenalectomy. A CT-guided biopsy of the left adrenal mass was performed and confirmed metastatic renal cell carcinoma. The neoplastic cells were positive for paired box gene 8 (PAX8) immunostain and negative for inhibin and human melanoma black 45 (HMB45).

TREATMENT AND FOLLOW-UP

The patient was initiated on hydrocortisone replacement therapy for primary adrenal insufficiency. The metastatic renal cell carcinoma was treated with

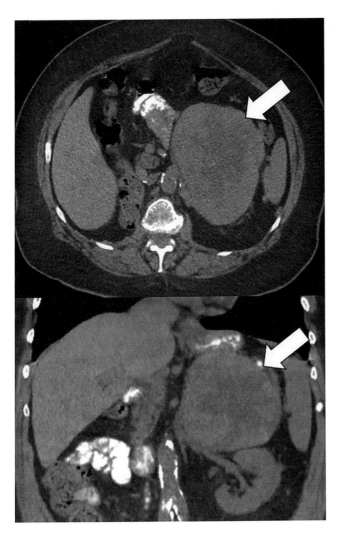

Fig. 3.1 Axial (*top*) and coronal (*bottom*) images from an unenhanced computed tomography (CT) scan demonstrated a large heterogeneous left adrenal mass measuring 12.3 × 8.3 × 9.1 cm. Measurement of CT attenuation within the nonnecrotic region was 41 Hounsfield units. CT also confirmed absence of the right kidney and right adrenal gland.

TABLE 3.1	Laboratory Tests	
Biochemical Test	**Result**	**Reference Range**
Sodium, mmol/L	134, 138	135–145
Potassium, mmol/L	5.0, 5.2	3.6–5.2
8 AM serum cortisol, mcg/dL	5.3, 8.0	7–25
ACTH, pg/mL	116	10–60
DHEA-S, mcg/dL	<15	15–157
Plasma metanephrine, nmol/L	<0.2	<0.5
Plasma normetanephrine, nmol/L	0.88	<0.9

ACTH, Corticotropin; *DHEA-S*, dehydroepiandrosterone-sulfate.

pazopanib. One year later, she was treated with surgical resection of the abdominal metastatic disease, which included resection of a 14-cm adrenal metastasis, distal pancreatectomy, and splenectomy. Fludrocortisone was added to hydrocortisone after the surgery. She continues to have a slowly progressive metastatic disease 3 years after initial presentation.

Discussion

Adrenal metastasis should be suspected in any patient with a history of extraadrenal malignancy who presents with an indeterminate adrenal mass. In a retrospective study of 579 patients with adrenal metastases, 59% were discovered during cancer staging imaging, 36% were incidentally discovered during workup performed for another reason, and 5% were detected due to other symptoms.[1] Adrenal metastases originated from the lung (39%), genitourinary (28%), gastrointestinal (14%), and other (20%) organ systems.[1] Notably, bilateral adrenal metastases were diagnosed at baseline, or developed during follow-up in 43% of patients. Primary adrenal insufficiency was not routinely tested for; however, it was diagnosed in 12.4% of patients with bilateral adrenal metastases and in 20% of patients with metastases >4 cm in diameter.[1]

Adrenal biopsy is a procedure that is rarely needed in the workup of adrenal masses.[2,3] It is reserved only for patients with indeterminate adrenal masses (e.g., unenhanced CT attenuation >10 Hounsfield units [HU]), after excluding pheochromocytoma, and in someone likely to have an adrenal metastasis.[2–4] Adrenal biopsy is not accurate in distinguishing between adrenocortical carcinoma and adrenocortical adenoma and should not be used with that intent.[5–7] The nondiagnostic rate for adrenal biopsy is around 5%, and complication rate is 3%.[5–7]

Key Points

- Adrenal biopsy should be performed only in patients with indeterminate adrenal masses (e.g., unenhanced CT attenuation >10 HU) and after excluding pheochromocytoma.
- Adrenal biopsy is not accurate in distinguishing between benign and malignant adrenocortical lesions; noninvasive diagnosis should be attempted in these cases[8] or adrenalectomy considered.[2]

- Primary adrenal insufficiency can occur in 12.4% of patients with bilateral adrenal metastases, and 20% of patients with large metastases >4 cm.[1]
- Primary adrenal insufficiency can occur in a patient with unilateral adrenal metastasis and history of contralateral adrenalectomy.

REFERENCES

1. Mao JJ, Dages KN, Suresh M, Bancos I. Presentation, disease progression and outcomes of adrenal gland metastases. *Clin Endocrinol (Oxf)*. 2020;93(5):546–554.
2. Fassnacht M, Arlt W, Bancos I, et al. Management of adrenal incidentalomas: European Society of Endocrinology Clinical Practice Guideline in collaboration with the European Network for the Study of Adrenal Tumors. *Eur J Endocrinol*. 2016;175(2):G1–G34.
3. Vaidya A, Hamrahian A, Bancos I, Fleseriu M, Ghayee HK. The evaluation of incidentally discovered adrenal masses. *Endocr Pract*. 2019;25(2):178–192.
4. Delivanis DA, Bancos I, Atwell TD, et al. Diagnostic performance of unenhanced computed tomography and (18) F-fluorodeoxyglucose positron emission tomography in indeterminate adrenal tumours. *Clin Endocrinol (Oxf)*. 2018;88(1):30–36.
5. Bancos I, Tamhane S, Shah M, et al. Diagnosis of endocrine disease: the diagnostic performance of adrenal biopsy: a systematic review and meta-analysis. *European Journal of Endocrinology*. 2016;175(2):R65–R80.
6. Delivanis DA, Erickson D, Atwell TD, et al. Procedural and clinical outcomes of percutaneous adrenal biopsy in a high-risk population for adrenal malignancy. *Clin Endocrinol (Oxf)*. 2016;85(5):710–716.
7. Zhang CD, Delivanis DA, Eiken PW, Atwell TD, Bancos I. Adrenal biopsy: performance and use. *Minerva Endocrinol*. 2019;44(3):288–300.
8. Bancos I, Taylor AE, Chortis V, et al. Urine steroid metabolomics for the differential diagnosis of adrenal incidentalomas in the EURINE-ACT study: a prospective test validation study. *Lancet Diabetes Endocrinol*. 2020;8(9):773–781.

Nonfunctioning Lipid-Rich Adrenocortical Adenoma: Role of Follow-Up

Any adrenal mass needs evaluation for adrenal hormonal excess and malignancy.[1,2] Imaging characteristics can be helpful to exclude malignancy.[3] Workup for adrenal hormone excess includes assessment for cortisol, aldosterone, and catecholamine excess. Here, we present a case of an incidentally discovered adrenal mass, which was determined to be benign and nonfunctioning and where further imaging and biochemical monitoring were not required.

Case Report

The patient was a 59-year-old woman who presented for evaluation of an incidentally discovered right adrenal mass on an abdominal computed tomography (CT) scan performed for investigation of left-sided abdominal pain. The right adrenal mass measured 1.6 × 2.0 × 1.2 cm with an unenhanced CT attenuation of 5.5 Hounsfield units (HU) (see Fig. 4.1). She had partial workup at home and was advised that she did not have a pheochromocytoma. She was referred to our institution for further evaluation.

She had a 6-year history of hypertension and type 2 diabetes mellitus. She was also diagnosed with dyslipidemia 4 years prior. Her bone mineral density performed several years prior was normal. Her medications included lisinopril, hydrochlorothiazide, glipizide, and insulin. She had no overt signs of adrenal dysfunction or past history of malignancy. She had no change in body weight. On physical examination her body mass index was 33.67 kg/m^2, blood pressure 132/82 mmHg, and

heart rate 94 beats per minute. She had no stigmata of Cushing syndrome.

INVESTIGATIONS

The baseline laboratory test results are shown in Table 4.1. The laboratory tests were normal.

OUTCOME AND FOLLOW-UP

The patient was counseled that the adrenal mass was a benign nonfunctioning adrenal adenoma. This was concluded based on imaging phenotype of the adrenal mass with low unenhanced CT attenuation. The patient was advised that no further endocrine follow-up was necessary.

Discussion

CT attenuation measurement on unenhanced CT can help clarify the etiology of an adrenal mass. Adrenocortical adenomas can be lipid rich (HU <10) in around 60% of cases, demonstrate indeterminate unenhanced CT attenuation of 10–20 HU in around 20%–25% of cases, and be lipid poor (>20 HU) in 15%–20% of cases.[4,5] Adrenocortical carcinomas, other malignant adrenal tumors (e.g., sarcomas, metastases), and pheochromocytomas usually demonstrate unenhanced CT attenuation >20–30 HU and infrequently in the indeterminate zone of 10–20 HU (around 2%–5%).[3–10] Thus, a homogeneous adrenal mass with an unenhanced CT attenuation of <10 HU excludes malignant adrenal tumors and pheochromocytomas, and imaging follow-up in these cases is not needed. In addition, workup for pheochromocytoma is not needed in adrenal tumors demonstrating unenhanced

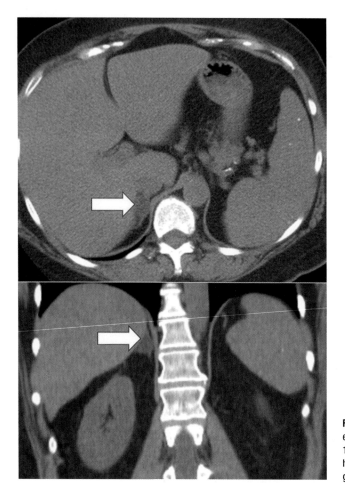

Fig. 4.1 Axial (*above*) and coronal (*below*) images from an unenhanced computed tomography (CT) scan demonstrated a 1.6 × 2.0 × 1.2 cm right adrenal mass (*arrows*) with an unenhanced CT attenuation of 5.5 Hounsfield units. The left adrenal gland was unremarkable.

TABLE 4.1	Laboratory Tests	
Biochemical Test	**Result**	**Reference Range**
4 PM serum cortisol, mcg/dL	2.5	1.4–7
1 mg DST serum cortisol, mcg/dL	<1	<1.8
ACTH, pg/mL	40	10–60
Aldosterone, ng/dL	8.5	≤21
Plasma renin activity, ng/mL/hr	15.3	≤0.6–3
DHEA-S, mcg/dL	95	16–195
Plasma metanephrine, nmol/L	0.1	<0.5
Plasma normetanephrine, nmol/L	0.56	<0.9

ACTH, Corticotropin; *DHEA-S*, dehydroepiandrosterone-sulfate, *DST*, dexamethasone suppression test.

CT attenuation with <10 HU.[5,7,9] As reported in a systematic review of 2023 patients with adrenal adenomas, 2.5% of adenomas may demonstrate growth >1 cm depending on when in relation to its natural history the tumor is first discovered.[11] However, the risk of malignant transformation was 0%.[11] In patients with either nonfunctioning adrenal adenomas (serum cortisol concentration after the 1-mg dexamethasone suppression test <1.8 mcg/dL) or those with mild autonomous cortisol secretion (MACS) (serum cortisol concentration after the 1-mg dexamethasone suppression test >1.8 mcg/dL), overt hormone excess (primary aldosteronism, catecholamine excess, or

Cushing syndrome) developed in approximately 0.2% (6 of 2745 patients).[11] The proportion of patients with nonfunctioning adrenal adenomas who developed new MACS during a mean follow-up of 20.3 months was 4.3% (149 of 2083).[11] Repeating dexamethasone suppression tests in patients with bilateral nodular disease or in those with new symptoms potentially related to MACS could be considered.

Key Points

- Unenhanced CT attenuation <10 HU in a homogeneous adrenal mass excludes malignancy and pheochromocytoma.
- Growth of >1 cm can be seen in 2.5% of adrenal adenomas; however, the risk of malignant transformation is 0%; thus imaging follow-up of homogeneous lipid-rich adenomas is not needed.
- The risk of new overt hormone excess in a patient with nonfunctioning unilateral adrenal adenoma is around 0.2%.
- The risk of new MACS is 4.3%; thus repeating dexamethasone suppression tests in selected patients could be considered, especially in those with bilateral adrenal adenomas, bilateral macronodular hyperplasia, or in those who develop comorbidities potentially related to MACS (e.g., osteoporosis, diabetes mellitus, hypertension, obesity).

REFERENCES

1. Fassnacht M, Arlt W, Bancos I, et al. Management of adrenal incidentalomas: European Society of Endocrinology Clinical Practice Guideline in collaboration with the European Network for the Study of Adrenal Tumors. *Eur J Endocrinol*. 2016;175(2):G1–G34.

2. Vaidya A, Hamrahian A, Bancos I, Fleseriu M, Ghayee HK. The evaluation of incidentally discovered adrenal masses. *Endocr Pract*. 2019;25(2):178–192.

3. Dinnes J, Bancos I, Ferrante di Ruffano L, et al. Management of endocrine disease: Imaging for the diagnosis of malignancy in incidentally discovered adrenal masses: a systematic review and meta-analysis. *Eur J Endocrinol*. 2016;175(2):R51–R64.

4. Ebbehoj A, Li D, Kaur RJ, et al. Epidemiology of adrenal tumours in Olmsted County, Minnesota, USA: a population-based cohort study. *Lancet Diabetes Endocrinol*. 2020;8(11):894–902.

5. Iniguez-Ariza NM, Kohlenberg JD, Delivanis DA, et al. Clinical, biochemical, and radiological characteristics of a single-center retrospective cohort of 705 large adrenal tumors. *Mayo Clin Proc Innov Qual Outcomes*. 2018;2(1):30–39.

6. Bancos I, Taylor AE, Chortis V, et al. Urine steroid metabolomics for the differential diagnosis of adrenal incidentalomas in the EURINE-ACT study: a prospective test validation study. *Lancet Diabetes Endocrinol*. 2020;8(9):773–781.

7. Canu L, Van Hemert JAW, Kerstens MN, et al. CT Characteristics of pheochromocytoma: relevance for the evaluation of adrenal incidentaloma. *J Clin Endocrinol Metab*. 2019;104(2):312–318.

8. Delivanis DA, Bancos I, Atwell TD, et al. Diagnostic performance of unenhanced computed tomography and (18) F-fluorodeoxyglucose positron emission tomography in indeterminate adrenal tumours. *Clin Endocrinol (Oxf)*. 2018;88(1):30–36.

9. Gruber LM, Strajina V, Bancos I, et al. Not all adrenal incidentalomas require biochemical testing to exclude pheochromocytoma: Mayo Clinic experience and a meta-analysis. *Gland Surg*. 2020;9(2):362–371.

10. Mao JJ, Dages KN, Suresh M, Bancos I. Presentation, disease progression and outcomes of adrenal gland metastases. *Clin Endocrinol (Oxf)*. 2020;93(5):546–554.

11. Elhassan YS, Alahdab F, Prete A, et al. Natural history of adrenal incidentalomas with and without mild autonomous cortisol excess: a systematic review and meta-analysis. *Ann Intern Med*. 2019;171(2):107–116.

54-Year-Old Woman With an Incidentally Discovered Adrenal Mass and Abnormal Dexamethasone Suppression Test: Role of Adrenalectomy

Mild autonomous cortisol secretion (MACS) is defined as an abnormal cortisol concentration following dexamethasone suppression test (post-DST cortisol >1.8 mcg/dL) and is detected in up to 50% of patients with adrenal cortical adenomas. Patients with MACS present with a higher prevalence of cardiovascular risk factors and events, osteopenia and osteoporosis, and increased risk of fractures. Adrenalectomy leads to improvement of comorbidities in 20%–70% of patients; however, estimating the degree of improvement prior to adrenalectomy is challenging.

Case Report

The patient was a 54-year-old woman who presented for evaluation of continuous weight gain of 50 pounds over 5–7 years. In addition, she had prediabetes (glycosylated hemoglobin = 6%, not on medications) and hypertension treated with metoprolol tartrate 25 mg twice a day and nifedipine 30 mg daily. Two years prior, she was diagnosed with osteoporosis. Several months prior, she was incidentally discovered with a 2.2-cm left adrenal mass initially visualized on chest computed tomography (CT) and further better characterized on abdominal CT (Fig. 5.1). Physical exam was positive for body mass index of 39.8 kg/m^2 and blood pressure of 138/86 mmHg, but no features of Cushing syndrome.

INVESTIGATIONS

On unenhanced CT of adrenal glands, the left adrenal mass was lipid rich (6 Hounsfield units [HU]), measuring 2.2 cm in the largest diameter (see Fig. 5.1). The right adrenal gland appeared normal. The baseline laboratory test results are shown in Table 5.1. The serum corticotropin (ACTH) and dehydroepiandrosterone-sulfate (DHEA-S) concentrations were low, and cortisol did not suppress normally with an overnight 1-mg dexamethasone suppression test (DST) (see Table 5.1). MACS was diagnosed.

TREATMENT

The patient was counseled that the adrenal mass was a benign adrenal adenoma that was producing cortisol autonomously. Malignancy was excluded based on the imaging phenotype (<10 HU). MACS was diagnosed based on an abnormal DST (cortisol >1.8 mcg/dL), as well as low ACTH and DHEA-S. The patient was counseled about possible relationship of MACS and cardiovascular comorbidities (e.g., hypertension, prediabetes, obesity), and conservative management versus adrenalectomy was discussed. A decision on adrenalectomy was made. Pathology demonstrated an adrenocortical adenoma forming a 3.1 × 2.5 × 1.7 cm adrenal nodule.

FOLLOW-UP

Postoperative adrenal insufficiency was diagnosed based on cortisol of 5.7 mcg/dL the morning after

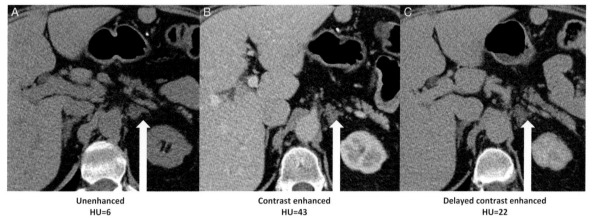

Fig. 5.1 Axial images from an unenhanced and contrast enhanced computed tomography (CT) scan showed a lipid-rich 2.2 × 1.4–cm left adrenal mass. (A) Unenhanced Hounsfield units (HU) of 6. (B) Contrast-enhanced HU of 43. (C) Delayed contrast-enhanced HU of 22.

surgery. Hydrocortisone supplementation was initiated with a plan to reassess adrenal function. At the 6-month follow-up, the patient's hypothalamic-pituitary-adrenal axis recovered and hydrocortisone was stopped. Clinically, the patient lost 15 pounds of body weight and her blood pressure measurements improved.

Discussion

As reported in a prospective study of 601 unselected patients undergoing CT scans, with a 7% prevalence of incidental adrenal tumors, MACS can be diagnosed in up to 50% of patients.[1] In a larger multicenter study of adrenal tumors evaluated in the adrenal practice,

TABLE 5.1 Laboratory Tests

Biochemical Test	Result	Reference Range
1-mg overnight DST, mcg/dL	2.3	<1.8
ACTH, pg/mL	<5	7.2–63
DHEA-S, mcg/dL	26	15–200
Aldosterone, ng/dL	8	<21
Plasma renin activity, ng/mL per hour	4.1	2.9–10.8
Urine metanephrines, mcg/24 h	236	<400
Urine normetanephrine, mcg/24 h	712	<900
Urine free cortisol, mcg/24 h	7.5	3.5–45

ACTH, Corticotropin; *DHEA-S,* dehydroepiandrosterone-sulfate; *DST,* dexamethasone suppression test.

48% of patients with adenoma and available DST had MACS.[2] Patients with MACS demonstrate higher prevalence of cardiovascular risk factors (hypertension, diabetes mellitus type 2, obesity, dyslipidemia), cardiovascular events and mortality, osteopenia, osteoporosis, and fractures.[3–5] In a systematic review and meta-analysis of adrenalectomy versus conservative management in MACS, patients undergoing adrenalectomy experienced improvement in hypertension and diabetes mellitus type 2.[6] However, studies included in this systematic review were of low to moderate quality and had heterogeneous definitions of both MACS and comorbidity improvement. Identifying patients most likely to experience improvement in long-term outcomes is challenging, and thus the decision regarding adrenalectomy needs to be individualized.

Key Points

- DST is required in any patient with adrenal mass, regardless of symptoms.
- MACS (DST >1.8 mcg/dL) is diagnosed in up to 50% of patients with adrenal adenoma.
- Patients with MACS have higher prevalence of cardiovascular risk factors, cardiovascular events, osteopenia, osteoporosis, and fractures.
- Adrenalectomy leads to improvement in cardiovascular risk factors; however, individual degree of improvement varies.
- Decision on adrenalectomy versus conservative managements needs to be individualized to the

patient's age, comorbidities, tumor imaging phenotype, local surgical expertise, and the patient's preference.

REFERENCES

1. Reimondo G, Castellano E, Grosso M, et al. Adrenal Incidentalomas are tied to increased risk of diabetes: findings from a prospective study. *J Clin Endocrinol Metab*. 2020:105.

2. Bancos I, Taylor AE, Chortis V, et al. Urine steroid metabolomics for the differential diagnosis of adrenal incidentalomas in the EURINE-ACT study: a prospective test validation study. *Lancet Diabetes Endocrinol*. 2020;8:773–781.

3. Elhassan YS, Alahdab F, Prete A, et al. Natural history of adrenal incidentalomas with and without mild autonomous cortisol excess: a systematic review and meta-analysis. *Ann Intern Med*. 2019;171:107–116.

4. Delivanis DA, Athimulam S, Bancos I. Modern management of mild autonomous cortisol secretion. *Clin Pharmacol Ther*. 2019;106:1209–1221.

5. Athimulam S, Bancos I. Evaluation of bone health in patients with adrenal tumors. *Curr Opin Endocrinol Diabetes Obes*. 2019;26:125–132.

6. Bancos I, Alahdab F, Crowley RK, et al. Therapy of endocrine disease: improvement of cardiovascular risk factors after adrenalectomy in patients with adrenal tumors and subclinical Cushing's syndrome: a systematic review and meta-analysis. *Eur J Endocrinol*. 2016;175:R283–R295.

Lipid-Poor Adrenal Masses: The Case for Aggressive Management

Lipid-poor adrenal masses are the landmines of adrenal disorders. Although lipid-poor adrenal masses may be benign nonfunctional cortical adenomas, it can be difficult to make the distinction from more concerning diagnoses such as a small adrenocortical carcinoma (ACC) (see Case 23) and prebiochemical pheochromocytoma (see Case 36). Choosing nonsurgical management can carry a clinically significant risk. Herein we present such a case.

Case Report

The patient was an 82-year-old woman who 5 months previously presented with community-acquired pneumonia. To exclude pulmonary embolism, a chest computed tomography (CT) angiogram was performed and a right adrenal mass was noted incidentally. An adrenal-dedicated CT scan showed the mass to measure 2.3 × 2.5 × 3.2 cm with an unenhanced CT attenuation of 28 Hounsfield units (HU) (Fig. 6.1). Follow-up CT scan was obtained 5 months later, and the right adrenal mass increased in size (2.8 × 2.5 × 3.5 cm) (see Fig. 6.1). She had a history of hypertension and type 2 diabetes mellitus. Her antihypertensive medications included a calcium channel blocker (amlodipine 10 mg daily) and a β-adrenergic blocker (metoprolol 12.5 mg twice daily). She had no overt signs of adrenal dysfunction or past history of malignancy. She had no change in body weight. On physical examination her body mass index was 32 kg/m², blood pressure 161/81 mmHg, and heart rate 81 beats per minute. She had no stigmata of Cushing syndrome.

INVESTIGATIONS

The baseline laboratory test results are shown in Table 6.1. The laboratory tests were normal with the exception of a positive case detection test for primary aldosteronism and minimal elevations in serum total testosterone and plasma normetanephrine.

TREATMENT

The patient was advised that she may have an adrenal malignancy, and right adrenalectomy was strongly recommended. However, her spouse was recovering from an illness, and she opted to care for the spouse over the subsequent months.

OUTCOME AND FOLLOW-UP

The patient did not return for medical evaluation for an additional 9 months. An abdominal CT without (see Fig. 6.1) and with contrast (Fig. 6.2) was obtained. The right adrenal mass had increased further in size (5.2 × 4.1 × 4.5 cm), and there was associated metastatic disease to the liver and lymph nodes (see Fig. 6.2). Biopsy of the liver confirmed metastatic adrenocortical carcinoma (ACC). The patient died 17 months after the first CT scan.

Key Points

- ACC is the most aggressive of all malignances seen by endocrinologists.
- All ACCs are small at the beginning.
- Lipid-poor adrenal masses should either be resected or followed closely with serial imaging.[1,2]
- Findings from F-18 fluorodeoxyglucose positron emission tomography and high-resolution accurate-mass mass spectrometry urine steroid

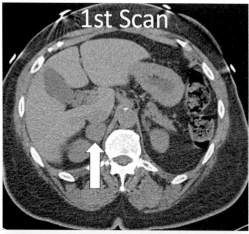

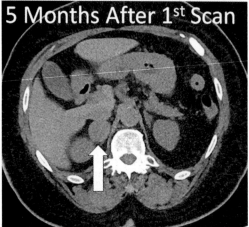

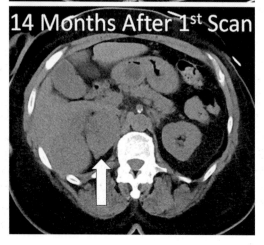

Fig. 6.1 Axial images from serial unenhanced computed tomography (CT) scans. *Top*, the initial scan showed a 2.3 × 2.5 × 3.2 cm right adrenal mass (*arrow*) with an unenhanced CT attenuation of 28 Hounsfield units (HU). *Middle*, the CT scan performed 5 months after the first scan showed that the adrenal mass (*arrow*) had increased in size (2.8 × 2.5 × 3.5 cm) and had an unenhanced CT attenuation of 34 HU. *Bottom*, the CT scan performed 14 months after the initial scan showed further enlargement of the right adrenal mass (*arrow*) (5.2 × 4.1 × 4.5 cm) and metastatic disease to the liver (see Fig. 6.2).

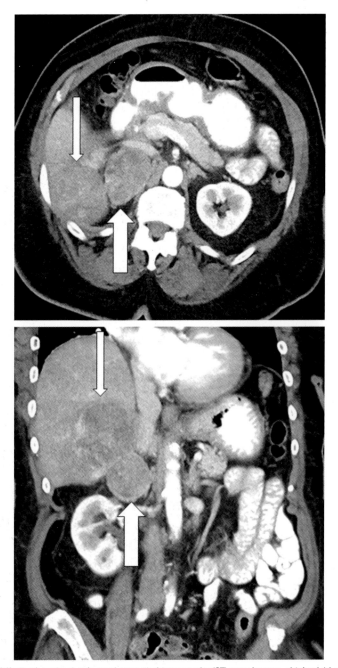

Fig. 6.2 Axial (*top*) and coronal (*bottom*) contrast-enhanced computed tomography (CT) scan images, obtained 14 months after the initial CT scan (see Fig. 6.1), showed an increased size of a large heterogeneous right adrenal mass (*large arrows*) and a large (9.8 × 8.6 cm) mass (*small arrows*) in the right hepatic lobe. In addition, there were multiple prominent retroperitoneal and mesenteric lymph nodes, including a right pericaval 1.5 × 0.8–cm retroperitoneal lymph node.

TABLE 6.1 Laboratory Tests

Biochemical Test	Result	Reference Range
Sodium, mmol/L	144	135–145
Potassium, mmol/L	3.6	3.6–5.2
Fasting plasma glucose, mg/dL	123	70–100
Creatinine, mg/dL	0.9	0.6–1.1
8 AM serum cortisol, mcg/dL	12	7–25
ACTH, pg/mL	23	10–60
Aldosterone, ng/dL	21	≤21
Plasma renin activity, ng/mL per hour	<0.6	≤0.6–3
DHEA-S, mcg/dL	47.3	15–157
Total testosterone, ng/dL	80	8–60
Androstenedione, ng/dL	172	30–200
Plasma metanephrine, nmol/L	0.35	<0.5
Plasma normetanephrine, nmol/L	1.0	<0.9
24-hour urine:		
Metanephrine, mcg	119	<400
Normetanephrine, mcg	396	<900
Norepinephrine, mcg	72	<80
Epinephrine, mcg	3.5	<20
Dopamine, mcg	170	<400
Cortisol, mcg	28	3.5–45

ACTH, Corticotropin; *DHEA-S,* dehydroepiandrosterone-sulfate.

profiling may help the clinician when there is uncertainty on whether to resect a lipid-poor adrenal mass.[3,4]

REFERENCES

1. Young Jr WF. Clinical practice. The incidentally discovered adrenal mass. *N Engl J Med.* 2007;356(6):601–610.

2. Young Jr WF. Conventional imaging in adrenocortical carcinoma: update and perspectives. *Horm Cancer.* 2011;2(6):341–347.

3. Delivanis DA, Bancos I, Atwell TD, et al. Diagnostic performance of unenhanced computed tomography and (18) F-fluorodeoxyglucose positron emission tomography in indeterminate adrenal tumours. *Clin Endocrinol (Oxf).* 2018;88(1):30–36.

4. Hines JM, Bancos I, Bancos C, et al. High-resolution, accurate-mass (HRAM) mass spectrometry urine steroid profiling in the diagnosis of adrenal disorders. *Clin Chem.* 2017;63(12):1824–1835.

Primary Aldosteronism

Hypertension, increased adrenal aldosterone secretion, and suppressed renin are the hallmarks of primary aldosteronism (PA). The prevalence of PA is approximately 5%–10% in people with hypertension and up to 20%–50% in those with treatment-resistant hypertension.[1–3] Cardiovascular and cerebrovascular morbidity and mortality rates in patients with PA are increased compared with patients with apparent essential hypertension when matched for age, sex, and blood pressure.[1] The early diagnosis of PA provides the opportunity to either cure hypertension or to direct targeted pharmacotherapy, both of which can prevent end-stage PA, which includes end-stage renal disease and irreversible cardiovascular damage.

Because hypokalemia is present in only 28% of patients with PA, all patients with hypertension are potential candidates for this disorder.[1,4] The degree of hypertension is typically moderate to severe and may be resistant to usual pharmacologic treatments. Aldosterone-producing adenoma (APA) and bilateral idiopathic hyperaldosteronism (IHA) are the two most common subtypes of PA (Table B.1). In general, patients with APA tend to have higher aldosterone levels and higher blood pressures than patients with IHA.[1] Several studies have demonstrated the negative impact of PA on quality of life and that surgical cure is more effective in normalizing quality-of-life metrics than chronic medical management is.[5]

The diagnosis of PA starts with case detection, followed by confirmatory tests and, finally, subtype evaluation (Fig. B.1).[1,3] As long as renin is suppressed, each step may be completed while the patient is taking antihypertensive medications. Although medications used to treat hypertension can potentially cause false-negative testing results in patients with mild PA, there is no medication that causes false-positive results, as long as a cut-off level for plasma aldosterone concentration (PAC) is used (e.g., >10 ng/dL).[1]

Case detection testing involves the measurement of PAC and plasma renin activity (PRA) (or plasma renin concentration [PRC]) in a random morning ambulatory blood sample. PA should be suspected if the PRA is suppressed to <1.0 ng/mL per hour (or PRC <8 mU/L) and the PAC is >10 ng/dL (see Fig. B.1).

Except for the clinical setting of spontaneous hypokalemia, suppressed PRA, and a PAC >20 ng/dL (where the diagnosis of PA is a certainty), all other patients should have PA confirmed by demonstration of aldosterone secretory autonomy with an aldosterone-suppression testing, which can be performed with (1) a high-sodium diet or orally administered sodium chloride and measurement of urinary aldosterone excretion; or (2) intravenous sodium chloride loading and measurement of PAC.[1,3]

The goal of subtype testing is to determine whether the source of aldosterone excess is from the right, left, or both adrenal glands. When localized to one adrenal gland, unilateral adrenalectomy results in normalization of hypokalemia in all patients; hypertension is improved in all patients and is cured in 30%–60%.[1] Adrenal-directed CT scan should be the first test in the subtype evaluation of PA (see Fig. B.1). However, because of the age-related prevalence of nonfunctioning adrenocortical nodules and the fact that APAs can be too small to be detected on CT, the reliability of CT in localizing APAs is poor. Adrenal CT is not able to distinguish accurately between APA and IHA.[1,3] Adrenal venous sampling (AVS) is the criterion standard test to distinguish unilateral from bilateral

TABLE B.1   Forms of Primary Aldosteronism

Subtype of Primary Aldosteronism	Estimated Proportion of All Patients With Primary Aldosteronism (%)
Aldosterone-producing adenoma (APA)	30
Bilateral idiopathic hyperplasia (IHA)	60
Unilateral (primary) adrenal hyperplasia (UAH/PAH)	4
Aldosterone-producing adrenocortical carcinoma	<1
Familial hyperaldosteronism (FH)	
Glucocorticoid-remediable aldosteronism (FH type I) (germline *CYP11B1/CYP11B2* chimeric gene)	<1
FH type II (APA or IHA) (germline *CLCN2* pathogenic variants)	<6
FH type III (germline *KCNJ5* pathogenic variants)	<1
FH type IV (germline *CACNA1H* pathogenic variants)	<0.1
Ectopic aldosterone-producing neoplasm	<0.1

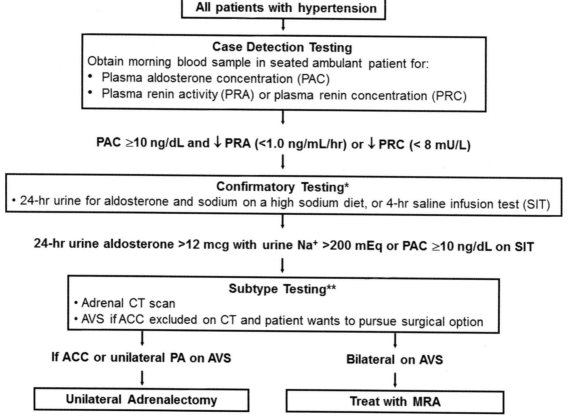

Fig. B.1 Algorithm for evaluation and treatment of primary aldosteronism (PA). *Formal confirmatory testing is not needed if the patient has spontaneous hypokalemia and a PAC >20 ng/dL. **AVS may not be needed in the young patient (<35 years of age) who has marked PA (e.g., spontaneous hypokalemia and PAC >30 ng/dL). *ACC,* Adrenocortical carcinoma; *AVS,* adrenal venous sampling; *CT,* computed tomography; *MRA,* mineralocorticoid receptor antagonist; *PAC,* plasma aldosterone concentration; *PRA,* plasma renin activity; *PRC,* plasma renin concentration; *SIT,* saline infusion test.

disease in patients with PA.[1,3] AVS is a technically demanding procedure because the right adrenal vein is small and may be difficult to locate and cannulate; the success rate depends on the expertise and the degree of engagement of the interventional radiologist.

The treatment objectives for patients with PA include (1) resolution of hypokalemia, (2) normal blood pressure, and (3) prevention of aldosterone-specific progressive chronic kidney disease and cardiovascular damage. The cause of PA dictates the optimal treatment option. It is essential for clinicians to understand that normalization of blood pressure is not the only goal. In the presence of sodium, excessive autonomous secretion of aldosterone is associated with an increased risk of cardiovascular disease and morbidity. Thus either curative surgery or optimized mineralocorticoid receptor blockade should be part of the management plan for all patients with PA.

REFERENCES

1. Young Jr WF. Diagnosis and treatment of primary aldosteronism: practical clinical perspectives. *J Intern Med.* 2019;285(2):126–148.

2. Brown JM, Siddiqui M, Calhoun DA, et al. The unrecognized prevalence of primary aldosteronism: a cross-sectional study. *Ann Intern Med.* 2020;173(1):10–20.

3. Funder JW, Carey RM, Mantero F, et al. The management of primary aldosteronism: case detection, diagnosis, and treatment: an Endocrine Society clinical practice guideline. *J Clin Endocrinol Metab.* 2016;101(5):1889–1916.

4. Mulatero P, Stowasser M, Loh KC, et al. Increased diagnosis of primary aldosteronism, including surgically correctable forms, in centers from five continents. *J Clin Endocrinol Metab.* 2004;89(3):1045–1050.

5. Velema M, Dekkers T, Hermus A, et al. Quality of life in primary aldosteronism: a comparative effectiveness study of adrenalectomy and medical treatment. *J Clin Endocrinol Metab.* 2018;103(1):16–24.

Primary Aldosteronism: When Adrenal Venous Sampling Is Not Needed Before Unilateral Adrenalectomy

There is a small subset of patients (≈5%) with primary aldosteronism (PA) in whom surgical management can proceed without the need for adrenal venous sampling (AVS). This subset includes those patients with the following characteristics: young (≤35 years), marked PA as demonstrated by spontaneous hypokalemia and plasma aldosterone concentration >30 ng/dL, and unilateral macroadenoma on adrenal computed tomography (CT) scan.

Case Report

The patient was a 35-year-old man with a 4-year history of hypertension. He was treated with a three-drug program: central α_2-agonist (clonidine 0.2 mg daily), calcium channel blocker (amlodipine 10 mg daily), and an angiotensin receptor blocker (valsartan 80 mg daily). Blood pressure control with these three medications was good. However, spontaneous hypokalemia had become a major problem requiring hospitalization on two occasions for potassium chloride infusions. At the time of referral to Mayo Clinic he was taking 80 mEq of potassium chloride daily to maintain a normal serum potassium concentration. Beyond hypertension and hypokalemia, the patient was healthy. He had no signs or symptoms of Cushing syndrome. He had no first-degree relatives who had been diagnosed with hypertension.

INVESTIGATIONS

The baseline laboratory test results are shown in Table 7.1. The patient had positive case detection testing for PA with a plasma aldosterone concentration (PAC) >10 ng/dL and plasma renin activity (PRA) <1.0 ng/mL per hour.[1] In addition, PA was confirmed because when a patient has spontaneous hypokalemia and the PAC >20 ng/dL, there are no other differential diagnostic possibilities beyond PA.[1,2] Thus formal confirmatory testing with oral sodium loading or a saline infusion test was not needed for this patient. The serum dehydroepiandrosterone sulfate (DHEA-S) concentration was mid-normal and cortisol suppressed normally with an overnight 1-mg dexamethasone suppression test (DST) (Table 7.1). Thus the adrenal adenoma was not cosecreting cortisol.

An unenhanced adrenal-dedicated CT scan showed a lipid-rich 2.0 × 1.0–cm right adrenal nodule (Fig. 7.1). The left adrenal gland appeared normal on CT.

The patient was informed that in view of his young age and severe PA, it was very likely (>95% probability) that his right adrenal nodule was indeed an aldosterone-producing adenoma (APA). This conclusion was based on the understanding that nonfunctioning adrenal nodules are uncommon in young people, and severe PA requires a large factory—typically an adrenal macroadenoma.[3,4] In a study from Mayo Clinic published in 2014, although the overall accuracy of CT and magnetic resonance imaging in detecting

TABLE 7.1 Laboratory Tests		
Biochemical Test	**Result**	**Reference Range**
Sodium, mmol/L	142	135–145
Potassium, mmol/L	4.1	3.6–5.2
Creatinine, mg/dL	1.2	0.8–1.3
Aldosterone, ng/dL	54	≤21 ng/dL
Plasma renin activity ng/mL per hour	<0.6	≤0.6–3
DHEA-S, mcg/dL	290	57–522
1-mg overnight DST	<1.0	<1.8

DHEA-S, Dehydroepiandrosterone-sulfate; *DST*, dexamethasone suppression test.

unilateral adrenal disease in patients with PA was poor at 58.6%, adrenal imaging performed well in those patients younger than 35 years of age, with 100% accuracy when an adrenal mass was detected.[4] The patient understood that a cure of his hypertension with surgery was a reasonable goal in view of his short duration of hypertension and lack of a family history of hypertension.[1,5]

TREATMENT

The optimal treatment of APA or unilateral hyperplasia is curative surgery, because hypertension control is improved in all patients and no blood pressure medications are required in 30%–60% of individuals.[4–6] In addition, quality-of-life outcomes are superior with surgical cure versus medical management with mineralocorticoid receptor blockade.[7] In a retrospective case series from 12 centers with data for 705 patients with PA who were treated surgically, 259 (37%) were cured of hypertension and 334 (47%) were improved; complete clinical success was more likely in female and younger patients.[8] Preoperative factors predictive of some degree of persistent hypertension after adrenalectomy include: more than one first-degree relative with hypertension, use of more than two antihypertensive agents, older age, increased serum creatinine level, and longer duration of hypertension.[5]

The patient underwent laparoscopic right adrenalectomy. The right adrenal gland weighed 7.9 g (normal adrenal gland weight is 4–5 g) and contained a 2.3 × 1.6 × 1.1 cm yellow cortical adenoma (Fig. 7.2). The PAC the day after surgery was 1.2 ng/dL and consistent with a surgical cure. Treatment with potassium chloride and losartan was stopped the day after surgery. The dosages of amlodipine and clonidine were decreased by 50%. The patient was advised to monitor his blood pressure daily and blood pressure medications adjusted as needed for high-normal blood pressure for the first month after surgery.

OUTCOME AND FOLLOW-UP

The patient's weekly blood potassium concentrations remained high-normal over 4 weeks after surgery. Serum creatinine remained normal. Two years postoperatively the patient had normal blood pressure without the need for antihypertensive medications.

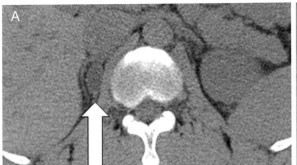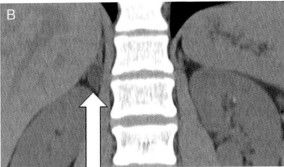

Fig. 7.1 Axial (A) and coronal (B) images from an unenhanced adrenal-dedicated computed tomography (CT) scan showed a lipid-rich (0.4 Hounsfield units) 1.0 × 2.0 cm right adrenal nodule (*arrow*). The left adrenal gland appeared normal on all images.

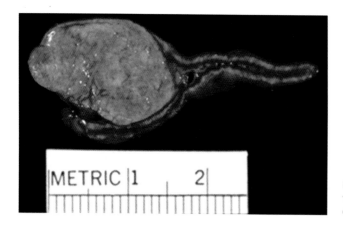

Fig. 7.2 The right adrenal gland weighed 7.9 g (normal adrenal weight is 4–5 g) and contained a 2.3 × 1.6 × 1.1 cm yellow cortical adenoma shown in the cut section.

Key Points

- Nearly all patients with PA who want to pursue the surgical option should undergo AVS. However, there are exceptions to this rule.
- In general, patients with PA due to an APA have more severe manifestations than those with bilateral idiopathic hyperplasia.
- There is an age-related prevalence of nonfunctional adrenal nodules: they are rare in individuals ≤35 years old but relatively common in those >70 years old.
- In the setting of a young (≤35 years) patient with PA who presents with severe PA (defined as spontaneous hypokalemia and PAC >30 ng/dL) and a unilateral adrenal macroadenoma (>1 cm) on CT scan, the clinician may consider bypassing AVS and proceeding to unilateral laparoscopic adrenalectomy (assuming that the contralateral adrenal gland is morphologically normal on CT).
- Preoperative factors in favor of a cure of hypertension following unilateral adrenalectomy in patients with PA include no family history of hypertension, use of two or fewer antihypertensive agents, younger age, normal serum creatinine level, and shorter duration of hypertension (e.g., <10 years).

REFERENCES

1. Young WF Jr. Diagnosis and treatment of primary aldosteronism: practical clinical perspectives. *J Intern Med.* 2019;285(2):126–148.
2. Funder JW, Carey RM, Mantero F, et al. The management of primary aldosteronism: case detection, diagnosis, and treatment: an Endocrine Society Clinical Practice Guideline. *J Clin Endocrinol Metab.* 2016;101(5):1889–1916.
3. Young WF Jr. Clinical practice. The incidentally discovered adrenal mass. *N Engl J Med.* 2007;356(6):601–610.
4. Lim V, Guo Q, Grant CS, et al. Accuracy of adrenal imaging and adrenal venous sampling in predicting surgical cure of primary aldosteronism. *J Clin Endocrinol Metab.* 2014;99(8):2712–2719.
5. Sawka AM, Young WF, Thompson GB, et al. Primary aldosteronism: factors associated with normalization of blood pressure after surgery. *Ann Intern Med.* 2001;135(4):258–261.
6. Benham JL, Eldoma M, Khokhar B, Roberts DJ, Rabi DM, Kline GA. Proportion of patients with hypertension resolution following adrenalectomy for primary aldosteronism: a systematic review and meta-analysis. *J Clin Hypertens* (Greenwich). 2016;18:1205–1212.
7. Velema M, Dekkers T, Hermus A, et al. Quality of life in primary aldosteronism: a comparative effectiveness study of adrenalectomy and medical treatment. *J Clin Endocrinol Metab.* 2018;103(1):16–24.
8. Williams TA, Lenders JWM, Mulatero P, et al. Outcomes after adrenalectomy for unilateral primary aldosteronism: an international consensus on outcome measures and analysis of remission rates in an international cohort. *Lancet Diabetes Endocrinol.* 2017;5:689–699.

Primary Aldosteronism With Unilateral Adrenal Nodule on Computed Tomography

Cross-sectional computed imaging lacks the necessary accuracy to determine if a patient has unilateral adrenal versus bilateral adrenal disease as the cause of primary aldosteronism (PA). If abdominal computed tomography (CT) does not reveal a large adrenal mass consistent with adrenocortical cancer, adrenal venous sampling (AVS) is an essential localization step in patients with confirmed PA who want to pursue surgical management. The only exception to this rule is the patient who is young, has marked PA, and a unilateral solitary adrenal macroadenoma is documented on adrenal CT (see Case 7).

Case Report

The patient was a 68-year-old woman who had been hypertensive for 40 years. However, she had accelerated hypertension and new-onset diuretic-induced hypokalemia over the past 6 months. Previously her blood pressure was under good control with an angiotensin-converting enzyme inhibitor and hydrochlorothiazide. Due to the hypokalemia, her local physician changed her antihypertensive program to metoprolol (12.5 mg twice daily) and amlodipine (5 mg daily). She took potassium 20 mEq twice daily to correct the hypokalemia. She had no signs or symptoms of Cushing syndrome.

INVESTIGATIONS

The baseline laboratory test results are shown in Table 8.1. The patient had positive case detection testing for PA with a plasma aldosterone concentration (PAC) >10 ng/dL and plasma renin activity

(PRA) <1.0 ng/mL per hour.[1] Due to lack of spontaneous hypokalemia, formal confirmatory testing with oral sodium loading was performed.[1,2] The patient was counseled on a high-sodium diet over 3 days, and the 24-hour urine was collected from day 3 to day 4. The patient monitored her blood pressure daily and serum potassium was checked daily. PA was confirmed with the 24-hour urinary aldosterone excretion of 20 mcg and a urinary sodium excretion of 190 mEq (the latter confirming compliance with the high-sodium diet). Clinicians frequently ask what to do if the 24-hour urine sodium is <200 mEq. The 200 mEq cutoff serves as a guide—it is not an absolute, and clinical judgment should be used. In this patient's case a 24-hour urine sodium of 190 mEq was "close enough" and a repeat test was not needed. The baseline dehydroepiandrosterone sulfate (DHEA-S) was normal, and cortisol suppressed normally with the 1-mg overnight dexamethasone suppression test (DST) (see Table 8.1).

An unenhanced adrenal-dedicated CT scan showed a lipid-rich 1.6-cm left adrenal nodule (Fig. 8.1).

After a thorough discussion with her, the patient was keen to pursue a surgical cure of hypokalemia and better control of her hypertension on less medication. She understood that a cure of her hypertension with surgery was not a reasonable goal in view of the duration of hypertension of >10 years.[1,3]

AVS was performed as the next step. AVS was successful based on adrenal vein-to-inferior vena cava (IVC) cortisol gradients of more than 5-to-1 (Box 8.1).[4,5] With the continuous cosyntropin infusion protocol (cosyntropin 50 mcg/h administered intravenously starting 30 minutes before AVS and continued throughout the procedure), the adrenal-to-IVC cortisol

TABLE 8.1 **Laboratory Tests**		
Biochemical Test	**Result**	**Reference Range**
Sodium	138	135–145
Potassium	4.2	3.6–5.2
Creatinine	0.8	0.8–1.3
eGFR	>60	>60 mL/min/BSA
Aldosterone	18	≤21 ng/dL
Plasma renin activity	<0.6	≤0.6–3 ng/mL per hour
DHEA-S	48.9	9.7–159 mcg/dL
1-mg overnight DST	<1.0	<1.8 mcg/dL
24-hour urine aldosterone	20	<12 mcg if 24-hour urine sodium >200 mEq
24-hour urine sodium	190	Goal for oral sodium loading >200 mEq

BSA, Body surface area; *DHEA-S,* dehydroepiandrosterone-sulfate; *DST,* dexamethasone suppression test; *eGFR,* estimated glomerular filtration rate.

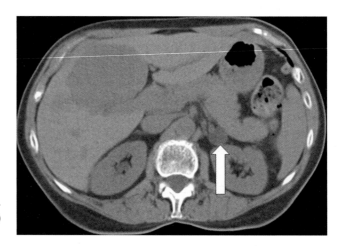

Fig. 8.1 An unenhanced adrenal-dedicated computed tomography scan (axial image) showed a lipid-rich (−1 Hounsfield unit) 1.6-cm left adrenal nodule (*arrow*).

gradients are typically well above the 5-to-1 cutoff (in this case, 25-to-1 on the right and 9.2-to-1 on the left). Each adrenal vein aldosterone (A) concentration is divided by the respective cortisol (C) concentration for the A/C ratio (see Box 8.1). The A/C ratio from the dominant adrenal is divided by the A/C ratio from the nondominant adrenal to determine the aldosterone lateralization ratio. In this case, an A/C ratio of 5.4 on the right is divided by an A/C ratio of 3.3 on the left, yielding an aldosterone lateralization ratio of 1.7-to-1 (right to left). When the aldosterone lateralization ratio is <3-to-1 and the A/C ratio from each adrenal vein is greater than the A/C ratio in the IVC, the patient is presumed to have bilateral idiopathic hyperplasia and medical management is advised.[1,4] Thus the 1.6-cm adrenal nodule in the left adrenal gland was not the source of aldosterone excess, and AVS prevented surgical mismanagement based on CT scan findings.

TREATMENT

The patient was advised to start treatment with spironolactone 50 mg daily. Treatments with potassium chloride and metoprolol were discontinued. The patient was advised to monitor blood pressure daily and follow up with her primary care physician for medication adjustments with a target average blood pressure of <135/85 mmHg. The dosage of spironolactone was not guided by blood pressure but rather by serum potassium concentration. She was advised to have serum potassium checked weekly and the dose of

BOX 8.1   ADRENAL VEIN SAMPLING[a]

	Right AV	IVC	Left AV
Aldosterone, ng/dL	3110	38	690
Cortisol, mcg/dL	576	23	212
A/C ratio[b]	5.4	1.7	3.3
Aldosterone lateralization ratio 1.7-to-1 (right-to-left)			
A/C ratios from both adrenal veins (5.4 on RT and 3.3 on LT) > A/C ratio in IVC (1.7)			

[a]Sequential AVS completed under continuous cosyntropin infusion 50 mcg/h.

[b]Each adrenal aldosterone concentration is divided by the respective cortisol concentration for the A/C ratio. The A/C ratio from the dominant adrenal is divided by the A/C ratio from the nondominant adrenal for the aldosterone lateralization ratio. In this case, 5.4 on the right is divided by 3.3 on the left, yielding an aldosterone lateralization ratio of 1.7-to-1 (right to left). When the aldosterone lateralization ratio is <3-to-1 and the A/C ratios from both adrenal veins are greater than the A/C ratio in the IVC, the data are consistent with bilateral idiopathic adrenal hyperplasia.

A, Aldosterone; *AV*, adrenal vein; *C*, cortisol; *LT*, left; *RT*, right; *IVC*, inferior vena cava.

spironolactone increased as needed for a target serum potassium concentration of 4.5 mEq/L.

OUTCOME AND FOLLOW-UP

To achieve a target serum potassium of 4.5 mEq/L, the patient's dose of spironolactone was increased to 100 mg daily. With improved blood pressure control, the dosage of amlodipine was decreased to 2.5 mg daily. CT without contrast and 1-mg DST performed 1 year later showed no change in the size of the left adrenal adenoma and normal cortisol suppression. The patient was advised to have no further imaging follow-up of the nonfunctioning lipid-rich left adrenal adenoma.

Key Points

- Computed cross-sectional imaging of the adrenal glands is not accurate in determining if PA is caused by unilateral or bilateral adrenal disease. Bottom line: don't trust CT!
- Use common sense in interpreting confirmatory testing for PA.
- The correct dosage of a mineralocorticoid antagonist is whatever it takes to achieve a target serum potassium of 4.5 mEq/L without the aid of potassium supplements.

REFERENCES

1. Young WF Jr. Diagnosis and treatment of primary aldosteronism: practical clinical perspectives. *J Intern Med.* 2019;285(2):126–148.
2. Funder JW, Carey RM, Mantero F, et al. The management of primary aldosteronism: case detection, diagnosis, and treatment: an Endocrine Society Clinical Practice Guideline. *J Clin Endocrinol Metab.* 2016;101(5):1889–1916.
3. Sawka AM, Young WF, Thompson GB, et al. Primary aldosteronism: factors associated with normalization of blood pressure after surgery. *Ann Intern Med.* 2001;135(4):258–261.
4. Young WF, Stanson AW, Thompson GB, Grant CS, Farley DR, van Heerden JA. Role for adrenal venous sampling in primary aldosteronism. *Surgery.* 2004;136(6):1227–1235.
5. Young WF, Stanson AW. What are the keys to successful adrenal venous sampling (AVS) in patients with primary aldosteronism? *Clin Endocrinol (Oxf).* 2009;70(1):14–17.

Primary Aldosteronism With Bilateral Adrenal Nodules on Computed Tomography

The differential diagnosis in a patient with primary aldosteronism (PA) when bilateral adrenocortical nodules are found on adrenal computed tomography (CT) scan includes bilateral idiopathic nodular hyperplasia, bilateral aldosterone-producing adrenal adenomas, unilateral aldosterone-producing adenoma and contralateral nonfunctioning nodule, and a mix of aldosterone- and cortisol-producing adrenal adenomas. All patients who have an adrenal nodule on CT should be evaluated for cortisol secretory autonomy with baseline blood dehydroepiandrosterone sulfate (DHEA-S) concentration and an overnight dexamethasone suppression test (DST). Whether to pursue subtype evaluation with adrenal venous sampling (AVS) is based on a shared decision-making discussion with the patient. If the patient would like to pursue the surgical treatment option and is a reasonable surgical candidate, then AVS is the best next step.

Case Report

The patient was a 69-year-old African American man with a 15-year history of hypertension. He was treated with a three-drug program: β-adrenergic blocker (carvedilol 25 mg twice daily), direct vasodilator (hydralazine 100 mg three times per day), and an angiotensin receptor blocker (losartan 50 mg daily). Blood pressure control was not optimal, with systolic blood pressures typically in the mid-150s mmHg. Spontaneous hypokalemia was first noted 7 years previously with serum potassium concentrations of 3.2 mmol/L and 3.1 mmol/L, but remarkably, he was not tested for PA until recently.

At the time of referral to Mayo Clinic he was taking 160 mEq of potassium chloride daily to maintain a normal serum potassium concentration. Beyond hypertension and chronic kidney disease (CKD), the patient was healthy. He had no signs or symptoms of Cushing syndrome.

INVESTIGATIONS

The baseline laboratory test results are shown in Table 9.1. The serum creatinine concentration was consistent with stage 3a CKD—likely the result of long-standing untreated PA.[1–3] The patient had positive case detection testing for PA with a plasma aldosterone concentration (PAC) >10 ng/dL and plasma renin activity (PRA) <0.6 ng/mL per hour.[1] In addition, PA was confirmed because when a patient has spontaneous hypokalemia and the PAC >20 ng/dL, there are no other differential diagnostic possibilities beyond PA.[1,2] Thus formal confirmatory testing with oral sodium loading or a saline infusion test was not needed. The low-normal levels of DHEA-S and corticotropin (ACTH) suggested that there may be a component of subclinical glucocorticoid secretory autonomy—a suggestion that was confirmed with lack of normal suppression of the serum cortisol concentration with the overnight 2-mg DST (see Table 9.1).

An unenhanced adrenal-dedicated CT scan showed a lipid-rich 1.2 × 1.6 cm right adrenal nodule and a lipid-poor 1.0-cm left adrenal nodule (Fig. 9.1).

After a thorough discussion with the patient, it was clear that the patient was keen to pursue a surgical cure of hypokalemia and better control of his hypertension on less medication. He understood that a cure of his hypertension with surgery was not a reasonable

TABLE 9.1	Laboratory Tests	
Biochemical Test	Result	Reference Range
Sodium	146	135–145
Potassium	4.5	3.6–5.2
Creatinine	1.6	0.8–1.3
eGFR	52	>60 mL/min per BSA
Aldosterone	71	≤21 ng/dL
Plasma renin activity	<0.6	≤0.6–3 ng/mL per hour
DHEA-S	37.3	25–131 mcg/dL
ACTH	12	7.2–63 pg/mL
2-mg overnight DST	2.6	<1.8 mcg/dL

ACTH, Corticotropin; *BSA*, body surface area; *DHEA-S*, dehydroepiandrosterone-sulfate; *DST*, dexamethasone suppression test; *eGFR*, estimated glomerular filtration rate.

goal in view of the duration of hypertension of >10 years and the presence of CKD.[1,4] He was also counseled that patients with PA hyperfiltrate at the kidney the degree of renal insufficiency is actually worse than it appears—PA "masks" the degree of underlying CKD.[1,5] This is not a reason to avoid effective therapy for a patient, but rather something that the patient and all of his or her physicians need to understand because

the serum creatinine will rise after effective treatment with either surgery or treatment with a mineralocorticoid receptor antagonist.[1,5]

AVS was performed as the next step. The patient was well hydrated with intravenously administered saline. In addition, care was taken to limit the use of contrast dye. AVS was successful based on adrenal vein-to-inferior vena cava (IVC) cortisol gradients of more than 5-to-1 (Box 9.1).[6,7] With the continuous cosyntropin infusion protocol (cosyntropin 50 mcg/h administered intravenously starting 30 minutes before AVS and continued throughout the procedure), the adrenal-to-IVC cortisol gradients are typically well above the 5-to-1 cutoff (in this case, 22.8-to-1 on the right and 13.1-to-1 on the left). Each adrenal aldosterone concentration is divided by the respective cortisol concentration for the A/C ratio (see Box 9.1). The A/C ratio from the dominant adrenal is divided by the A/C ratio from the nondominant adrenal for the aldosterone lateralization ratio. In this case, 46.8 on the left is divided by 1.9 on the right, yielding an aldosterone lateralization ratio of 24.6-to-1 (left-to-right). When the aldosterone lateralization ratio is >4-to-1, unilateral adrenalectomy will be curative.[1,6] It is also

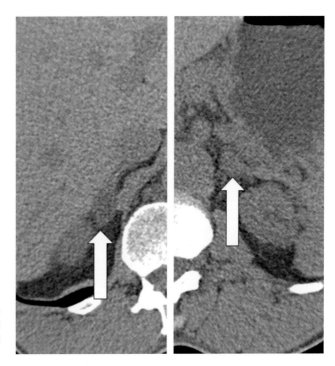

Fig. 9.1 An unenhanced adrenal-dedicated computed tomography scan showed a lipid-rich (−1.9 Hounsfield units [HU]) 1.2 × 1.6 cm right adrenal nodule (*arrow*) and a lipid-poor (22.2 HU) 1.0-cm left adrenal nodule (*arrow*).

BOX 9.1   ADRENAL VEIN SAMPLING[a]

	Right AV	IVC	Left AV
Aldosterone, ng/dL	790	170	11,000
Cortisol, mcg/dL	411	18	235
A/C ratio[b]	1.9	9.4	46.8
Aldosterone lateralization ratio			24.6-to-1
Contralateral suppression index 0.2			

[a]Sequential AVS completed under continuous cosyntropin infusion 50 mcg/h.
[b]Each adrenal aldosterone concentration is divided by the respective cortisol concentration for the A/C ratio. The A/C ratio from the dominant adrenal is divided by the A/C ratio from the nondominant adrenal for the aldosterone lateralization ratio. In this case, 46.8 on the left is divided by 1.9 on the right, yielding an aldosterone lateralization ratio of 24.6-to-1 (left to right). When the aldosterone lateralization ratio is >4-to-1, unilateral adrenalectomy will be curative. An additional predictor of unilateral disease is when the nondominant adrenal vein A/C ratio is less than that in the IVC and this is termed the contralateral suppression index.
AV, Adrenal vein; *IVC,* inferior vena cava.

reassuring to confirm relative suppression of aldosterone secretion from the nondominant adrenal by dividing the A/C ratio from the nondominant adrenal by the A/C ratio from the IVC.[1,6] In this case, the A/C ratio of 1.9 on the right was divided by 9.4 from the IVC, yielding a value of 0.2. Contralateral adrenal suppression is confirmed when this value is <1.0. Thus the larger adrenal nodule in the right adrenal gland was not the source of aldosterone excess.

TREATMENT

The patient underwent laparoscopic left adrenalectomy. The left adrenal gland weighed 9 g and contained a 1.5 × 1.0 × 0.9 cm yellow cortical adenoma (Fig. 9.2). The PAC the day after surgery was <4 ng/dL and consistent with a surgical cure. In view of the mild degree of glucocorticoid secretory autonomy, he was given perioperative glucocorticoid coverage and was sent home on prednisone 5 mg every morning with the plan to check a morning serum cortisol 2 weeks later. Treatment with potassium chloride and losartan was stopped the day after surgery. The patient was advised to monitor his blood pressure daily and blood pressure medications adjusted as needed for high-normal blood pressure for the first month after surgery.

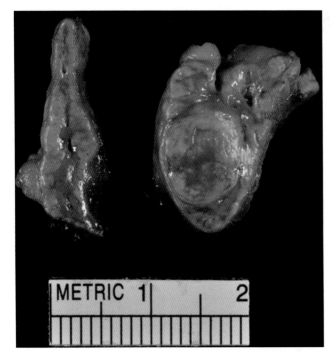

Fig. 9.2 The left adrenal gland weighed 9 g (normal adrenal weight is 4 g) and contained a 1.5 × 1.0 × 0.9–cm yellow cortical adenoma shown in the cut section on the right.

OUTCOME AND FOLLOW-UP

The patient's weekly blood potassium concentrations remained normal (3.7, 4.4, 4.4, and 4.2 mmol/L), and treatment with fludrocortisone was not needed. The 8 AM serum cortisol was checked before his morning dose of prednisone 2 weeks after surgery and was normal (15.2 mcg/dL). Prednisone was discontinued. One month after surgery, as predicted, the serum creatinine rose to 1.9 mg/dL with an estimated glomerular filtration rate (eGFR) of 43 (stage 3b CKD). One year postoperatively the adrenal magnetic resonance imaging scan showed no change in the right adrenal nodule. Two years postoperatively the patient had good blood pressure control on amlodipine 10 mg daily, carvedilol 6.25 mg daily, and hydralazine 50 mg twice daily. His serum potassium concentration remained normal at 4.1 mmol/L and the serum creatinine was slightly higher at 2.15 mg/dL (eGFR 37). The 1-mg overnight DST was normal.

Key Points

- Most patients with PA remain undiagnosed for years. What was remarkable in this case was that despite chronic hypokalemia, it was 7 years before case detection testing for PA was performed for this patient.
- To prevent PA-related cardiac disease and renal dysfunction, all patients with hypertension should have case detection testing for PA at least once.
- In the setting of spontaneous hypokalemia, PAC >20 ng/dL, and PRA <1 ng/mL per hour, formal confirmatory testing for PA is not needed.
- All patients with PA who have an adrenal nodule on CT should be screened for subclinical glucocorticoid secretory autonomy with a baseline DHEA-S and an overnight DST.
- Subclinical glucocorticoid secretory autonomy, when mild, does not interfere with the interpretation of AVS.

- When a patient with PA has bilateral adrenal nodules, AVS is mandatory if the patient wants to pursue a surgical cure.
- Due to the hyperfiltration associated with untreated PA, renal function appears better than it is and serum creatinine will rise with effective treatment of PA.
- Reasonable surgical treatment goals in those patients with PA who have had hypertension for more than 10 years are resolution of hypokalemia and improved hypertension control on 50% less medication.

REFERENCES

1. Young WF Jr. Diagnosis and treatment of primary aldosteronism: practical clinical perspectives. *J Intern Med.* 2019;285(2):126–148.
2. Funder JW, Carey RM, Mantero F, et al. The management of primary aldosteronism: case detection, diagnosis, and treatment: an endocrine society clinical practice guideline. *J Clin Endocrinol Metab.* 2016;101(5): 1889–1916.
3. Nishiyama A. Pathophysiological mechanisms of mineralocorticoid receptor-dependent cardiovascular and chronic kidney disease. *Hypertens Res.* 2019;42(3):293–300.
4. Sawka AM, Young WF, Thompson GB, et al. Primary aldosteronism: factors associated with normalization of blood pressure after surgery. *Ann Intern Med.* 2001;135(4):258–261.
5. Kim IY, Park IS, Kim MJ, et al. Change in kidney function after unilateral adrenalectomy in patients with primary aldosteronism: identification of risk factors for decreased kidney function. *Int Urol Nephrol.* 2018;50(10):1887–1895.
6. Young WF, Stanson AW, Thompson GB, Grant CS, Farley DR, van Heerden JA. Role for adrenal venous sampling in primary aldosteronism. *Surgery.* 2004;136(6):1227–1235.
7. Young WF, Stanson AW. What are the keys to successful adrenal venous sampling (AVS) in patients with primary aldosteronism? *Clin Endocrinol (Oxf).* 2009;70(1):14–17.

Primary Aldosteronism Caused by Unilateral Adrenal Hyperplasia

There are six subtypes of primary aldosteronism (PA). The most common subtype of PA is bilateral idiopathic adrenal hyperplasia (IHA) ($\approx$60% of patients) (see Case 8). The second most common subtype of PA, in approximately 30% of patients, is caused by a unilateral aldosterone-producing adenoma (APA) (see Cases 7, 9, 12, 13, 14, and 15). The third most common subtype of PA is unilateral or primary adrenal hyperplasia (referred to as UAH or PAH). The diagnosis of UAH is based on (1) unilateral adrenal localization with adrenal venous sampling (AVS), (2) lack of an adrenal adenoma and the presence of zona glomerulosa hyperplasia on pathology, and (3) long-term cure of PA with unilateral adrenalectomy.

Case Report

The patient was a 65-year-old man who had been hypertensive for 20 years. He had spontaneous hypokalemia for the past 4 years. He was treated with 60 mEq of potassium chloride per day along with five antihypertensive drugs including clonidine (0.3 mg twice daily), doxazosin (8 mg daily), lisinopril (40 mg daily), verapamil (240 mg twice daily), and hydralazine (100 mg three times per day). He had a subarachnoid hemorrhage 6 years previously that left him with left-sided weakness. He had no signs or symptoms of Cushing syndrome.

INVESTIGATIONS

The baseline laboratory test results are shown in Table 10.1. The patient had positive case detection testing for PA with a plasma aldosterone concentration (PAC) >10 ng/dL and plasma renin activity (PRA) <1.0 ng/mL per hour.[1] Because the patient had spontaneous hypokalemia and a PAC >20 ng/dL,

formal confirmatory testing was not needed.[1,2] The baseline dehydroepiandrosterone sulfate (DHEA-S) was normal (see Table 10.1). An enhanced adrenal-dedicated CT scan showed nodular thickening of the left adrenal gland (Fig. 10.1).

After a thorough discussion with him, the patient was keen to pursue a surgical cure of hypokalemia and better control of his hypertension on less medication. He understood that a cure of his hypertension with surgery was not a reasonable goal in view of the duration of hypertension of >10 years.[1,3]

AVS was performed as the next step (Fig. 10.2). AVS was successful based on adrenal vein-to–inferior vena cava (IVC) cortisol gradients of more to 5-to-1 (Box 10.1).[4,5] With the continuous cosyntropin infusion protocol (cosyntropin 50 mcg/h administered intravenously starting 30 minutes before AVS and continued throughout the procedure), the adrenal-to-IVC cortisol gradients are typically well above the 5-to-1 cutoff (in this case, 55.5-to-1 on the right and 30-to-1 on the left). Each adrenal vein aldosterone (A) concentration is divided by the respective cortisol (C) concentration for the A/C ratio (see Box 10.1). The A/C ratio from the dominant adrenal is divided by the A/C ratio from the nondominant adrenal to determine the aldosterone lateralization ratio. In this case, an A/C ratio of 13.8 on the left is divided by an A/C ratio of 0.5 on the right, yielding an aldosterone lateralization ratio of 25.5-to-1 (left to right). When the aldosterone lateralization ratio is >4-to-1, unilateral adrenalectomy will be curative.[1,6] It is also reassuring to confirm relative suppression of aldosterone secretion from the nondominant adrenal by dividing the A/C ratio from the nondominant adrenal by the A/C ratio from the IVC.[1,6] In this case, the A/C ratio of 0.2 on the right was divided by 2.4 from the IVC, yielding a value

TABLE 10.1	Laboratory Tests	
Biochemical Test	**Result**	**Reference Range**
Sodium	146	135–145
Potassium	3.8	3.6–5.2
Creatinine	1.0	0.8–1.3
eGFR	>60	>60 mL/min per BSA
Aldosterone	36	≤21 ng/dL
Plasma renin activity	<0.6	≤0.6–3 ng/mL per hour
DHEA-S	146	12–227 mcg/dL

BSA, Body surface area; *DHEA-S*, dehydroepiandrosterone sulfate; *eGFR*, estimated glomerular filtration rate.

of 0.08. Contralateral adrenal suppression is confirmed when this value is <1.0.

TREATMENT

The patient underwent laparoscopic left adrenalectomy. The left adrenal gland weighed 13.2 g (normal, 4–5 g), and the cut surface of the adrenal gland was uniform yellow-brown in color, soft, and no adenoma was present. Microscopic examination showed cortical hyperplasia (Table 10.2). The PAC the day after surgery was <4 ng/dL and consistent with a surgical cure. His home-going medications included clonidine (0.3 mg twice daily), doxazosin (8 mg daily), lisinopril (20 mg daily), verapamil (240 mg twice daily), and hydralazine (50 mg three times per day). Treatment with potassium chloride and doxazosin was discontinued. The patient was advised to monitor his blood pressure daily and blood pressure medications adjusted as needed for high-normal blood pressure for the first month after surgery.

OUTCOME AND FOLLOW-UP

The patient's weekly blood potassium concentrations over 4 weeks were normal, and treatment with fludrocortisone was not needed. The underlying pathophysiology of UAH is unknown. In our Mayo Clinic series of 203 patients with PA published in 2004, UAH was diagnosed in 8 patients (4%).[4] Postoperatively, with a mean follow-up of 6.2 years, six of the eight patients (75%) were normotensive without the aid of antihypertensive drugs, and none had recurrent PA.[4] In a more recent surgical series from Mayo Clinic published in 2019, UAH was diagnosed in 33 of 206 patients with PA who were sent to surgery.[6] Patients with UAH were more likely to be male, undergo left-sided adrenalectomy, and had lower median AVS

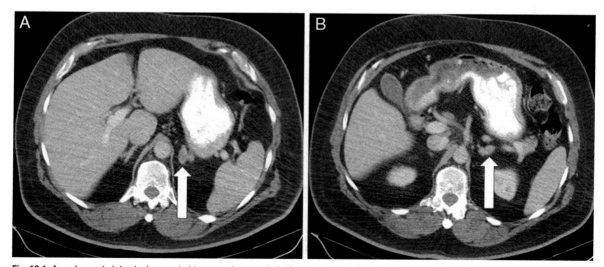

Fig. 10.1 An enhanced abdominal computed tomography scan (axial image) showed nodular thickening of the left adrenal gland. A, Superior limb of the left adrenal gland is thickened (*arrow*). B, Inferior limb of the left adrenal gland is also thickened (*arrow*).

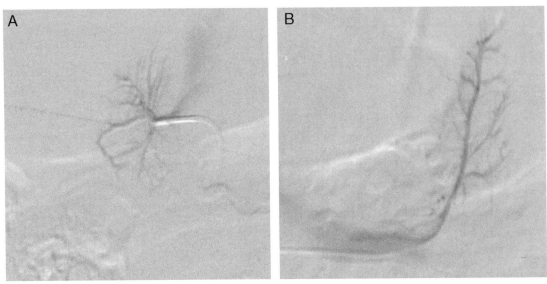

Fig. 10.2 Radiographs from adrenal venous sampling. A, Right adrenal venous anatomy is shown with contrast administration. B, Left adrenal vein venous anatomy is shown.

BOX 10.1 ADRENAL VEIN SAMPLING[a]

	Right AV	IVC	Left AV
Aldosterone, ng/dL	654	53	9280
Cortisol, mcg/dL	1220	22	673
A/C ratio[b]	0.5	2.4	13.8
Aldosterone lateralization ratio			25.5-to-1
Contralateral suppression index 0.2			

[a]Sequential AVS completed under continuous cosyntropin infusion 50 mcg/h.
[b]Each adrenal aldosterone concentration is divided by the respective cortisol concentration for the A/C ratio. The A/C ratio from the dominant adrenal is divided by the A/C ratio from the nondominant adrenal for the aldosterone lateralization ratio. In this case, 13.8 on the left is divided by 0.5 on the right, yielding an aldosterone lateralization ratio of 25.5-to-1 (left to right). When the aldosterone lateralization ratio is >4-to-1, unilateral adrenalectomy will be curative. An additional predictor of unilateral disease is when the nondominant adrenal vein A/C ratio is less than that in the IVC and this is termed the contralateral suppression index. A, Aldosterone; AV, adrenal vein; C, cortisol; IVC, inferior vena cava; LT, left; RT, right.

TABLE 10.2 Forms of Primary Aldosteronism

Subtype of Primary Aldosteronism (PA)	Estimated Proportion of All Patients with PA
Aldosterone-producing adenoma (APA)	30%
Bilateral idiopathic hyperplasia (IHA)	60%
Unilateral (primary) adrenal hyperplasia (UAH/PAH)	4%
Aldosterone-producing adrenocortical carcinoma	<1%
Familial hyperaldosteronism (FH)	
Glucocorticoid-remediable aldosteronism (FH type I) (germline CYP11B1/CYP11B2 chimeric gene)	<1%
FH type II (APA or IHA) (germline CLCN2 pathogenic variants)	<6%
FH type III (germline KCNJ5 pathogenic variants)	<1%
FH type IV (germline CACNA1H pathogenic variants)	<0.1%
Ectopic aldosterone-producing neoplasm	<0.1%

aldosterone lateralization ratios (9.8 versus 19.8, $P = .04$) compared to patients with APA. No significant differences in the rates of hypertension cure or improvement were observed between patients with

UAH versus APA.[6] Thus detecting and surgically managing UAH is just as important and successful as that for APAs. Five years after surgery our patient was normokalemic, and hypertension was well controlled on only two antihypertensive medications (lisinopril and verapamil).

Key Points

- Although UAH is less common than IHA or APA, it is important to identify patients with UAH because they have a long-term cure with unilateral adrenalectomy (see Table 10.2).
- The diagnosis of UAH is made postoperatively and is based on (1) localization to one adrenal gland with AVS, (2) lack of an adrenal adenoma and the presence of zona glomerulosa hyperplasia on pathology, and (3) long-term cure of PA with unilateral adrenalectomy.

REFERENCES

1. Young WF Jr. Diagnosis and treatment of primary aldosteronism: practical clinical perspectives. *J Intern Med.* 2019;285(2):126–148.
2. Funder JW, Carey RM, Mantero F, et al. The management of primary aldosteronism: case detection, diagnosis, and treatment: an Endocrine Society Clinical Practice Guideline. *J Clin Endocrinol Metab.* 2016;101(5):1889–1916.
3. Sawka AM, Young WF, Thompson GB, et al. Primary aldosteronism: factors associated with normalization of blood pressure after surgery. *Ann Intern Med.* 2001;135(4):258–261.
4. Young WF, Stanson AW, Thompson GB, Grant CS, Farley DR, van Heerden JA. Role for adrenal venous sampling in primary aldosteronism. *Surgery.* 2004;136(6):1227–1235.
5. Young WF, Stanson AW. What are the keys to successful adrenal venous sampling (AVS) in patients with primary aldosteronism? *Clin Endocrinol* (Oxf). 2009;70(1):14–17.
6. Shariq OA, Mehta K, Thompson GB, et al. Primary aldosteronism: does underlying pathology impact clinical presentation and outcomes following unilateral adrenalectomy? *World J Surg.* 2019;43(10):2469–2476.

Primary Aldosteronism in a Patient With Bilateral Macronodular Adrenal Hyperplasia and Associated Clinically Important Cortisol Cosecretion

Bilateral macronodular adrenal hyperplasia (BMAH) is typically a computed tomography (CT)-based diagnosis. When patients present with primary aldosteronism (PA) and BMAH is found on the CT scan, the aldosterone hypersecretion is bilateral and usually associated with cortisol cosecretion, resulting in either clinically evident Cushing syndrome or subclinical Cushing syndrome (also referred to as "mild autonomous cortisol secretion"). Adrenal venous sampling (AVS) is usually not needed in this setting because, by definition, the disorder is bilateral. Treatment is surgical. If the patient has subclinical Cushing syndrome (mild autonomous cortisol secretion), then there is the opportunity to resect the larger adrenal gland to debulk the disease. If the patient has clinically overt Cushing syndrome, bilateral adrenalectomy is the best treatment option.

Case Report

The patient was a 69-year-old man with a 34-year history of hypertension; PA was diagnosed 9 years previously when he presented with spontaneous hypokalemia. His visit to Mayo Clinic was triggered by accelerated hypertension 6 months prior. He was treated with a four-drug program: calcium channel blocker (nifedipine 30 mg daily), β-adrenergic blocker (carvedilol 12.5 mg twice daily), an angiotensin receptor blocker (losartan 100 mg daily), and a diuretic (chlorthalidone 25 mg daily). Blood pressure control was not optimal. At the time of referral to Mayo Clinic he was taking 40 mEq of potassium chloride daily in an effort to maintain a normal serum potassium concentration. Beyond hypertension and hypokalemia, the patient was healthy. He had no signs or symptoms of overt Cushing syndrome. He did not have diabetes mellitus or osteoporosis. He had one first-degree relative who had been diagnosed with hypertension.

INVESTIGATIONS

The baseline laboratory test results are shown in Table 11.1. The patient had positive case detection testing for PA with plasma aldosterone concentration (PAC) >10 ng/dL and plasma renin activity (PRA) <1.0 ng/mL per hour.[1] In addition, PA was confirmed because when a patient has spontaneous hypokalemia (noted prior to diuretic therapy) and PAC >20 ng/dL, there are no other differential diagnostic possibilities beyond PA.[1,2] Thus formal confirmatory testing with oral sodium loading or a saline infusion test was not needed for this patient. The diagnosis of glucocorticoid secretory autonomy was based on low serum corticotropin (ACTH) concentration, low-normal serum dehydroepiandrosterone sulfate (DHEA-S) concentration, mild elevation in 24-hour urinary free cortisol excretion, and lack of complete suppression in serum

TABLE 11.1   Laboratory Tests

Biochemical Test	Result	Reference Range
Sodium, mmol/L	144	135–145
Potassium, mmol/L	4.0	3.6–5.2
Creatinine, mg/dL	1.0	0.8–1.3
Aldosterone, ng/dL	24	≤21 ng/dL
Plasma renin activity, ng/mL per hour	<0.6	≤0.6–3
DHEA-S, mcg/dL	39	12–227
ACTH, pg/mL	13	10–60
1-mg overnight DST, mcg/dL	2.5	<1.8
8-mg overnight DST, mcg/dL	3.6	<1.0
24-hour urine cortisol, mcg	84	<45

ACTH, Corticotropin; *DHEA-S*, dehydroepiandrosterone sulfate; *DST*, dexamethasone suppression test.

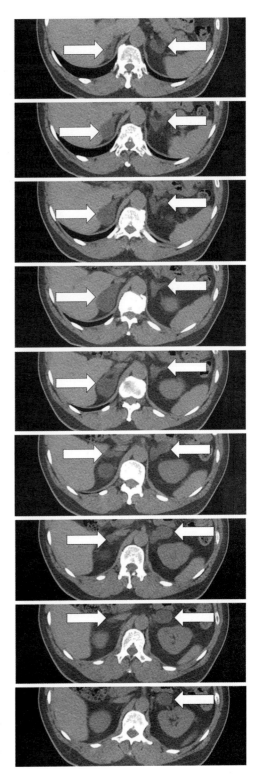

cortisol with an overnight 8-mg dexamethasone suppression test (DST) (see Table 11.1).[3] An unenhanced abdominal CT scan showed bilateral macronodular hyperplasia (Fig. 11.1).

The patient was informed that both adrenal glands were producing aldosterone and cortisol. He understood that because he had subclinical Cushing syndrome (mild autonomous cortisol excess), we had the opportunity to start with a debulking operation by resecting his larger right adrenal gland, and if that did not provide a clinically significant remission, completion adrenalectomy would be needed.

TREATMENT

With perioperative glucocorticoid coverage (100 mg hydrocortisone administered intravenously on call to the operating room and again 8 hours later), the patient underwent laparoscopic right adrenalectomy.

Fig. 11.1 Serial axial images of the adrenal glands (cranial images at *top* and caudal images at *bottom*) from an unenhanced abdominal computed tomography (CT) scan. Bilateral multinodular adrenal glands are shown (*arrows*). The largest nodule in the right adrenal gland was 5.3 cm in diameter and had an unenhanced CT attenuation of –4 Hounsfield units (HU). The largest nodule in the left adrenal gland was 4.2 cm in diameter and had an unenhanced CT attenuation of 9 HU.

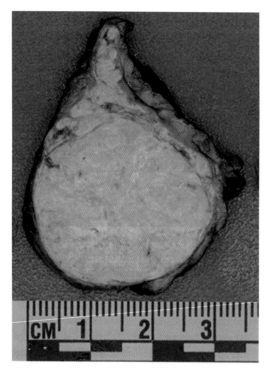

Fig. 11.2 Gross pathology cut section of the right adrenal gland shows diffuse nodular hyperplasia.

The right adrenal gland weighed 39 g (normal, 4–5 g) and on serial sectioning it had a golden-yellow multinodular cut surface (nodules ranging from 0.3 to 3.0 cm in greatest dimension) (Fig. 11.2). The PAC the day after surgery was <4 ng/dL and consistent with a surgical cure. Treatment with potassium chloride, losartan, nifedipine, and chlorthalidone was stopped the day after surgery. On discharge from the hospital the patient was prescribed carvedilol and advised to monitor his blood pressure daily, and blood pressure medications were adjusted as needed for high-normal blood pressure for the first month after surgery. The patient was discharged from the hospital with instructions to take 20 mg of hydrocortisone every morning and to decrease the dosage to 15 mg every morning in 2 weeks.

OUTCOME AND FOLLOW-UP

The patient's serum cortisol was normal 2 weeks after surgery, and hydrocortisone was discontinued. Fourteen months after surgery the patient had excellent blood pressure control on a three-drug program: β-adrenergic blocker (carvedilol 12.5 mg twice daily), an angiotensin receptor blocker (valsartan 160 mg daily), and a mineralocorticoid receptor antagonist (eplerenone 50 mg daily). His serum potassium concentrations were high-normal. Measurements of aldosterone and cortisol were normal, and the patient was extremely pleased with the surgical outcome.

Key Points

- When a patient with PA has a CT-based diagnosis of BMAH, the aldosterone hypersecretion is uniformly bilateral and AVS is not needed.
- The 8-mg overnight DST has a role to absolutely confirm glucocorticoid secretory autonomy in patients with an abnormal 1-mg overnight DST. A normal serum cortisol concentration following 8-mg of dexamethasone is undetectable.
- Autonomous cortisol cosecretion is present in most patients PA who have BMAH. If the patient has ACTH-independent Cushing syndrome, bilateral adrenalectomy is the treatment of choice, whereas if the patient has subclinical Cushing syndrome (mild autonomous cortisol excess), a debulking operation by resecting the larger adrenal gland is a reasonable first operation—recognizing that completion adrenalectomy may be needed in the future.
- Patients with BMAH who have aldosterone and cortisol cosecretion should have perioperative stress glucocorticoid coverage and on discharge should be prescribed a morning dose of hydrocortisone until the hypothalamic-pituitary-adrenal axis recovers.

REFERENCES

1. Young WF Jr. Diagnosis and treatment of primary aldosteronism: practical clinical perspectives. *J Intern Med.* 2019;285(2):126–148.
2. Funder JW, Carey RM, Mantero F, et al. The management of primary aldosteronism: case detection, diagnosis, and treatment: an Endocrine Society Clinical Practice Guideline. *J Clin Endocrinol Metab.* 2016;101(5):1889–1916.
3. Tokumoto M, Onoda N, Tauchi Y, et al. A case of Adrenocoricotrophic hormone-independent bilateral adrenocortical macronodular hyperplasia concomitant with primary aldosteronism. *BMC Surg.* 2017;17(1):97.

Primary Aldosteronism in a Patient With an Adrenal Macroadenoma and Clinically Important Cortisol Cosecretion

Unlike aldosterone-producing adenomas (APAs) that can be <1 cm in diameter and cause the full syndrome of primary aldosteronism (PA), clinically important cortisol-secreting adenomas require a "big factory" (e.g., typically >2 cm in diameter). Thus when a patient with PA has a large adrenal adenoma (>1.5 cm), clinicians should screen for cortisol cosecretion. If autonomous cortisol cosecretion is present in a patient with PA who has a unilateral adrenal macroadenoma, then adrenal venous sampling (AVS) is not needed. Usually in this setting the macroadenoma is cosecreting aldosterone and cortisol. However, even if the patient has PA caused by bilateral idiopathic hyperplasia (IHA) or a contralateral adrenal microadenoma, we do not have a good long-term viable medical treatment option for hypercortisolism, whereas mineralocorticoid receptor antagonists are an excellent treatment option for PA if it proves to persist following unilateral adrenalectomy. Thus if AVS is performed in the setting described in the preceding text, the findings do not guide surgical management.

Case Report

The patient was a 46-year-old man with a 15-year history of hypertension, which accelerated 10 years ago. He was treated with a three-drug program: calcium channel blocker (amlodipine 10 mg daily), combined β- and α-adrenergic blocker (labetalol 400 mg twice daily), and an angiotensin-converting enzyme inhibitor (enalapril 10 mg daily). Blood pressure control was not optimal. He was referred to Mayo Clinic for AVS. At the time of referral to Mayo Clinic he was taking 40 mEq of potassium chloride daily in an effort to maintain a normal serum potassium concentration. Beyond hypertension and hypokalemia, the patient was healthy. His body mass index was 29.2 kg/m^2. He had no signs or symptoms of overt Cushing syndrome. He did not have diabetes mellitus or osteoporosis. He had two first-degree relatives who had been diagnosed with hypertension.

INVESTIGATIONS

The baseline laboratory test results are shown in Table 12.1. The patient had positive case detection testing for PA with plasma aldosterone concentration (PAC) >10 ng/dL and plasma renin activity (PRA) <1.0 ng/mL per hour.[1] In addition, PA was confirmed because when a patient has spontaneous hypokalemia and a PAC >20 ng/dL, there are no other differential diagnostic possibilities beyond PA.[1,2] Thus formal confirmatory testing with oral sodium loading or a saline infusion test was not needed for this patient. A baseline 24-hour urine for sodium showed that this patient was on a daily high sodium diet, which was contributing to his resistant hypertension and hypokalemia. Serum corticotropin (ACTH) was undetectable and the serum dehydroepiandrosterone sulfate (DHEA-S) concentration was low-normal, and cortisol did not suppress with an overnight 8-mg dexamethasone suppression test (DST) (see Table 12.1).

TABLE 12.1 Laboratory Tests		
Biochemical Test	Result	Reference Range
Sodium, mmol/L	141	135–145
Potassium, mmol/L	3.3	3.6–5.2
Creatinine, mg/dL	1.3	0.8–1.3
Aldosterone, ng/dL	26	≤21 ng/dL
Plasma renin activity, ng/mL per hour	<0.6	≤0.6–3
DHEA-S, mcg/dL	62.9	48–244
ACTH, pg/mL	<5.0	10–60
8-mg overnight DST, mcg/dL	5.9	<1.0
24-hour urine sodium, mmol	343	40–217
24-hour urine aldosterone, mcg	28	<12 if urine sodium >200 mmol

ACTH, Corticotropin; *DHEA-S*, dehydroepiandrosterone-sulfate; *DST*, dexamethasone suppression test.

An unenhanced adrenal-dedicated CT scan showed an indeterminate 4.2-cm left adrenal mass (Fig. 12.1). The right adrenal gland appeared atrophic on CT.

The patient was informed that the left adrenal mass was the source of glucocorticoid secretory autonomy, and that it was also likely the source of aldosterone hypersecretion. He understood that regardless of what an AVS study might show, the left indeterminate adrenal mass should be resected with the goal curing the glucocorticoid secretory autonomy and hopefully PA too.

TREATMENT

With perioperative glucocorticoid coverage (40 mg of methylprednisolone administered intramuscularly on call to the operating room and again 12 hours later), the patient underwent laparoscopic left adrenalectomy. The left adrenal weighed 36.3 g (normal, 4–5 g) and contained a 3.5 × 3.5 × 2.2–cm yellow cortical adenoma. The PAC the day after surgery was <4 ng/dL and consistent with a surgical cure. Treatment with potassium chloride and enalapril was stopped the day after surgery. The patient was advised to monitor his blood pressure daily and blood pressure medications adjusted as needed for high-normal blood pressure for the first month after surgery. On discharge from the hospital the patient was prescribed 20 mg of hydrocortisone every morning with instructions to decrease the dosage to 15 mg every morning in 2 weeks.

OUTCOME AND FOLLOW-UP

The patient's weekly blood potassium concentrations remained high-normal weekly for 4 weeks after surgery. Serum creatinine remained normal. He had good blood pressure control on lower dosages of amlodipine and labetalol. The 8 AM serum cortisol concentration obtained before his morning dose of hydrocortisone

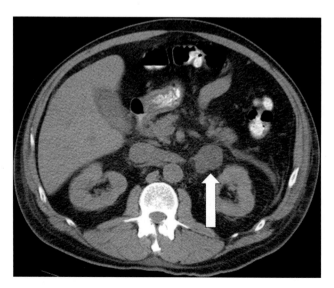

Fig. 12.1 Axial image from an unenhanced adrenal-dedicated computed tomography (CT) scan showed an indeterminate (15.6 Hounsfield units [HU]) 4.2-cm left adrenal mass (*arrow*). The right adrenal gland appeared atrophic.

was >10 mcg/dL at 6 weeks after surgery, and hydrocortisone was discontinued.

Key Points

- When a patient with PA has a large (>1.5 cm) adrenal adenoma, clinicians should screen for cortisol cosecretion with baseline DHEA-S and overnight DST.
- The 8-mg overnight DST has a role to absolutely confirm glucocorticoid secretory autonomy in patients with an abnormal 1-mg overnight DST. A normal serum cortisol concentration following 8-mg of dexamethasone is undetectable.
- If autonomous cortisol cosecretion is present in a patient with PA who has a unilateral adrenal macroadenoma, then adrenal venous sampling (AVS) is not needed. Usually in this setting the macroadenoma is cosecreting aldosterone and cortisol.
- Patients with aldosterone and cortisol cosecreting adenomas should have perioperative stress glucocorticoid coverage and on discharge from the hospital prescribed a morning dose of hydrocortisone until the hypothalamic-pituitary-adrenal axis recovers.

REFERENCES

1. Young WF Jr. Diagnosis and treatment of primary aldosteronism: practical clinical perspectives. *J Intern Med*. 2019;285(2):126–148.
2. Funder JW, Carey RM, Mantero F, et al. The management of primary aldosteronism: case detection, diagnosis, and treatment: an Endocrine Society Clinical Practice Guideline. *J Clin Endocrinol Metab*. 2016;101(5):1889–1916.

Primary Aldosteronism in a Patient Treated With Spironolactone

Mineralocorticoid receptor antagonists (MRAs) (e.g., spironolactone and eplerenone) prevent aldosterone from activating the receptor, resulting, sequentially, in sodium loss, a decrease in plasma volume, and an elevation in renin. If plasma renin activity (PRA) or plasma renin concentration (PRC) is not suppressed in a patient treated with a MRA, then no further primary aldosteronism (PA)-related testing can be performed, and the MRA should be discontinued for 6 weeks before retesting. However, if the patient is hypokalemic despite treatment with a MRA, then the mineralocorticoid receptors are not fully blocked, and PRA or PRC should be suppressed in such a patient with PA. In addition, most patients with PA are treated with suboptimal dosages of MRAs, and the mineralocorticoid receptors are not fully blocked. Thus for case detection testing, blood pressure medications, including MRAs, should not be discontinued. In the setting of suppressed PRA or PRC, clinicians can proceed with case detection testing in all patients treated with MRAs, and the MRA does not need to be discontinued for confirmatory or subtype testing with adrenal venous sampling (AVS).

Case Report

The patient was a 57-year-old woman with an 11-year history of hypertension. She was treated with a four-drug program: β-adrenergic blocker (atenolol 50 mg daily), calcium channel blocker (nifedipine extended release 60 mg per day), an angiotensin-converting enzyme inhibitor (lisinopril 20 mg daily), and a mineralocorticoid receptor antagonist (spironolactone 100 mg daily). She was also taking 60 mEq of potassium chloride twice daily. Hypokalemia was first noted 1 year previously when her serum potassium level was 2.2 mEq/L. Her home blood pressures averaged 117/72 mmHg. Before the hypokalemia was treated, she had frequent nocturia, which improved with restoration of her serum potassium to normal. She had been treated with spironolactone for the past 1 year. There was a strong family history of hypertension in both parents and her son, as well as the paternal aunts and uncles. She had no other major medical health issues. She had no signs or symptoms of Cushing syndrome.

INVESTIGATIONS

The baseline laboratory test results are shown in Table 13.1. The patient had positive case detection testing for PA with a PAC >10 ng/dL and the PRA <0.6 ng/mL per hour.[1] In addition, PA was confirmed because when a patient has spontaneous hypokalemia and the PAC >20 ng/dL, there are no other differential diagnostic possibilities beyond PA.[1,2] Thus formal confirmatory testing with oral sodium loading or a saline infusion test was not needed.

An unenhanced adrenal-dedicated computed tomography (CT) scan showed an indeterminate attenuation 1.2-cm right adrenal nodule and a 0.3-cm left adrenal nodule (Fig. 13.1).

After a thorough discussion with the patient, she was keen to pursue a surgical cure of hypokalemia and better control of her hypertension on less medication. She understood that a complete cure of her hypertension with surgery was not a reasonable goal in view of the duration of hypertension of >10 years.[1]

AVS was already attempted elsewhere and the right adrenal vein was not successfully catheterized. The aldosterone and cortisol values from the left adrenal vein and inferior vena cava (IVC) were not provided in the outside records. Repeat AVS at Mayo Clinic was

TABLE 13.1   Laboratory Tests

Biochemical Test	Result	Reference Range
Sodium	138	135–145
Potassium	3.5	3.6–5.2
Creatinine	0.9	0.8–1.3
eGFR	>60	>60 mL/min per BSA
Aldosterone	75	≤21 ng/dL
Plasma renin activity	<0.6	≤0.6–3 ng/mL per hour
DHEA-S	112	16–195 mcg/dL

BSA, Body surface area; *DHEA-S*, dehydroepiandrosterone sulfate; *eGFR*, estimated glomerular filtration rate.

performed as the next step. The results from AVS are reliable in patients treated with MRAs as long as PRA or PRC are suppressed.[1,3–5] AVS was successful based on adrenal vein-to-IVC cortisol gradients of more to 5-to-1 (Box 13.1). With continuous cosyntropin infusion protocol (cosyntropin 50 mcg/h administered intravenously starting 30 minutes before AVS and continued throughout the procedure), the adrenal vein-to-IVC cortisol gradients are typically well above the 5-to-1 cutoff (in this case, 32.3-to-1 on the right and 14.7-to-1 on the left). Each adrenal aldosterone (A) concentration is divided by the respective cortisol (C) concentration for the A/C ratio (see Box 13.1).

The A/C ratio from the dominant adrenal is divided by the A/C ratio from the nondominant adrenal for the aldosterone lateralization ratio. In this case, an A/C ratio of 20.8 on the right was divided by an A/C ratio of 0.7 on the left, yielding an aldosterone lateralization ratio of 32.1-to-1 (right to left). When the aldosterone lateralization ratio is >4-to-1, unilateral adrenalectomy will be curative.[1] It is also reassuring to confirm relative suppression of aldosterone secretion from the nondominant adrenal by dividing the A/C ratio from the nondominant adrenal by the A/C ratio from the IVC.[1] In this case, the A/C ratio of 0.7 on the left was divided by 2.8 from the IVC, yielding a value of 0.3. Contralateral adrenal suppression is confirmed when this value is <1.0.

TREATMENT

The patient underwent laparoscopic right adrenalectomy. The right adrenal gland weighed 6.13 g (normal, 4–5 g) and contained a 1.1 × 1.0 × 0.9–cm nodule. The PAC the day after surgery was <2 ng/dL and consistent with a surgical cure. Treatment with potassium chloride, spironolactone, and lisinopril was stopped the day after surgery. The patient was advised to monitor her blood pressure daily and blood pressure medications adjusted as needed for high-normal blood pressure for the first month after surgery.

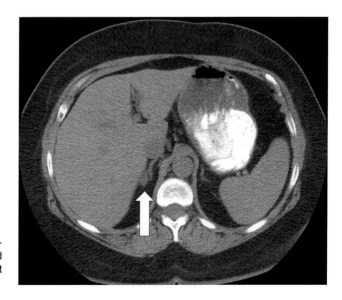

Fig. 13.1 An unenhanced adrenal-dedicated computed tomography scan showed an indeterminate attenuation (15.4 Hounsfield units) 1.2-cm right adrenal nodule (*arrow*) and a 0.3-cm left adrenal nodule.

BOX 13.1   ADRENAL VENOUS SAMPLING[a]

	Right AV	IVC	Left AV
Aldosterone, ng/dL	17,500	74	247
Cortisol, mcg/dL	840	26	382
A/C ratio[b]	20.8	2.8	0.7
Aldosterone lateralization ratio 32.1-to-1			
Contralateral suppression index			0.3

[a]Sequential AVS completed under continuous cosyntropin infusion 50 mcg/h.

[b]Each adrenal aldosterone concentration is divided by the respective cortisol concentration for the A/C ratio. The A/C ratio from the dominant adrenal is divided by the A/C ratio from the nondominant adrenal for the aldosterone lateralization ratio. In this case, 20.8 on the right is divided by 0.7 on the left, yielding an aldosterone lateralization ratio of 32.1-to-1 (right to left). When the aldosterone lateralization ratio is >4-to-1, unilateral adrenalectomy will be curative. An additional predictor of unilateral disease is when the nondominant AV A/C ratio is less than that in the IVC and this is termed the contralateral suppression index.

A, Aldosterone; *AV*, adrenal vein; *AVS*, adrenal venous sampling; *C*, cortisol; *IVC*, inferior vena cava.

OUTCOME AND FOLLOW-UP

The patient's blood potassium concentrations, obtained weekly for 4 weeks, remained normal, and treatment with fludrocortisone was not needed. Twelve years postoperatively the patient had good blood pressure control on two antihypertensive medications (enalapril 10 mg daily and metoprolol 50 mg daily). Her serum potassium concentration remained normal without the need for potassium supplementation.

Key Points

- If PRA or PRC are not suppressed in a patient treated with a MRA, then no further PA-related testing can be performed, and the MRA should be discontinued for 6 weeks before retesting.
- Most patients with PA are treated with suboptimal dosages of MRAs, and the mineralocorticoid receptors are not fully blocked.
- If the patient is hypokalemic despite treatment with a MRA, then the mineralocorticoid receptors are not fully blocked, and PRA or PRC should be suppressed in such a patient with PA. In the clinical setting of suppressed PRA or PRC, the MRA does not need to be discontinued for subtype testing with AVS.

REFERENCES

1. Young WF Jr. Diagnosis and treatment of primary aldosteronism: practical clinical perspectives. *J Intern Med*. 2019;285(2):126–148.

2. Funder JW, Carey RM, Mantero F, et al. The management of primary aldosteronism: case detection, diagnosis, and treatment: an Endocrine Society Clinical Practice Guideline. *J Clin Endocrinol Metab*. 2016;101(5):1889–1916.

3. Haase M, Riester A, Kropil P, et al. Outcome of adrenal vein sampling performed during concurrent mineralocorticoid receptor antagonist therapy. *J Clin Endocrinol Metab*. 2014;99:4397–4402.

4. Nanba AT, Wannachalee T, Shields JJ, et al. Adrenal vein sampling lateralization despite mineralocorticoid receptor antagonists exposure in primary aldosteronism. *J Clin Endocrinol Metab*. 2019;104(2):487–492.

5. Nagasawa M, Yamamoto K, Rakugi H, et al. Influence of antihypertensive drugs in the subtype diagnosis of primary aldosteronism by adrenal venous sampling. *J Hypertens*. 2019;37(7):1493–1499.

Failed Catheterization of the Right Adrenal Vein: When Incomplete Adrenal Venous Sampling Data Can Be Used to Direct a Surgical Cure

Adrenal venous sampling (AVS) is technically demanding. The success rate of sampling both adrenal veins is ≈95% at centers of excellence. However, at medical centers with low AVS case volume or where multiple interventional radiologists perform AVS, the success rate can be as low at 30%. When AVS is not successful, it is almost always due to lack of successful sampling of the right adrenal vein. The right adrenal vein is small and enters the inferior vena cava (IVC) at an acute angle. When the right adrenal vein is not sampled, but the left adrenal production of aldosterone is suppressed, it can be inferred that the right adrenal gland is the source of aldosterone hypersecretion.

Case Report

The patient was a 58-year-old man with a 20-year history of hypertension that accelerated over the past 1 year. Two months previously he was admitted to the hospital with a blood pressure of 240/113 mmHg and a serum potassium level of 2.6 mEq/L. He was treated with a two-drug program: β-adrenergic blocker (nebivolol 5 mg twice daily) and a calcium channel blocker (nifedipine 60 mg extended release twice daily). Blood pressure control was not optimal, with systolic blood pressures typically in the 140–150 mmHg range. At the time of referral to Mayo Clinic he was taking 80 mEq of potassium chloride daily. He was recently diagnosed with type 2 diabetes mellitus. He had no signs or symptoms of Cushing syndrome.

INVESTIGATIONS

The baseline laboratory test results are shown in Table 14.1. The patient had positive case detection testing for primary aldosteronism (PA) with plasma aldosterone concentration (PAC) >10 ng/dL and plasma renin activity (PRA) <0.6 ng/mL per hour.[1] In addition, PA was confirmed because when a patient has spontaneous hypokalemia and the PAC >20 ng/dL, there are no other differential diagnostic possibilities beyond PA.[1,2] Thus formal confirmatory testing (e.g., oral sodium loading or a saline infusion test) was not needed (see Table 14.1).

A contrast-enhanced abdominal computed tomography (CT) scan showed a 1.4-cm nodule in the lateral limb of the right adrenal gland (Fig. 14.1); some mild thickening and micronodular changes were seen in the left adrenal gland.

After a thorough discussion with the patient about his treatment options, he chose to pursue a surgical cure of hypokalemia and better control of his hypertension on less medication. He understood that a cure of his hypertension with surgery was not a reasonable goal in view of the duration of hypertension of >10 years.[1] AVS was performed as the next step. Bilateral adrenal vein catheterization was not successful (Box 14.1). With the continuous cosyntropin infusion protocol (cosyntropin 50 mcg/h administered intravenously starting 30 minutes before AVS

TABLE 14.1	Laboratory Tests	
Biochemical Test	**Result**	**Reference Range**
Sodium	140	135–145
Potassium	3.0	3.6–5.2
Creatinine	1.2	0.8–1.3
eGFR	>60	>60 mL/min per BSA
Aldosterone	23.8	≤21 ng/dL
Plasma renin activity	<0.6	≤0.6–3 ng/mL per hour

BSA, Body surface area; *eGFR,* estimated glomerular filtration rate.

and continued throughout the procedure), the adrenal vein-to-IVC cortisol gradients are typically well above the 5-to-1 cutoff that defines successful adrenal vein catheterization (in this case, 1.1-to-1 on the right and 18.7-to-1 on the left). Thus an aldosterone lateralization ratio could not be calculated. The IVC and left adrenal aldosterone (A) concentrations were divided by the respective cortisol (C) concentration for A/C ratios (see Box 14.1). The A/C ratio of 0.25 on the left was divided by an A/C ratio of 1.95 from the IVC, yielding a value of 0.13. Contralateral adrenal suppression is confirmed when this value is <1.0, and when ≤0.5, it can be used as proof that the left adrenal gland is not the source of aldosterone hypersecretion. We studied this concept of contralateral suppression in 150 patients with PA (61 with bilateral and 89 with

unilateral disease).[3] A contralateral suppression index cutoff of ≤0.5 to predict contralateral disease would have not led to any inappropriate adrenalectomies and would have missed 19% of patients with unilateral disease.[3]

TREATMENT

We discussed with the patient that the left adrenal gland was clearly not the source of aldosterone excess and that he either had right adrenal disease or an ectopic aldosterone-producing tumor.[4–6] Recognizing that ectopic aldosterone-producing tumors are exceedingly rare and that he did have a nodule in this right adrenal gland on CT, it was decided to proceed with laparoscopic right adrenalectomy. The right adrenal gland weighed 11.5 g (normal, 4–5 g) and contained a 1.4 × 0.9 × 0.8–cm yellow cortical adenoma. The PAC the day after surgery was <4 ng/dL, consistent with a surgical cure. Treatment with potassium chloride was stopped the day after surgery. The patient was advised to monitor his blood pressure daily and blood pressure medications adjusted as needed for high-normal blood pressure for the first month after surgery.

OUTCOME AND FOLLOW-UP

The patient's weekly blood potassium concentrations over 4 weeks remained high-normal, and treatment with fludrocortisone was not needed. Three years after surgery his potassium levels remained normal. Blood

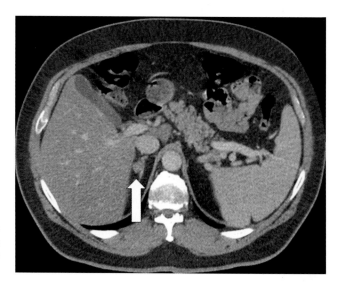

Fig. 14.1 Contrast-enhanced adrenal-dedicated computed tomography scan showed a 1.4-cm nodule in the lateral limb of the right adrenal (*arrow*) and some mild thickening and micronodular changes in the left adrenal gland (*not shown*).

BOX 14.1   **ADRENAL VENOUS SAMPLING**[a]

	Right AV	IVC	Left AV
Aldosterone, ng/dL	37	39	94
Cortisol, mcg/dL	21	20	373
A/C ratio[b]		1.95	0.25
Aldosterone lateralization ratio			
Contralateral suppression index			0.13

[a]Sequential AVS completed under continuous cosyntropin infusion 50 mcg/h.
[b]To document bilateral successful AVS, the cortisol concentration from each adrenal vein must be at least fivefold higher than the cortisol concentration in the IVC (i.e., the IVC cortisol concentration is 20 mcg/dL and each adrenal vein cortisol concentration should be >100 mcg/dL). However, in this case, there is no gradient in cortisol coming from the "right adrenal vein," and thus it was not successfully catheterized. The aldosterone concentrations in the IVC and left adrenal vein were divided by the respective cortisol concentration for the A/C ratio. The A/C ratio from the left adrenal vein of 0.25 was then divided by the A/C ratio of 1.95 from the IVC for a contralateral suppression index of 0.13; when this index is less than 0.5, it indicates that the adrenal gland is not the source of aldosterone hypersecretion.[3]
A, Aldosterone; *AV,* adrenal vein; *AVS,* adrenal venous sampling; *C,* cortisol; *IVC,* inferior vena cava.

pressure was 90–115/70–78 mmHg on nifedipine 60 mg twice daily and nebivolol 10 mg daily. He was very pleased with the surgical outcome.

Key Points

- When AVS is not successful, it is almost always due to lack of successful sampling of the right adrenal vein.

- When the right adrenal vein is not sampled but the left adrenal production of aldosterone is suppressed, it can be inferred that the source of aldosterone hypersecretion is either the right adrenal gland (almost always) or an ectopic aldosterone-producing tumor (exceedingly rare).

REFERENCES

1. Young WF Jr. Diagnosis and treatment of primary aldosteronism: practical clinical perspectives. *J Intern Med.* 2019;285(2):126–148.

2. Funder JW, Carey RM, Mantero F, et al. The management of primary aldosteronism: case detection, diagnosis, and treatment: an Endocrine Society Clinical Practice Guideline. *J Clin Endocrinol Metab.* 2016;101(5):1889–1916.

3. Strajina V, Al-Hilli Z, Andrews JC, et al. Primary aldosteronism: making sense of partial data sets from failed adrenal venous sampling-suppression of adrenal aldosterone production can be used in clinical decision making. *Surgery.* 2018;163(4):801–806.

4. Todesco S, Mantero F, Terribile V, Guarnieri GF, Borsatti A. Ectopic aldosterone production. *Lancet.* 1973;2(7826):443.

5. Flanagan MJ, McDonald JH. Heterotopic adrenocortical adenoma producing primary aldosteronism. *J Urol.* 1967;98(2):133–139.

6. Ehrlich EN, Dominguez OV, Samuels LT, Lynch D, Oberhelman H Jr, Warner NE. Aldosteronism and precocious puberty due to an ovarian androblastoma (Sertoli cell tumor). *J Clin Endocrinol Metab.* 1963;23(4):358–367.

Primary Aldosteronism: When Adrenal Venous Sampling Shows Suppressed Aldosterone Secretion From Both Adrenal Glands

It is a curious conundrum when adrenal venous sampling (AVS) is performed in a patient with primary aldosteronism (PA) and the aldosterone concentrations from both successfully sampled adrenal veins are low. This clinical circumstance raises the exceedingly rare possibility of an ectopic aldosterone-producing tumor in a gonad or kidney. However, at Mayo Clinic, every time this conundrum on AVS has occurred over the past 30 years, it proved to be due to a technical issue with AVS itself. Herein, we share such a case.

Case Report

The patient was a 34-year-old man who had been hypertensive for 6 years. He had spontaneous hypokalemia for the past 5 years. He was treated with 120 mEq of potassium chloride per day along with four antihypertensive drugs including betaxolol (10 mg daily), amlodipine (10 mg daily), valsartan (320 mg daily), and hydrochlorothiazide (25 mg daily). Blood pressure was poorly controlled and averaged 165/95 mmHg. His lowest serum potassium concentration was 2.2 mEq/L. He had no signs or symptoms of Cushing syndrome. He had a family history of hypertension in his father and brother.

INVESTIGATIONS

The baseline laboratory test results are shown in Table 15.1. The patient had positive case detection testing for PA with a plasma aldosterone concentration (PAC) >10 ng/dL and plasma renin activity (PRA) <1.0 ng/mL per hour.[1] Although the patient was taking a diuretic when he came to Mayo Clinic, because of the previously documented spontaneous hypokalemia, formal confirmatory testing was not needed.[1,2]

MRI scan of the abdomen demonstrated a 1-cm nodule in the lateral aspect of the right adrenal gland and micronodularity in the left adrenal gland (Fig. 15.1).

After a thorough discussion with the patient, he was keen to pursue a surgical cure of hypokalemia and either cure or achieve better control of his hypertension on less medication.

AVS was performed as the next step (Fig. 15.2). AVS was successful based on adrenal vein-to-IVC cortisol gradients of more to 5-to-1 (Box 15.1).[1] With the continuous cosyntropin infusion protocol (cosyntropin 50 mcg/h administered intravenously starting 30 minutes before AVS and continued throughout the procedure), the adrenal vein-to-IVC cortisol gradients are typically well above the 5-to-1 cutoff (in this case, 31.4-to-1 on the right and 23.0-to-1 on the left). Each adrenal vein aldosterone (A) concentration was divided by the respective cortisol (C) concentration for the A/C ratio (see Box 15.1). In this case, the A/C ratio from each adrenal was markedly less than the A/C ratio in the IVC (0.17 on the right versus 0.14 on the left versus 3.1 in the IVC). When an A/C ratio from an adrenal vein is >50% less than that in the IVC, it is termed *contralateral suppression*.

TABLE 15.1 Laboratory Tests

Biochemical Test	Result	Reference Range
Sodium	141	135–145
Potassium	3.4	3.6–5.2
Creatinine	0.9	0.8–1.3
eGFR	>60	>60 mL/min per BSA
Aldosterone	35	≤21 ng/dL
Plasma renin activity	<0.6	≤0.6–3 ng/mL per hour

BSA, Body surface area; *eGFR,* estimated glomerular filtration rate.

In this patient aldosterone secretion from both adrenal glands appeared to be suppressed, raising the possibility of an ectopic aldosterone-producing neoplasm in a kidney or gonad.[3–5] As a result of these findings, AVS was repeated, and the renal and gonadal veins were also sampled. The IVC aldosterone concentration was 85 ng/dL. The aldosterone concentrations from the right and left renal veins were 68 ng/dL and 75 ng/dL, respectively (thus excluding an ectopic source from the kidneys). The aldosterone concentrations from the right and left gonadal veins were 71 ng/dL and 68 ng/dL, respectively (excluding an ectopic source from the testicles). Taking great care on the right side to have

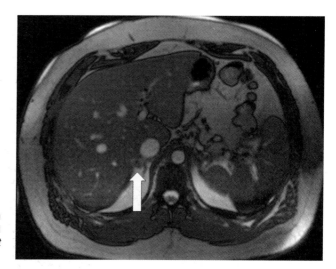

Fig. 15.1 Axial magnetic resonance image of the abdomen showed a 1-cm nodule in the lateral aspect of the right adrenal gland (*arrow*) and micronodularity in the left adrenal gland (*not shown*).

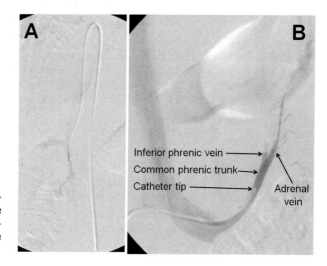

Fig. 15.2 Radiographs from adrenal venous sampling. (A) Right adrenal venous anatomy is shown with contrast administration. The sample was taken directly from the right adrenal vein. (B) Left adrenal vein venous anatomy is shown. The sample was taken from the common phrenic trunk.

BOX 15.1   INITIAL ADRENAL VENOUS SAMPLING[a]

	Right AV	IVC	Left AV
Aldosterone, ng/dL	110	65	67
Cortisol, mcg/dL	660	21	482
A/C ratio[b]	0.17	3.1	0.14
Contralateral suppression index	0.06		0.05

[a]Sequential AVS completed under continuous cosyntropin infusion 50 mcg/hr.
[b]Each adrenal aldosterone concentration was divided by the respective cortisol concentration for the A/C ratio. The A/C ratio from the dominant adrenal was divided by the A/C ratio from the nondominant adrenal for the aldosterone lateralization ratio. In this case, the A/C ratio from each adrenal was dramatically less than that in the IVC (0.17 on the RT versus 0.14 on the LT versus 3.1 in the IVC). When an A/C ratio from an adrenal vein is less than that in the IVC, it is termed the *contralateral suppression*. In this patient aldosterone secretion from both adrenal glands appeared to be suppressed.
A, Aldosterone; *AV*, adrenal vein; *AVS*, adrenal venous sampling; *C*, cortisol; *IVC*, inferior vena cava; *LT*, left; *RT*, right.

BOX 15.2   REPEAT ADRENAL VENOUS SAMPLING[a]

	Right AV	IVC	Left AV
Aldosterone, ng/dL	5000	85	107
Cortisol, mcg/dL	726	20	768
A/C ratio[b]	6.89	4.25	0.14
Aldosterone lateralization ratio 49.2-to-1			
Contralateral suppression index			0.03

[a]Sequential AVS completed under continuous cosyntropin infusion 50 mcg/h.
[b]Each adrenal aldosterone concentration was divided by the respective cortisol concentration for the A/C ratio. The A/C ratio from the dominant adrenal was divided by the A/C ratio from the nondominant adrenal for the aldosterone lateralization ratio. In this case, and A/C ratio of 6.89 on the right was divided by 0.14 on the left, yielding an aldosterone lateralization ratio of 49.2-to-1 (right to left). When the aldosterone lateralization ratio is >4-to-1, unilateral adrenalectomy will be curative. An additional predictor of unilateral disease is when the nondominant adrenal vein A/C ratio is less than that in the IVC and this is termed the contralateral suppression index.
A, Aldosterone; *AV*, adrenal vein; *AVS*, adrenal venous sampling; *C*, cortisol; *IVC*, inferior vena cava.

TREATMENT

The patient underwent laparoscopic right adrenalectomy. The right adrenal gland weighed 9 g (normal, 4–5 g) and contained a 1.0 × 0.9 × 0.8–cm yellow cortical adenoma. The PAC the day after surgery was <4 ng/dL and consistent with a surgical cure. Treatment with potassium chloride was discontinued, and the dosages of valsartan and amlodipine were cut in half. The patient was advised to monitor his blood pressure daily and blood pressure medications adjusted as needed for high-normal blood pressure for the first month after surgery.

OUTCOME AND FOLLOW-UP

The patient's weekly blood potassium concentrations over 4 weeks were normal, and treatment with fludrocortisone was not needed. Eight years after surgery he was normokalemic, and hypertension was well controlled (average <135/<85 mmHg) on a calcium channel blocker (nifedipine 60 mg/d) and a β-adrenergic blocker (betaxolol 10 mg daily). He is very pleased with the outcome.

Key Points

• When AVS is performed in a patient with PA and the aldosterone concentrations from both

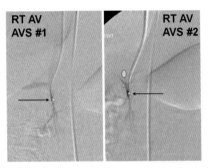

Fig. 15.3 Radiographs from adrenal venous sampling (AVS) of the right adrenal vein on two separate occasions. Catheterization of the right adrenal vein with the first AVS is shown on the *left* (RT AV – AVS 1) and the image from the second AVS is shown on the *right* (RT AV – AVS 2). Arrows document catheter tip placement. With AVS 1 the catheter tip was imbedded deeper into the main right adrenal vein and bypassed the venous effluent from the APA. With AVS 2 the catheter tip was kept at the orifice of the right adrenal vein as can be seen with more venous anatomy visualized and the venous effluent from the proximal APA (depicted in yellow) was successfully sampled.

the catheter tip in the proximal right adrenal vein the right adrenal gland proved to be the source of aldosterone hypersecretion (Fig. 15.3 and Box 15.2). Based on cases like this one, a coaxial guide wire-catheter technique was developed to facilitate successful right adrenal venous sampling by positioning the catheter tip at the orifice of the right adrenal vein.[6]

successfully sampled adrenal veins are low, it raises the exceedingly rare possibility of an ectopic aldosterone-producing tumor in the gonad or kidney.

- However, atypical findings on AVS are almost always due to technical issues with AVS.
- The interventional radiologist needs to take great care to not imbed the catheter tip too far into the right adrenal vein—in doing so the venous effluent from an aldosterone-producing adenoma may be bypassed.

REFERENCES

1. Young WF Jr. Diagnosis and treatment of primary aldosteronism: practical clinical perspectives. *J Intern Med*. 2019;285(2):126–148.

2. Funder JW, Carey RM, Mantero F, et al. The management of primary aldosteronism: case detection, diagnosis, and treatment: an Endocrine Society Clinical Practice Guideline. *J Clin Endocrinol Metab*. 2016;101(5):1889–1916.

3. Todesco S, Mantero F, Terribile V, Guarnieri GF, Borsatti A. Ectopic aldosterone production. *Lancet*. 1973;2(7826):443.

4. Flanagan MJ, McDonald JH. Heterotopic adrenocortical adenoma producing primary aldosteronism. *J Urol*. 1967;98(2):133–139.

5. Ehrlich EN, Dominguez OV, Samuels LT, Lynch D, Oberhelman H Jr, Warner NE. Aldosteronism and precocious puberty due to an ovarian androblastoma (Sertoli cell tumor). *J Clin Endocrinol Metab*. 1963;23(4):358–367.

6. Andrews JC, Thompson SM, Young WF. A coaxial guide wire-catheter technique to facilitate right adrenal vein sampling: evaluation in 76 patients. *J Vasc Interv Radiol*. 2015;26(12):1871–1873.

Corticotropin-Independent Cushing Syndrome

Corticotropin-Independent Hypercortisolism

Corticotropin (ACTH)-independent hypercortisolism can present with overt features of Cushing syndrome (CS) or as mild autonomous cortisol secretion (MACS)[1–3] (Table C.1).

ACTH-independent CS is relatively rare, diagnosed in <5% of patients with adrenal tumors or hyperplasia, while MACS is common, affecting up to 50% of patients with adrenal adenomas.[3] Patients with ACTH-independent hypercortisolism usually present with unilateral adrenal adenoma, bilateral macronodular hyperplasia or adenomas, micronodular hyperplasia, or adrenal cortical carcinoma (Table C.2).

Once ACTH-independent cortisol excess is confirmed (Table C.3) cross-sectional adrenal imaging should be obtained to identify the cause.[3] Unenhanced computed tomography is the best imaging modality to localize and characterize the culprit lesion. Adrenalectomy is the treatment of choice for a unilateral adrenal mass.[1,2,4] In patients with bilateral adrenal adenomas of similar size, adrenal venous sampling (AVS) can be used to identify the site with dominant cortisol secretion.[5,6] In macronodular hyperplasia, unilateral or bilateral adrenalectomy can be used depending on the severity of hypercortisolism.[7] In micronodular adrenal hyperplasia, adrenal glands are generally not enlarged and may appear normal on the cross-sectional imaging. Diagnostic workup in these situations should include evaluation for exogenous glucocorticoid

TABLE C.1 Clinical Presentation of Corticotropin-Independent Hypercortisolism[10]	
Overt Cushing Syndrome	**Mild Autonomous Cortisol Secretion**
Obesity, weight gain	Obesity, weight gain
Abdominal fat redistribution	
Dorsocervical fat pads	
Supraclavicular pads	
Striae (e.g., abdomen, arms, hips)	
Proximal myopathy	
Thinning of the skin	
Easy bruising	
Hypertension	Hypertension
Prediabetes, diabetes mellitus type 2	Prediabetes, diabetes mellitus type 2
Dyslipidemia	Dyslipidemia
Cardiovascular events	Cardiovascular events
Osteoporosis, fragility fractures	Osteoporosis, fragility fractures
Depression, anxiety	Depression, anxiety

use, evaluation for other features of Carney complex, and possibly genetic testing for *PRKAR1A* mutations.[8]

Curative surgery for ACTH-independent hypercortisolism results in adrenal insufficiency that needs to be properly treated. In addition, most patients report symptoms of glucocorticoid withdrawal that may last months and is characterized by fatigue, arthralgias, myalgias, headaches, insomnia, anxiety, and depression.[9] All patients need appropriate

TABLE C.2 **Etiology of Corticotropin-Independent Hypercortisolism**

Etiology	Prevalence (%)	Demographic Presentation	Features
Adrenal adenoma (unilateral or bilateral)	90	Age: 30–70 years Women: 60%–70%	Most patients present with MACS, diagnosed during hormonal work-up for an incidentally discovered adrenal mass
Bilateral macronodular adrenal hyperplasia (sporadic or familial)	5	Age: 40–70 years Women: 60%–70%	Commonly coproducing cortisol and aldosterone. Usually progressive disease. May demonstrate autocrine and paracrine ACTH production
Bilateral micronodular adrenal hyperplasia Primary pigmented nodular adrenocortical disease, isolated or a part of Carney complex Isolated micronodular adrenocortical disease	1	Age: 5–30 years Women: 40%–60%	Adrenal size often normal Paradoxical increase of urine free cortisol with Liddle's oral dexamethasone suppression test Nonpigmented adrenal micronodules
Adrenal carcinoma (unilateral)	4	Age: first decade, and 40–60 years Women: 60%–70%	Commonly cortisol and androgen cosecretion
Ectopic cortisol-producing mass	<0.1	N/A	Extremely rare, i.e., steroid ovarian mass

ACTH, Corticotropin; *DHEA-S*, dehydroepiandrosterone sulfate; *MACS*, mild autonomous cortisol secretion.

TABLE C.3 **Tests Used in Diagnosis of Corticotropin-Independent Hypercortisolism**

Establishing Diagnosis of Hypercortisolism	Comments
1-mg overnight dexamethasone suppression test	First-line testing
8-mg overnight dexamethasone suppression test	
24-Hour urinary free cortisol excretion	Usually within normal ranges in MACS
Late-night salivary cortisol	May be normal in MACS
Establishing Subtype of Hypercortisolism	**Comments**
Plasma ACTH	Undetectable or low, may be mid-normal in bilateral macronodular hyperplasia
Serum DHEA-S	Undetectable or low
Localization of Hypercortisolism	**Comments**
Computed tomography of adrenal glands	Indicated only after confirmation of ACTH independence
Adrenal venous sampling for hypercortisolism (very rare)	Useful in bilateral adrenal adenomas of similar size

ACTH, Corticotropin; *DHEA-S*, dehydroepiandrosterone sulfate; *MACS*, mild autonomous cortisol secretion.

counseling in regard to both adrenal insufficiency management and symptoms of glucocorticoid withdrawal syndrome.

REFERENCES

1. Fassnacht M, Arlt W, Bancos I, et al. Management of adrenal incidentalomas: European Society of Endocrinology Clinical Practice Guideline in collaboration with the European Network for the Study of Adrenal Tumors. *Eur J Endocrinol*. 2016;175(2):G1–G34.
2. Vaidya A, Hamrahian A, Bancos I, Fleseriu M, Ghayee HK. The evaluation of incidentally discovered adrenal masses. *Endocr Pract*. 2019;25(2):178–192.
3. Nieman LK, Biller BM, Findling JW, et al. The diagnosis of Cushing's syndrome: an Endocrine Society Clinical Practice Guideline. *J Clin Endocrinol Metab*. 2008;93(5):1526–1540.

4. Nieman LK, Biller BM, Findling JW, et al. Treatment of Cushing's syndrome: an Endocrine Society Clinical Practice Guideline. *J Clin Endocrinol Metab*. 2015;100(8):2807–2831.

5. Young WF, Jr. du Plessis H, Thompson GB, et al. The clinical conundrum of corticotropin-independent autonomous cortisol secretion in patients with bilateral adrenal masses. *World J Surg*. 2008;32(5):856–862.

6. Ueland GA, Methlie P, Jossang DE, et al. Adrenal venous sampling for assessment of autonomous cortisol secretion. *J Clin Endocrinol Metab*. 2018;103(12):4553–4560.

7. Vassiliadi DA, Tsagarakis S. Diagnosis and management of primary bilateral macronodular adrenal hyperplasia. *Endocr Relat Cancer*. 2019;26(10):R567–R581.

8. Bertherat J, Horvath A, Groussin L, et al. Mutations in regulatory subunit type 1A of cyclic adenosine 5′-monophosphate-dependent protein kinase (*PRKAR1A*): phenotype analysis in 353 patients and 80 different genotypes. *J Clin Endocrinol Metab*. 2009;94(6):2085–2091.

9. Hurtado MD, Cortes T, Natt N, Young WF, Jr. Bancos I. Extensive clinical experience: Hypothalamic-pituitary-adrenal axis recovery after adrenalectomy for corticotropin-independent cortisol excess. *Clin Endocrinol (Oxf)*. 2018;89(6):721–733.

10. Elhassan YS, Alahdab F, Prete A, et al. Natural history of adrenal incidentalomas with and without mild autonomous cortisol excess: a systematic review and meta-analysis. *Ann Intern Med*. 2019;171(2):107–116.

28-Year-Old Woman With a Remote History of Adrenal Mass Presenting With New-Onset Hypertension and Weight Gain

Workup for corticotropin (ACTH)-independent hypercortisolism is required in any patient with an adrenal mass, regardless of symptoms of hormone excess. Adrenalectomy is the treatment of choice for a unilateral cortisol-secreting adrenal mass. Secondary adrenal insufficiency develops in 50%–100% of patients after adrenalectomy and needs to be properly treated. Glucocorticoid withdrawal syndrome occurs in the majority of patients; its severity depends on the degree and duration of hypercortisolism

CASE REPORT

A 28-year-old woman was referred for the evaluation of elevated blood pressure, episodic diaphoresis, and tachycardia. One year before the current visit, she was initiated on lisinopril, and several months ago, metoprolol was added. As she continued to have episodic hypertension and diaphoresis, workup for secondary causes of hypertension was performed, including workup for catecholamine excess and primary aldosteronism (both negative). She was referred to endocrinology to investigate the reason for her unexplained symptoms.

Her medical history was positive for fibromyalgia and hypertension. In addition, she reported an incidental finding of adrenal adenoma 3 years ago. She did not recall any particular evaluation at that time. Medications at the time of referral included lisinopril 5 mg daily, metoprolol 50 mg daily, and duloxetine 60 mg daily. She also reported

a 40-pound weight gain over the last several years, noted easier bruising, hair loss, and irregular menses. She denied hirsutism or acne.

On physical examination, her blood pressure was 126/87 mmHg and body mass index (BMI) was 28.68 kg/m^2. She had no striae or proximal myopathy but did have a mild dorsocervical pad, supraclavicular pads, and mild rounding of the face.

INVESTIGATIONS

Unenhanced computed tomography (CT) of the abdomen was performed and demonstrated a 1.6-cm left adrenal mass consistent with a diagnosis of adrenal cortical adenoma (unenhanced CT attenuation was 6 Hounsfield units [HU]) (Fig. 16.1). The right adrenal gland was slightly atrophic. Hormonal workup for hypercortisolism was performed, including morning measurement of ACTH and dehydroepiandrosterone sulfate (DHEA-S), 1-mg overnight dexamethasone suppression test, and 24-hour urinary free cortisol (UFC) excretion. The laboratory data were consistent with ACTH-independent hypercortisolism (Table 16.1). Laparoscopic adrenalectomy was recommended.

TREATMENT

The patient was treated with a laparoscopic left adrenalectomy, with pathologic analysis showing a 1.6 × 2.0–cm adenoma (Fig. 16.2). She was educated on adrenal insufficiency, and hydrocortisone therapy was initiated. Anticipating glucocorticoid withdrawal syndrome, the initial dose of hydrocortisone was

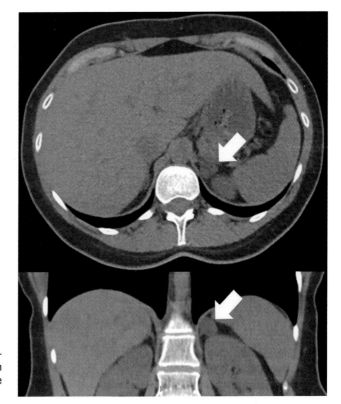

Fig. 16.1 Axial (top) and coronal (bottom) images from an unenhanced computed tomography scan showed a lipid-rich (6 Hounsfield units) 1.6 × 2–cm left adrenal nodule (*arrow*). The right adrenal gland appeared normal on all images.

TABLE 16.1 Laboratory Tests		
Biochemical Test	**Result**	**Reference Range**
1-mg overnight DST, mcg/dL	11	<1.8
Morning cortisol, mcg/dL	13	7–25
ACTH, pg/mL	<5	7.2–63
DHEA-S, mcg/dL	<15	18–284
Urine free cortisol, mcg/24 h	108	3.5–45

ACTH, Corticotropin; *DHEA-S*, dehydroepiandrosterone sulfate; *DST*, dexamethasone suppression test.

supraphysiologic at 30 mg in the morning and 20 mg at noon. The patient was advised to decrease hydrocortisone by 5 mg each week until she reached a total daily hydrocortisone dose of 20 mg daily (15 mg in the morning, 5 mg at noon). Despite this hydrocortisone regimen, she developed clinically significant fatigue, arthralgias, and myalgias. Because of the severity of withdrawal symptoms, at 3 weeks after surgery (when total daily hydrocortisone dose was 35 mg a day), she

was advised to increase hydrocortisone to 40 mg daily for 1 week before trying to decrease again. She was eventually able to decrease total daily hydrocortisone dose to 20 mg at 3 months after adrenalectomy. She had regular reassessment of adrenal function. Her serum cortisol concentration remained undetectable (24-hour after hydrocortisone dosing) 19 months after adrenalectomy. She continues to take daily hydrocortisone and follow sick day rules.

Discussion

The patient presented with unrecognized, longstanding ACTH-independent hypercortisolism due to a unilateral adrenal adenoma. It is unclear whether workup for hypercortisolism was performed at the time of adrenal incidentaloma discovery. Assuming another diagnosis is not obvious (e.g., pheochromocytoma), a dexamethasone suppression test should be performed in any patient with an adrenal mass, regardless of symptoms of hormone excess. Our patient was

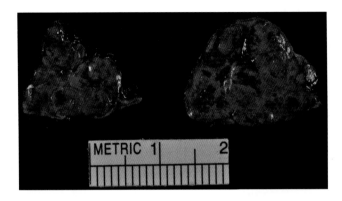

Fig. 16.2 Gross anatomy: left adrenal cortical adenoma forming a 2.0 × 1.8 × 1.6–cm mass. The mass was encapsulated, yellow-brown, and firm; located in the cortex; and did not extend beyond the adrenal gland.

diagnosed with overt Cushing syndrome (CS), as she presented with clinical features of hypercortisolism on examination (Table C.1). Biochemical workup was consistent with ACTH-independent hypercortisolism with undetectable ACTH and DHEA-S, abnormal DST, and elevated 24-hour UFC. With confirmation of ACTH-independent hypercortisolism, the unilateral adrenal mass was considered the culprit lesion, and adrenalectomy was recommended. Adrenal insufficiency occurs in almost 100% of patients with overt adrenal-dependent CS and around 50% of patients with mild autonomous cortisol secretion (MACS) after curative adrenalectomy.[1] Thus it is important to ensure that steroids are administered perioperatively, and patients are initiated and educated on glucocorticoid replacement therapy after adrenalectomy. Recovery of the hypothalamic-pituitary-adrenal (HPA) axis likely depends on the duration and degree of untreated hypercortisolism before curative surgery.[2–4] Factors such as age, gender, BMI, subtypes of CS, duration of symptoms, clinical and biochemical severity, and postoperative glucocorticoid dosing have been reported to affect the duration of HPA recovery.[1–5] Regular reassessment of the HPA axis should be performed in all patients with adrenal insufficiency. Recovery of the HPA axis takes months to years.[2,4,5]

Glucocorticoid withdrawal syndrome (GWS) is a withdrawal reaction that occurs due to a decrease in supraphysiologic glucocorticoid concentrations.[6] The mechanism of GWS is multifactorial and is mediated by the central noradrenergic and dopaminergic system, decrease in pro-opiomelanocortin-related peptides due to chronic suppression of HPA axis, and rebound increase in cytokines such as interleukin

(IL)-6, tumor necrosis factor-α (TNF-α), and IL-1b and prostaglandins, which occur with decreased serum cortisol concentrations.[6] Patients often feel unwell with flu-like symptoms including anorexia, nausea, emesis, lethargy, somnolence, arthralgia, myalgia, fever, and postural hypotension.[6] The symptoms and signs may be prolonged, and despite the glucocorticoid replacement, restoration of physical well-being and quality of life may take months or years.[7] Overall prevalence of GWS was 57% in patients undergoing unilateral adrenalectomy for mild or overt ACTH-independent hypercortisolism, higher in those with overt CS.[5]

Key Points

- Unless another diagnosis is obvious (e.g., pheochromocytoma), workup for ACTH-independent hypercortisolism is recommended in any patient with an adrenal mass, regardless of symptoms.
- Unilateral adrenalectomy is the treatment of choice for a cortisol-secreting adenoma.
- Adrenal insufficiency develops in 50% of patients with MACS and in almost 100% of patients with overt CS.
- Following curative adrenal surgery, all patients need to be educated on adrenal insufficiency management.
- GWS is characterized by fatigue, myalgias, arthralgias, nausea, and other symptoms that occur due to a decrease in supraphysiologic glucocorticoid concentrations following curative surgery for CS.
- GWS is treated with a titration of glucocorticoid dose and supportive therapy.

REFERENCES

1. Di Dalmazi G, Berr CM, Fassnacht M, Beuschlein F, Reincke M. Adrenal function after adrenalectomy for subclinical hypercortisolism and Cushing's syndrome: a systematic review of the literature. *J Clin Endocrinol Metab*. 2014;99(8):2637–2645.

2. Berr CM, Di Dalmazi G, Osswald A, et al. Time to recovery of adrenal function after curative surgery for Cushing's syndrome depends on etiology. *J Clin Endocrinol Metab*. 2015;100(4):1300–1308.

3. Klose M, Jorgensen K, Kristensen LO. Characteristics of recovery of adrenocortical function after treatment for Cushing's syndrome due to pituitary or adrenal adenomas. *Clin Endocrinol (Oxf)*. 2004;61(3):394–399.

4. Prete A, Paragliola RM, Bottiglieri F, et al. Factors predicting the duration of adrenal insufficiency in patients successfully treated for Cushing disease and nonmalignant primary adrenal Cushing syndrome. *Endocrine*. 2017;55(3):969–980.

5. Hurtado MD, Cortes T, Natt N, Young WF Jr, Bancos I. Extensive clinical experience: hypothalamic-pituitary-adrenal axis recovery after adrenalectomy for corticotropin-independent cortisol excess. *Clin Endocrinol (Oxf)*. 2018;89(6):721–733.

6. Hochberg Z, Pacak K, Chrousos GP. Endocrine withdrawal syndromes. *Endocr Rev*. 2003;24(4):523–538.

7. Dorn LD, Burgess ES, Friedman TC, Dubbert B, Gold PW, Chrousos GP. The longitudinal course of psychopathology in Cushing's syndrome after correction of hypercortisolism. *J Clin Endocrinol Metab*. 1997;82(3):912–919.

26-Year-Old Woman With a Discrepant Workup for Cushing Syndrome Subtype

Establishing corticotropin (ACTH) dependence is a crucial step in the diagnostic evaluation of hypercortisolism and relies on measurement of ACTH.[1] In ACTH-dependent hypercortisolism, pituitary magnetic resonance imaging (MRI) is the first localization test, whereas in ACTH-independent hypercortisolism, computed cross-sectional adrenal imaging is recommended. Discordant findings in the diagnostic evaluation should raise suspicion for a laboratory error.

Case Report

A 26-year-old woman was referred for the evaluation of Cushing syndrome (CS). For 2 years before the diagnosis of CS, she noticed development of striae, weight gain of 25 pounds, headaches, and hypertension. She was referred to a local endocrinologist who suspected and confirmed hypercortisolism with elevated levels of 24-hour urinary free cortisol and midnight salivary cortisol. ACTH-dependent hypercortisolism was diagnosed after the plasma ACTH was found to be elevated. MRI of pituitary gland was performed and was negative for pituitary lesions. The patient was referred to a tertiary center for further evaluation. On physical examination, she was noted to have facial rounding, facial erythema, supraclavicular pads, and dorsocervical pad. Oral examination demonstrated thrush. She had several abdominal striae. Her body mass index was 26.6 kg/m^2, and blood pressure was 142/95 mmHg. Her only medical therapy at the time of evaluation was spironolactone, 100 mg daily.

INVESTIGATIONS

Hypercortisolism was confirmed at our institution (Table 17.1). However, baseline testing revealed discrepant workup for ACTH dependence: whereas ACTH was elevated at 119 pg/mL (normal, 10–60), dehydroepiandrosterone sulfate (DHEA-S) was low-normal at 53 mcg/dL (normal, 44–332), suggestive of ACTH-independent hypercortisolism. This discrepancy prompted further communication with our laboratory medicine team, and it was decided to reanalyze ACTH with an alternate assay, suspecting an interference affecting the Siemens Immulite ACTH assay. When reanalyzed with the Roche Elecsys assay, ACTH was undetectable (Table 17.1). After confirmation of ACTH-independent hypercortisolism, adrenal imaging was obtained. MRI of abdomen revealed a 4.2-cm well-circumscribed, homogeneously enhancing mass arising from the left adrenal gland (Fig. 17.1). Adrenalectomy was recommended.

TREATMENT

Patient was treated with a laparoscopic left adrenalectomy, and pathologic analysis showed a 5.1 × 4.4 × 2.9-cm adrenal cortical adenoma. After adrenalectomy, she was treated for adrenal insufficiency. The hypothalamic-pituitary-adrenal axis recovered 14 months after curative adrenalectomy, and hydrocortisone was discontinued.

Discussion

This case illustrates a rare situation when a discrepant workup (nonconcordant ACTH and DHEA-S)

TABLE 17.1   Laboratory Tests

Biochemical Test	Result	Reference Range
Midnight salivary cortisol, ng/dL	620	<100
Midnight salivary cortisol, ng/dL	927	<100
Morning serum cortisol, mcg/dL	26	7–25
ACTH, pg/mL (Siemens Immulite assay)	119	10–60
ACTH, pg/mL, reanalyzed by a different assay (Roche Elecsys assay)	<5	7.2–63
DHEA-S, mcg/dL	53	44–332
Aldosterone, ng/dL (on spironolactone)	22	<21
Plasma renin activity, ng/mL per hour (on spironolactone)	8.4	2.9–10.8
Plasma metanephrine, nmol/L	0.22	<0.5
Plasma normetanephrine, nmol/L	0.25	<0.9
Urine free cortisol, mcg/24 h	120	3.5–45

ACTH, Corticotropin, *DHEA-S*, dehydroepiandrosterone sulfate.

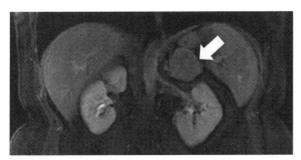

Fig. 17.1 Coronal image from magnetic resonance imaging showing a 4.2 × 3.3 × 3.8–cm well-circumscribed, homogeneously enhancing mass arising from the left adrenal gland (*arrow*). The right adrenal gland appeared normal.

identified an interference in the ACTH assay by the heterophile antibodies. Such interferences lead to erroneous interpretation of results, unnecessary procedures (MRI of pituitary gland in this case), and even unnecessary invasive procedures.[2] As ACTH-dependent CS due to pituitary origin frequently presents with a negative MRI, pursuing this diagnosis would have also led to unnecessary inferior petrosal sinus sampling and even pituitary exploration. The low serum DHEA-S concentration in this case raised the possibility of laboratory error, and further collaboration with the laboratory medicine team helped confirm it.

In addition to assay interference, other causes of laboratory errors may be inappropriate handling of specimens, hemolysis, and delay in the processing of specimens.[2]

Key Points

- Establishing ACTH dependence guides localization studies and management decisions in patients with CS.
- Discordance of blood concentrations of ACTH and DHEA-S should prompt reconsideration of the subtype diagnosis of CS and investigation of the discordance.
- Assay interference, inappropriate handling or processing of specimens, and hemolysis may lead to laboratory errors.

REFERENCES

1. Nieman LK, Biller BM, Findling JW, et al. The diagnosis of Cushing's syndrome: an Endocrine Society Clinical Practice Guideline. *J Clin Endocrinol Metab.* 2008;93(5):1526–1540.
2. Donegan DM, Algeciras-Schimnich A, Hamidi O, et al. Corticotropin hormone assay interference: a case series. *Clin Biochem.* 2019;63:143–147.

45-Year-Old Woman With Corticotropin-Independent Cushing Syndrome and Bilateral Adrenal Adenomas

Management of corticotropin (ACTH)-independent hypercortisolism in patients with bilateral adrenal nodules depends on imaging findings (adenomas versus macronodular hyperplasia) and tumor size. Adrenal venous sampling (AVS) is useful in patients with bilateral adrenal adenomas of similar size to guide surgical management.

Case Report

A 45-year-old woman presented for evaluation of self-diagnosed Cushing syndrome (CS). Over the prior 2 years, she progressively gained weight with abdominal fat redistribution, developed striae over her abdomen, supraclavicular and dorsocervical fat pads, hair loss, mood swings, anxiety, depression, insomnia, and signs of proximal myopathy (that she noticed on climbing up the stairs). She had also noticed facial rounding and erythema. Despite working out in the gym, she was unable to lose weight. In addition, she reported a new-onset hypertension and a new-onset diabetes mellitus type 2 (hemoglobin A1C, 6.7%) diagnosed 6 months previously. Medications included lisinopril, hydrochlorothiazide, and metformin. The patient researched her constellation of symptoms and suspected CS. Further workup at home confirmed hypercortisolism. On physical examination, her blood pressure was 172/105 mmHg and body mass index was 34.2 kg/m². She had abdominal striae, facial rounding and erythema, dorsocervical pad, and supraclavicular pads.

INVESTIGATIONS

After confirmation of ACTH-independent hypercortisolism (Table 18.1), abdominal imaging was obtained. Abdominal computed tomography demonstrated bilateral adrenal nodules, 2.6 cm on the right and 2.8 cm on the left (Fig. 18.1). As imaging phenotype was not consistent with bilateral macronodular hyperplasia, AVS was performed to identify the source of autonomous cortisol secretion. In preparation for the AVS procedure, dexamethasone 0.5 mg was initiated on the morning the day prior, and every 6 hours, including the morning of AVS. Cosyntropin (which is commonly infused during AVS in patients with primary aldosteronism) was not administered. Concentrations of cortisol and epinephrine were measured in inferior vena cava (IVC) and both adrenal veins (Box 18.1). Based on the left adrenal vein-to-IVC cortisol ratio of 17.2 and the left adrenal vein to right adrenal vein cortisol ratio of 3.9, ACTH-independent hypercortisolism due to the dominant left adrenal adenoma was diagnosed, and left adrenalectomy was recommended. However, the patient was advised that she may continue to demonstrate a mild autonomous cortisol secretion from the right adrenal adenoma, given the right adrenal vein to inferior vena cava ratio of 4.4 (see Box 18.1).

TABLE 18.1   Laboratory Tests

Biochemical Test	Result	Reference Range
Morning cortisol, mcg/dL	22	7–25
ACTH, pg/mL	<5	7.2–63
DHEA-S, mcg/dL	<15	18–284
Aldosterone, ng/dL	4	<21
Plasma renin activity, ng/mL per hour	<0.6	2.9–10.8
Plasma metanephrine, nmol/L	0.21	<0.5
Plasma normetanephrine, nmol/L	0.6	<0.9
Urine free cortisol, mcg/24 h	373	3.5–45

ACTH, Corticotropin; *DHEA-S*, dehydroepiandrosterone sulfate.

BOX 18.1   ADRENAL VENOUS SAMPLING[a]

	Right AV	IVC	Left AV
Epinephrine, pg/dL[b]	3905	69	1796
Cortisol, mcg/dL	74	17	292
Cortisol AV/IVC ratio	4.4		17.2
Cortisol RAV/LAV ratio	3.9		

[a]AVS completed under continuous dexamethasone suppression of 0.5 mg every 6 hours started 24 hours before the AVS.
[b]Adrenal vein epinephrine concentrations of at least 100 pg/mL more than concentrations in the inferior vena cava were used to confirm successful adrenal vein cannulation.
Interpretation: Cortisol AV/IVC ratio >6.5 confirms autonomous cortisol secretion from the adrenal gland, while cortisol AV/IVC ratio <3.3 excludes it. Cortisol LAV/RAV >2.3 confirms predominantly unilateral autonomous cortisol secretion.
AVS, Adrenal venous sampling; *IVC*, inferior vena cava; *LAV*, left adrenal vein; *RAV*, right adrenal vein.

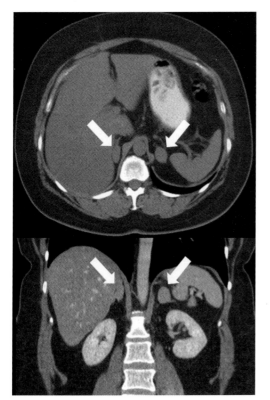

Fig. 18.1 Axial (*top*) and coronal (*bottom*) images from a contrast-enhanced computed tomography scan showed bilateral adrenal masses, 2.6 cm on the right and 2.8 cm on the left (*arrows*).

TREATMENT

Patient was treated with a laparoscopic left adrenalectomy that revealed a 2.6-cm pigmented adrenal cortical adenoma (Fig. 18.2). Following adrenalectomy, she developed secondary adrenal insufficiency that resolved 15 months later, at which point she discontinued hydrocortisone. She was very pleased with resolution of diabetes mellitus type 2 and hypertension, weight loss of 20 pounds, and a significant improvement in anxiety. Two years after left adrenalectomy, abdominal imaging was repeated and redemonstrated a right 2.6-cm stable adrenal adenoma. While the features of overt CS resolved, repeat workup demonstrated mild glucocorticoid autonomy (cortisol after the 1-mg overnight dexamethasone suppression test was 3.2 mcg/dL [normal <1.8]). Clinical monitoring was implemented.

Discussion

Causes of the ACTH-independent hypercortisolism due to bilateral adrenal disease include bilateral adenomas, bilateral macronodular hyperplasia, and bilateral micronodular hyperplasia (Table C.2). Bilateral adrenal cortical carcinoma is extremely rare and is unlikely to occur outside of a genetic syndrome. Imaging can frequently distinguish a single adenoma from a macronodular hyperplasia, though this may not always

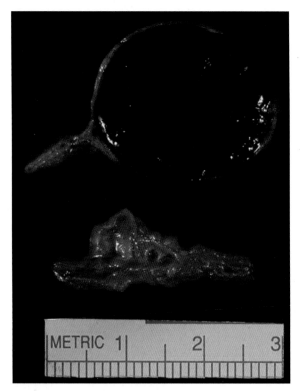

Fig. 18.2 Gross anatomy of left adrenal gland: well-circumscribed pigmented adrenal cortical adenoma measuring 2.8 × 2.3 cm.

be straightforward. While macronodular hyperplasia presents with bilateral cortisol secretion, this may not be the case in a patient with bilateral adenomas (when one adrenal adenoma may be cortisol-secreting, while the other one is nonfunctioning). AVS in these situations can be useful, as illustrated in this case.[1,2] Adrenal vein cortisol ratio >2.3 in these cases identifies the culprit lesion.[2] Notably, in patients with bilateral adenomas of unequal size, cortisol secretion usually originates from the much larger adrenal mass, and in these cases, AVS may not be needed.

Key Points

- Adrenal imaging is the first step to determine the etiology of ACTH-independent hypercortisolism.
- AVS under dexamethasone suppression, with cortisol and epinephrine measurements, is useful in patients with ACTH-independent hypercortisolism and imaging suggestive of bilateral adrenal adenomas.
- AVS is not indicated in patients with unilateral adenoma, bilateral micronodular hyperplasia, or macronodular hyperplasia.
- AVS may not be useful in patients with bilateral adenomas with significant differences in size (>2 cm), as cortisol secretion usually originates from the larger adrenal mass.

REFERENCES

1. Ueland GA, Methlie P, Jossang DE, et al. Adrenal venous sampling for assessment of autonomous cortisol secretion. *J Clin Endocrinol Metab.* 2018;103(12):4553–4560.
2. Young WF Jr, du Plessis H, Thompson GB, et al. The clinical conundrum of corticotropin-independent autonomous cortisol secretion in patients with bilateral adrenal masses. *World J Surg.* 2008;32(5):856–862.

Corticotropin-Independent Cushing Syndrome in a Patient With "Normal" Adrenal Imaging

The diagnosis of corticotropin (ACTH)-independent hypercortisolism with adrenal imaging that does not demonstrate unilateral or bilateral nodules should prompt consideration of bilateral micronodular hyperplasia (Table C.2). Primary pigmented nodular adrenocortical disease (PPNAD) may be isolated or part of Carney complex.

Case Report

The patient was a 20-year-old woman who has been referred to endocrinology after developing unexplained avascular necrosis of the hips. On interview, she reported a progressive weight gain of 75 pounds over 18 months; development of striae over her arms, abdomen, back, and hips, development of dorsocervical and supraclavicular pads; rounding and erythema of the face; and intensification of anxiety. In addition, she noticed difficulties keeping up with her training in the nursing school due to progressive fatigue and decrease in concentration. She reported a remote exogenous glucocorticoid use history (two hip injections 3 years prior). Medical history was positive for low bone mass on bone mineral density testing (T scores of –1.3), avascular necrosis of the hips, and anxiety. The family history was negative for adrenal disorders. On physical examination, her body mass index was 32 kg/m^2 and blood pressure was 136/87 mmHg. Physical examination demonstrated abdominal fat redistribution with obesity, prominent supraclavicular and dorsocervical pads, facial rounding, and

striae. Skin examination revealed several café-au-lait lesions on the neck.

INVESTIGATIONS

Owing to a high clinical suspicion for Cushing syndrome (CS), laboratory workup was initiated, which confirmed glucocorticoid autonomy (Table 19.1). An unenhanced adrenal-dedicated computed tomography (CT) scan was initially interpreted as normal, although on closer examination it showed micronodular thickening of both adrenal glands (Fig. 19.1). PPNAD was suspected, and bilateral adrenalectomy was recommended.

TREATMENT

The patient underwent laparoscopic bilateral adrenalectomy. Macroscopic examination showed adrenal glands of normal size and weight, with multiple brown nodules (Fig. 19.2). On microscopic examination,

TABLE 19.1 Laboratory Tests		
Biochemical Test	Result	Reference Range
1-mg overnight DST, mcg/dL	9	<1.8
8-mg overnight DST, mcg/dL	13	<1
Morning serum cortisol, mcg/dL	8	7–25
ACTH, pg/mL	<5	7.2–63
DHEA-S, mcg/dL	37	44–332
Urine free cortisol, mcg/24 h	22	3.5–45
Midnight salivary cortisol, ng/dL	60	<100

ACTH, Corticotropin; *DHEA-S,* dehydroepiandrosterone sulfate; *DST,* dexamethasone suppression test.

nodules contained brown pigment, consistent with PPNAD. Treatment with hydrocortisone and fludrocortisone was initiated, and the patient was educated on adrenal insufficiency management. Symptoms and signs of cortisol excess eventually improved, and she lost approximately 50 pounds in the 12 months after the adrenalectomy.

A medical genetics service was consulted. Although a detailed family history was negative for Carney complex, genetic testing did demonstrate a pathogenic variant in the *PRKARIA* gene. Evaluation for other components of Carney complex did not reveal myxomas, acromegaly, or other tumors. Monitoring was implemented.

Discussion

Carney complex is a rare syndrome characterized by multiple neoplasia, including endocrine tumors and myxomas.[1] Patients may have skin pigmentations on physical examination, including blue nevi and pigmented lentiginous lesions.[2] PPNAD occurs in up to 60% of patients with Carney complex and usually presents with overt ACTH-independent hypercortisolism. Adrenal imaging is frequently interpreted as normal. Timely diagnosis and regular monitoring for other manifestations of Carney complex ensure early intervention. Surveillance usually includes echocardiogram

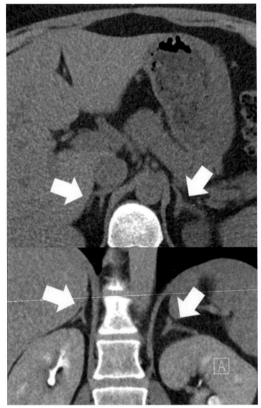

Fig. 19.1 Unenhanced abdominal computed tomography scan images, axial (*top*) and coronal (*bottom*), showed micronodular thickening of both adrenal glands (*arrows*).

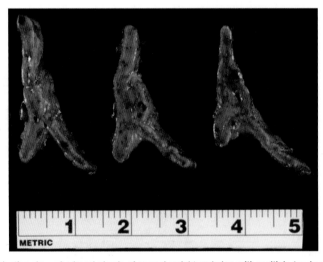

Fig. 19.2 Gross pathology examination showed adrenal glands of normal weight and size, with multiple tan-brown nodules seen on the capsule and within the cortex.

(to assess for cardiac myxoma), skin evaluation, pituitary and thyroid imaging, and measurements of insulin-like growth factor 1 and prolactin.[3]

Key Points

- ACTH-independent hypercortisolism due to bilateral micronodular adrenal hyperplasia is rare and should prompt consideration of Carney complex.
- Surveillance for endocrine and nonendocrine manifestations of Carney complex should be instituted to ensure early diagnosis and treatment of cardiac myxomas and endocrine neoplasia.

REFERENCES

1. Zhang CD, Pichurin PN, Bobr A, Lyden ML, Young WF, Bancos I. Cushing syndrome: uncovering Carney complex due to novel PRKAR1A mutation. *Endocrinol Diabetes Metab Case Rep*. 2019;2019.

2. Bertherat J, Horvath A, Groussin L, et al. Mutations in regulatory subunit type 1A of cyclic adenosine 5'-monophosphate-dependent protein kinase (PRKAR1A): phenotype analysis in 353 patients and 80 different genotypes. *J Clin Endocrinol Metab*. 2009;94(6):2085–2091.

3. Stratakis CA, Kirschner LS, Carney JA. Clinical and molecular features of the Carney complex: diagnostic criteria and recommendations for patient evaluation. *J Clin Endocrinol Metab*. 2001;86(9):4041–4046.

66-Year-Old Woman With Corticotropin-Independent Hypercortisolism and Bilateral Macronodular Adrenal Hyperplasia

Bilateral macronodular adrenal hyperplasia (BMAH) is an uncommon cause of adrenal hypercortisolism. It is a progressive disease that may present with a spectrum of cortisol and aldosterone secretion. BMAH can be sporadic or familial, usually due to germline pathogenic variants in armadillo repeat containing 5 (*ARMC5*).[1,2]

Case Report

A 66-year-old woman presented for evaluation of corticotropin (ACTH)-independent hypercortisolism. She was initially discovered with bilateral adrenal nodules during abdominal imaging performed for appendicitis. Following this incidental discovery, she was referred to a local endocrinologist who performed workup for adrenal hormone excess and diagnosed autonomous cortisol secretion.

Over the preceding 8–12 months, she had gained 30 pounds in weight, and her hypertension was more difficult to control, necessitating addition of another medication. Her hypertension was treated with lisinopril, hydrochlorothiazide, metoprolol, and amlodipine. In addition, she took 60 mEq of potassium per day for hypokalemia. She had dyslipidemia that was treated with simvastatin. On physical examination, her blood pressure was 142/72 mmHg and body mass index was 39.6 kg/m². She had abdominal obesity but no supraclavicular or dorsocervical pads, no striae, no facial rounding, and no proximal myopathy.

INVESTIGATIONS

Autonomous cortisol secretion was confirmed, and case detection testing for primary aldosteronism was positive (Table 20.1). Confirmatory testing for primary aldosteronism was not pursued. Abdominal computed tomography (CT) demonstrated bilateral macronodular adrenal hyperplasia (Fig. 20.1).

TREATMENT

The patient was counseled about the natural history of BMAH and treatment options for bilateral cortisol (and likely aldosterone) hypersecretion. She opted for bilateral adrenalectomy. Pathology demonstrated bilateral

TABLE 20.1 Laboratory Tests

Biochemical Test	Result	Reference Range
1 mg DST, mcg/dL	14.7	<1.8
8 mg DST, mcg/dL	11.2	<1
ACTH, pg/mL	<5	7.2–63
DHEA-S, mcg/dL	26	<15–157
Aldosterone, ng/dL	11, 13	<21
Plasma renin activity, ng/mL per hour	<0.6	2.9–10.8
Urine metanephrines, mcg/24 h	51	<400
Urine normetanephrines, mcg/24 h	273	<900
Urine free cortisol, mcg/24 h	8	3.5–45
Midnight salivary cortisol, ng/dL	172	<100

ACTH, Corticotropin; *DHEA-S,* dehydroepiandrosterone sulfate; *DST,* dexamethasone suppression test.

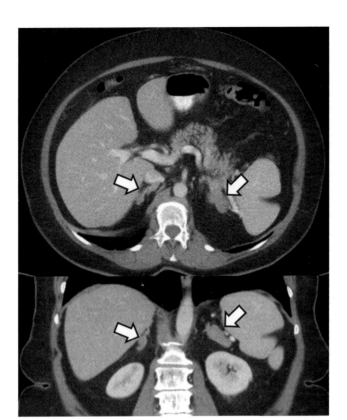

Fig. 20.1 Axial (*top*) and coronal (*bottom*) images from a contrast-enhanced computed tomography scan showed bilateral macronodular hyperplasia, 6.5 × 3.4 × 2.0 cm on the right and 7.1 × 4.0 × 1.6 cm on the left (*arrows*).

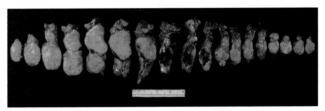

Fig. 20.2 Gross anatomy of the left adrenal gland demonstrating nodular hyperplasia with numerous nodules ranging from 0.2 cm to 3.5 cm. The right adrenal gland is not shown.

nodular adrenocortical hyperplasia with the left adrenal gland weighing 20 g (7.5 × 4.2 × 1.6 cm in size) and the right adrenal gland weighing 19 g (7.0 × 3.8 × 2.2 cm in size). Both adrenal glands contained numerous nodules ranging in size from 0.2 to 3.5 cm (Fig. 20.2). Following bilateral adrenalectomy, she developed permanent adrenal insufficiency and was initiated on hydrocortisone and fludrocortisone therapy. At the 1-month follow-up, her hypertension improved, allowing for

a decrease in the intensity of her antihypertensive management.

Discussion

Causes of the ACTH-independent hypercortisolism due to bilateral adrenal disease include bilateral adenomas, BMAH, and bilateral micronodular hyperplasia (Box C.2). Patients with BMAH present with a spectrum of hypercortisolism severity, with most diagnosed with mild autonomous cortisol secretion. A workup for primary aldosteronism should be performed in any patient with BMAH and hypertension. Combined cortisol and aldosterone secretion is common.[3,4] Imaging findings usually include multiple nodules that can be as large as several centimeters in diameter, and in some cases, diffuse enlargement of bilateral adrenal glands can be seen. Management options include bilateral adrenalectomy, unilateral adrenalectomy (for milder forms of hypercortisolism), or a conservative approach (with treatment of comorbidities, lifestyle intervention, and medical therapy).

Key Points

- Adrenal imaging is the first step to determining the etiology of ACTH-independent hypercortisolism.
- Adrenal venous sampling is not useful in patients with BMAH, as hormone excess is bilateral.
- Patients with BMAH may present with both hypercortisolism and primary aldosteronism.

- The management approach to BMAH may include bilateral or unilateral adrenalectomy or conservative management and depends on the severity of hormone excess.

REFERENCES

1. Bourdeau I, Oble S, Magne F, et al. *ARMC5* mutations in a large French-Canadian family with cortisol-secreting β-adrenergic/vasopressin responsive bilateral macronodular adrenal hyperplasia. *Eur J Endocrinol.* 2016;174(1):85–96.
2. Espiard S, Drougat L, Libe R, et al. *ARMC5* mutations in a large cohort of primary macronodular adrenal hyperplasia: clinical and functional consequences. *J Clin Endocrinol Metab.* 2015;100(6):E926–E935.
3. Mamedova EO, Vasilyev EV, Petrov VM, et al. [Hereditary Cushing's syndrome caused by primary bilateral macronodular adrenal hyperplasia due to *ARMC5* mutation with concomitant primary hyperparathyroidism: the first known case in Russia]. *Probl Endokrinol (Mosk).* 2019;65(2):89–94.
4. Tokumoto M, Onoda N, Tauchi Y, et al. A case of adrenocoricotrophic hormone-independent bilateral adrenocortical macronodular hyperplasia concomitant with primary aldosteronism. *BMC Surg.* 2017;17(1):97.

35-Year-Old Woman With Low Bone Density and Fractures

Symptoms of overt glucocorticoid excess should prompt appropriate biochemical and imaging workup. In this case, despite imaging characteristics of myelolipoma and contralateral adrenal gland without abnormalities, ipsilateral adrenal adenoma was suspected in a patient with confirmed corticotropin (ACTH)-independent hypercortisolism.

Case Report

A 35-year-old woman was referred for the evaluation of low bone mineral density (L1-L4: z score of −2.5, left hip: z score of −2.0) discovered during workup of recurrent bilateral metatarsal fractures. Her medical history included obesity, hypertension (treated with hydrochlorothiazide and metoprolol), dyslipidemia, anxiety, and depression. She also complained of fatigue, generalized weakness, easy bruising, and nausea.

On physical examination, her blood pressure was 140/89 mmHg and body mass index was 40.55 kg/m^2. She had no striae or proximal myopathy but did have a mild dorsocervical pad, supraclavicular pads, and mild rounding of the face.

INVESTIGATIONS

Cushing syndrome (CS) was not suspected during the initial evaluation. However, during investigation of secondary causes of osteoporosis, the 1-mg overnight dexamethasone suppression test (DST) was performed and was abnormal with a next-day serum cortisol concentration of 13 mcg/dL (normal <1.8 mcg/dL). Further testing included morning measurement of serum ACTH and dehydroepiandrosterone sulfate (DHEA-S), 8 mg overnight DST, and 24-hour urine cortisol excretion. The workup was consistent with ACTH-independent

hypercortisolism (Table 21.1). Unenhanced computed tomography (CT) of the abdomen was performed and demonstrated a 5.8-cm left adrenal mass with typical imaging characteristics of myelolipoma (unenhanced CT attenuation was −64 Hounsfield units [HU]) (Fig. 21.1). The right adrenal gland was slightly atrophic. Despite the imaging findings pathognomonic for myelolipoma, evidence of ACTH-independent hypercortisolism and a contralateral adrenal gland without an adrenal mass led to the decision to proceed with left adrenalectomy. A collision tumor was suspected.

TREATMENT

The patient was treated with a laparoscopic left adrenalectomy, with pathology showing a 5.8 × 4.4 × 3.4–cm yellow-brown, soft, fatty mass located in the adrenal cortex with final pathologic diagnosis of adrenocortical adenoma with lipomatous metaplasia (Fig. 21.2).

TABLE 21.1 Laboratory Tests

Biochemical Test	Result	Reference Range
1-mg overnight DST, mcg/dL	13	<1.8
8-mg overnight DST, mcg/dL	12	<1.0
Morning cortisol, mcg/dL	13	7–25
ACTH, pg/mL	9.2	7.2–63
DHEA-S, mcg/dL	<15	18–284
Aldosterone, ng/dL	11	<21
Plasma renin activity, ng/mL per hour	<0.6	2.9–10.8
Plasma metanephrine, nmol/L	0.22	<0.5
Plasma normetanephrine, nmol/L	0.7	<0.9
Urine free cortisol, mcg/24 h	34	3.5–45

ACTH, Corticotropin; *DHEA-S*, dehydroepiandrosterone sulfate; *DST*, dexamethasone suppression test.

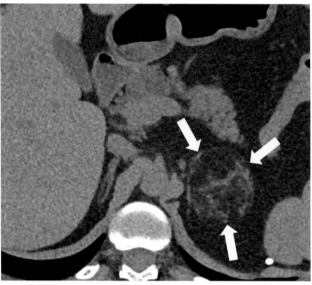

Fig. 21.1 Axial image from an unenhanced computed tomography (CT) scan showed a lipid-rich (CT attenuation −64 Hounsfield units [HU]) 4.9 × 3.2–cm left adrenal nodule, with areas of macroscopic fat (*arrow*). The right adrenal gland appeared normal on all images.

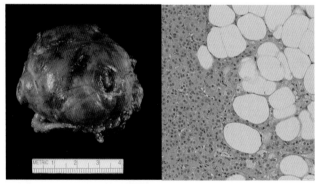

Fig. 21.2 Gross anatomy (*left*): well-circumscribed soft yellow mass measuring 5.8 × 4.4 × 3.4 cm. Microscopic (*right*): adenoma 20×. The adrenal cortical adenoma forms a well-circumscribed lesion composed of cords and nests of pale eosinophilic cells with small dark nuclei and interspersed groups of adipose cells.

The morning after surgery, cortisol was measured and was undetectable (<1.0 mcg/dL). She was educated on adrenal insufficiency and treated with hydrocortisone therapy until recovery of the hypothalamic-pituitary-adrenal axis occurred 12 months later.

Discussion

Myelolipomas are benign nonfunctioning adrenal tumors that represent 6% of all adrenal tumors and present with pathognomonic radiographic features of macroscopic fat[1] (see Case 65). The etiology of myelolipomas remains uncertain. One postulated theory[2] is that the fat component of adrenal myelolipomas derives from mesenchymal stem cells of stromal fat of the adrenal cortex, with subsequent mature adipocytes possibly releasing stimulating factors to recruit circulating hematopoietic progenitors. Myelolipomas are not capable of steroidogenesis; however, adrenal hormone excess has reported in patients with myelolipomas, including primary hyperaldosteronism and hypercortisolism.[1] It is possible that so-called functioning myelolipomas are adrenocortical adenomas with lipomatous metaplasia (as in this case) or a collision tumor.

Key Points

- Myelolipomas are benign adrenal tumors that are not capable of steroidogenesis. Myelolipomas exhibit pathognomonic features on imaging with areas of macroscopic fat.
- In rare cases of adrenal adenomas with lipomatous metaplasia, the imaging presentation is similar to that of myelolipomas.

- This case illustrates the importance of physical examination and appropriate workup in patients with features suggestive of adrenal hormonal excess.

REFERENCES

1. Hamidi O, Raman R, Lazik N, et al. Clinical course of adrenal myelolipoma: a long-term longitudinal follow-up study. *Clin Endocrinol (Oxf)*. 2020;93(1):11–18.
2. Feng C, Jiang H, Ding Q, Wen H. Adrenal myelolipoma: a mingle of progenitor cells? *Med Hypotheses*. 2013;80(6):819–822.

Carney Triad (Pentad) and Adrenal Adenoma With Clinically Important Cortisol Secretory Autonomy

Carney triad (described in 1977) is a rare, nonfamilial, multitumoral syndrome, with three tumors in the initial description: gastrointestinal stromal tumor (GIST), pulmonary chondroma, and extraadrenal paraganglioma. Subsequently, two other tumors, adrenal cortical adenoma and esophageal leiomyoma, were added as components—thus Carney triad is actually a "pentad." Although it is rare, it is important for endocrinologists to be aware of this disorder because of the links to paraganglioma and adrenocortical tumors. The adrenocortical tumors are usually nonfunctioning adenomas. However, as highlighted in the case described herein, the adrenocortical tumor can secrete cortisol autonomously and lead to a perioperative catastrophe if not recognized before surgery.

Case Report

The patient was a 46-year-old woman referred for evaluation of recurrent gastric GISTs and an incidentally discovered left adrenal mass. At 11 years of age she had a 3.5-cm left carotid body tumor resected. At age 24 she presented with massive gastrointestinal bleeding and was treated with a partial gastrectomy for multiple gastric GISTs; it was also at that time that a posterior mediastinal paraganglioma was resected and multiple calcified pulmonary chondromas were noted on chest radiograph (Fig. 22.1). She proved to be the index case for Dr. Aidan Carney's original description of Carney triad.[1,2] No surgeries had been performed between ages 24 and 46 years. The current visit to Mayo Clinic was for evaluation of recurrent gastric

GIST and a left adrenal mass. Esophageal leiomyomas and adrenocortical adenomas had recently been recognized to also be linked to Carney triad.[3,4]

INVESTIGATIONS

A recent abdominal magnetic resonance imaging (MRI) scan showed two masses in the upper stomach (4 cm and 2.7 cm) and a 2 × 3–cm inhomogeneous left adrenal mass (Fig. 22.2). She was asymptomatic. Her weight was stable (body mass index, 18.9 kg/m^2) and she had regular menses. Her blood pressure was normal and she had no symptoms of catecholamine or glucocorticoid excess. The 24-hour urine for fractionated catecholamines and metanephrines was normal. Plasma fractionated metanephrines were normal. The 24-hour urinary free cortisol excretion was normal at 28.2 mcg (normal <45 mcg).

TREATMENT

The patient underwent an open abdominal exploration for completion gastrectomy to treat multifocal GISTs. In addition, hepatic GIST metastases and the left adrenal gland were resected. The left adrenal contained two cortical adenomas (2.0 cm and 1.7 cm) and there was marked cortical atrophy (Fig. 22.3).

OUTCOME AND FOLLOW-UP

Because of the marked adrenocortical atrophy noted by Dr. Carney, who was in the operating room, the patient received 100 mg of intravenously administered hydrocortisone intraoperatively. Six days after surgery and 24 hours after her previous dose of hydrocortisone, the serum cortisol concentration was low at 4.8 mcg/dL (normal, 7–25 mcg/dL) and consistent with

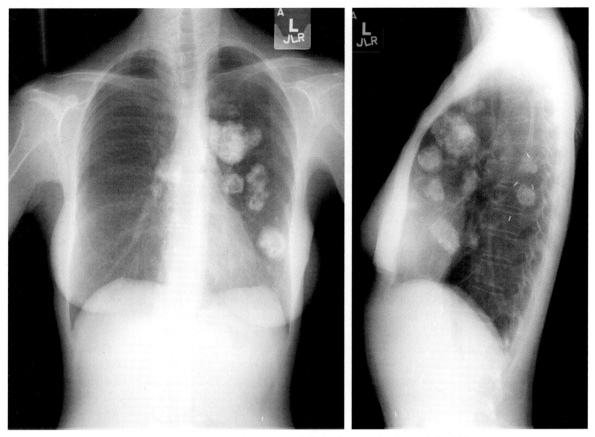

Fig. 22.1 Chest radiograph showing multiple calcified pulmonary chondromas in the left lung.

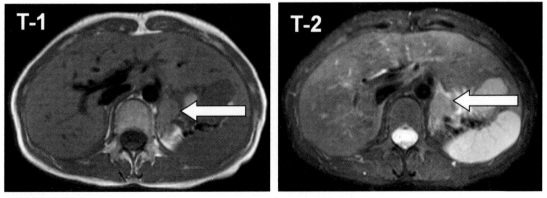

Fig. 22.2 Axial magnetic resonance images show a poorly defined, somewhat inhomogeneous 2 × 3–cm left adrenal mass (*arrows*).

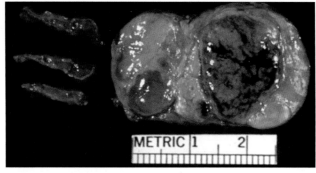

Fig. 22.3 Gross pathology image showing two juxtaposed adenomas measuring 2.0 and 1.7 cm in diameter. One nodule had a variegated pattern, predominantly yellow but with dark brown and black streaks and a tan area. The extratumoral cortex (see cut sections on left side of the figure) showed marked atrophy with no zona reticularis visible.

a partially suppressed hypothalamic-pituitary-adrenal (HPA) axis. She was discharged from the hospital on hydrocortisone replacement. One month later the HPA axis was recovering based on a morning serum cortisol concentration of 9 mcg/dL. Three months after surgery the serum cortisol was 14 mcg/dL, and the partial replacement with hydrocortisone was discontinued. It was an error to not screen this patient for glucocorticoid secretory autonomy before surgery. All patients with adrenal tumors (unless an alternate pathology is obvious, e.g., pheochromocytoma) should have case detection testing for subclinical Cushing syndrome (mild autonomous cortisol secretion) with baseline serum dehydroepiandrosterone sulfate and overnight dexamethasone suppression testing.

The adrenal surgery was performed in January 1999. She died 15 years later due to progressive and metastatic GIST at 63 years of age, more than 50 years after recognition of her first tumor.[5] At autopsy her right adrenal gland weighed 8.7 g (normal, 4–5 g). There were two cortical nodules (1.5 cm and 1.1 cm) without associated cortical atrophy. In a series of 14 patients with Carney triad and an adrenal neoplasm we found that the cortical neoplasm was uniformly asymptomatic.[3] In addition, results of adrenocortical function tests were usually normal. Unenhanced computed tomography attenuation typically showed low-density adrenal masses consistent with cortical adenomas.[3]

Carney triad is a rare multitumoral syndrome of uncertain etiology. Approximately 150 cases have been identified.[4] The disorder occurs almost exclusively in young women and is not familial. Only one patient has had tumors in all five organs (see Case 49). Most patients have two-organ involvement. Thus Carney triad is usually only partially expressed. The gastric tumors are malignant and metastasize to the liver, peritoneum, and lymph nodes. The lung, adrenal, and esophageal tumors are benign. The paragangliomas are usually benign. Long-term follow-up shows that the syndrome is a chronic, persistent, and generally indolent condition whose outcome is largely dependent on the behavior of the metastases from the GIST.

The findings from one study suggested that a DNA hypermethylation pattern was correlated to a reduced mRNA expression of *SDHC* and concurrent loss of the SDHC subunit on the protein level.[6] These data suggested epigenetic inactivation of the *SDHC* gene locus with functional impairment of the succinate dehydrogenase complex as a plausible mechanism of tumorigenesis in Carney triad.[6]

Key Points

- Although rare, endocrinologists should be aware of the five components of Carney triad, which include paraganglioma, adrenal cortical adenoma, pulmonary chondromas, esophageal leiomyoma, and GIST.

- When adrenalectomy is planned, all patients' adrenal adenomas >1-cm diameter should have case detection testing for subclinical glucocorticoid secretory autonomy preoperatively.
- When glucocorticoid secretory autonomy is documented, the patient should have perioperative stress glucocorticoid coverage and on discharge prescribed a morning dose of hydrocortisone until the HPA axis recovers.

REFERENCES

1. Carney JA, Sheps SG, Go VL, et al. The triad of gastric leiomyosarcoma, functioning extra-adrenal paraganglioma and pulmonary chondroma. *N Engl J Med*. 1977;296:1517–1518.

2. Carney JA. The triad of gastric epithelioid leiomyosarcoma, functioning extra-adrenal paraganglioma, and pulmonary chondroma. *Cancer*. 1979;43:374–382.

3. Carney JA, Stratakis CA, Young WF Jr. Adrenal cortical adenoma: the fourth component of the Carney triad and an association with subclinical Cushing syndrome. *Am J Surg Pathol*. 2013;37(8):1140–1149 .

4. Carney JA. Carney triad. *Front Horm Res*. 2013;41:92–110.

5. Juskewich JE, Carney JA, Alexander MP. The case of index patient of Carney Triad: a clinical puzzle and an epigenetic solution. *Am J Surg Pathol: Reviews and Reports*. 2017;22:54–57.

6. Haller F, Moskalev EA, Faucz FR, et al. Aberrant DNA hypermethylation of SDHC: a novel mechanism of tumor development in Carney triad. *Endocr Relat Cancer*. 2014;21(4):567–577.

Adrenal Cortical Carcinoma and Oncocytic Neoplasm

Adrenal Cortical Carcinoma

Adrenal cortical carcinoma (ACC) is a rare malignancy with an incidence of 1–2 cases per million population per year.[1] ACC represents only 0.4% of all adrenal tumors diagnosed in a population setting.[2] In endocrine practice, ACC may be diagnosed in approximately 5% of patients presenting with adrenal tumors overall, and in 13% of patients with adrenal tumors >4 cm.[3]

ACC affects women more than men (1.5–2:1 ratio) and follows a bimodal age distribution usually developing in young children and adults 40–50 years old. Most cases are sporadic; however, association with several hereditary syndromes was reported, including Li-Fraumeni, Beckwith-Wiedemann, neurofibromatosis type 1, multiple endocrine neoplasia type 1 (see Case 32), and Lynch syndromes (see Case 31).[4–6]

ACC can be diagnosed incidentally (40%–45%) on imaging performed for reasons other than adrenal mass, present with symptoms of hormone excess (30%–40%), or symptoms of mass effect (20%).[3] On imaging, ACC is most frequently a unilateral large adrenal mass with a median tumor size of approximately 10 cm, reflective of a relatively rapid tumor growth. Imaging characteristics include unenhanced computed tomography (CT) attenuation > 20 Hounsfield units (HU) (median of 35 HU), lack of chemical shift on magnetic resonance imaging (MRI), positive uptake on F-18 fluorodeoxyglucose positron emission tomography, and frequently heterogeneous on CT and MRI—reflective of the underlying necrosis.[3,7,8] Infrequently, ACC can be detected at a smaller tumor size (see Case 23), providing an opportunity to ensure an excellent prognosis if managed properly.[9]

All patients with ACC should undergo a comprehensive workup for hormonal excess.[10,11] ACCs frequently demonstrate a combined hormone excess (i.e., cortisol and androgen excess).[4,6,12,13] Urine steroid profiling (see Case 24) was recently validated as an accurate noninvasive diagnostic test and is likely to gain more popularity in the diagnosis of indeterminate adrenal tumors in the future.[14–16]

Initial stage of ACC (Table D.1) as well as the possibility of complete resection are the most important prognostic factors in patients with ACC.[6,12] Surgical resection with open adrenalectomy is the mainstay of management for ACC and the only potentially curative therapy. Mitotic rate and the Ki-67 labeling index have also been shown to have prognostic implications, with higher numbers associated with worse prognosis. Postoperative mitotane therapy is usually recommended for patients at highest risk of recurrence (Ki-67>10%, mitotic rate >20/50 high-power fields, and tumors with vascular or capsular invasion).[6,12] Monitoring includes periodic imaging and biochemical reassessment with steroid markers.[6,12,17]

Stage	ENSAT	Comments
TABLE D.1	**European Network for the Study of Adrenal Tumors (ENSAT) Classification[6]**	
I	T1, N0, M0	T1: tumor ≤5 cm
II	T2, N0, M0	T2: tumor >5 cm
III	T3 or T4, N0, M0	T3: tumor infiltration in surrounding tissue
		T4: tumor invasion in adjacent organs, venous tumor thrombus in vena cava or renal vein
IV	Any with M1	N0: no positive lymph nodes
		N1: positive lymph nodes
		M0: no distance metastases
		M1: presence of distant metastasis

From Fassnacht M, Dekkers OM, Else T, et al. European Society of Endocrinology Clinical Practice Guidelines on the management of adrenocortical carcinoma in adults, in collaboration with the European Network for the Study of Adrenal Tumors. *Eur J Endocrinol.* 2018;179(4):G1-G46.

Mitotane is an adrenolytic drug that is used in treatment of ACC. All studies investigating mitotane to date are retrospective.[6–8] Mitotane therapy has been associated with a longer recurrence-free survival, a better 5-year survival, but not a better overall survival.[6–8] The dose of mitotane is usually approximately 3–6 g per day. Mitotane concentrations can be helpful in deciding on the dose (goal of 14–20 mg/L). The patient's tolerance to mitotane and side effects also contribute to the decision on dosing (see Case 26). Mitotane-induced adrenal insufficiency should be anticipated and properly treated. Patients require an increased dose of hydrocortisone while on mitotane therapy (30–60 mg daily in divided doses) because of the mitotane-induced increase in cortisol metabolism. Other common side effects include fatigue, nausea, diarrhea, gynecomastia, and, less commonly, confusion, dizziness, and ataxia. In addition to clinical evaluation for signs and symptoms of cortisol excess or deficiency, and other side effects to mitotane, all patients require biochemical monitoring with serum electrolytes, liver function tests, thyroid function tests, cholesterol, and tests for mineralocorticoid deficiency.[4,5]

For advanced ACC, cytotoxic chemotherapy with or without mitotane has been used, with the most common regimen including etoposide, doxorubicin, and cisplatin.[6,12] New therapies are currently under investigation or have been tried, including immunotherapy.[6,12,18]

REFERENCES

1. Kerkhofs TM, Verhoeven RH, Van der Zwan JM, et al. Adrenocortical carcinoma: a population-based study on incidence and survival in the Netherlands since 1993. *Eur J Cancer.* 2013;49(11):2579–2586.

2. Ebbehoj A, Li D, Kaur RJ, et al. Epidemiology of adrenal tumours in Olmsted County, Minnesota, USA: a population-based cohort study. *Lancet Diabetes Endocrinol.* 2020;8(11):894–902.

3. Iniguez-Ariza NM, Kohlenberg JD, Delivanis DA, et al. Clinical, biochemical, and radiological characteristics of a single-center retrospective cohort of 705 large adrenal tumors. *Mayo Clin Proc Innov Qual Outcomes.* 2018;2(1):30–39.

4. Kaur RJ, Pichurin PN, Hines JM, Singh RJ, Grebe SK, Bancos I. Adrenal cortical carcinoma associated with lynch syndrome: a case report and review of literature. *J Endocr Soc.* 2019;3(4):784–790.

5. Koch CA, Pacak K, Chrousos GP. The molecular pathogenesis of hereditary and sporadic adrenocortical and adrenomedullary tumors. *J Clin Endocrinol Metab.* 2002;87(12):5367–5384.

6. Fassnacht M, Dekkers OM, Else T, et al. European Society of Endocrinology Clinical Practice Guidelines on the management of adrenocortical carcinoma in adults, in collaboration with the European Network for the Study of Adrenal Tumors. *Eur J Endocrinol.* 2018;179(4):G1–G46.

7. Dinnes J, Bancos I, Ferrante di Ruffano L, et al. management of endocrine disease: imaging for the diagnosis of malignancy in incidentally discovered adrenal masses: a systematic review and meta-analysis. *Eur J Endocrinol.* 2016;175(2):R51–R64.

8. Delivanis DA, Bancos I, Atwell TD, et al. Diagnostic performance of unenhanced computed tomography and (18) F-fluorodeoxyglucose positron emission tomography in indeterminate adrenal tumours. *Clin Endocrinol (Oxf).* 2018;88(1):30–36.

9. Gagnon N, Boily P, Alguire C, et al. Small adrenal incidentaloma becoming an aggressive adrenocortical carcinoma in a patient carrying a germline APC variant. *Endocrine*. 2020;68(1):203–209.

10. Vaidya A, Hamrahian A, Bancos I, Fleseriu M, Ghayee HK. The evaluation of incidentally discovered adrenal masses. *Endocr Pract*. 2019;25(2):178–192.

11. Fassnacht M, Arlt W, Bancos I, et al. Management of adrenal incidentalomas: European Society of Endocrinology Clinical Practice Guideline in collaboration with the European Network for the Study of Adrenal Tumors. *Eur J Endocrinol*. 2016;175(2):G1–G34.

12. Kiseljak-Vassiliades K, Bancos I, Hamrahian A, et al. American Association of Clinical Endocrinology disease state clinical review on the evaluation and management of adrenocortical carcinoma in an adult: a practical approach. *Endocrine Practice*. 2020;26(11):1366–1383.

13. Sada A, Asaad M, Bews KA, et al. Comparison between functional and non-functional adrenocortical carcinoma. *Surgery*. 2020;167(1):216–223.

14. Bancos I, Arlt W. Diagnosis of a malignant adrenal mass: the role of urinary steroid metabolite profiling. *Curr Opin Endocrinol Diabetes Obes*. 2017;24(3):200–207.

15. Bancos I, Taylor AE, Chortis V, et al. Urine steroid metabolomics for the differential diagnosis of adrenal incidentalomas in the EURINE-ACT study: a prospective test validation study. *Lancet Diabetes Endocrinol*. 2020;8(9):773–781.

16. Hines JM, Bancos I, Bancos C, et al. High-resolution, accurate-mass (HRAM) Mass Spectrometry Urine Steroid Profiling in the Diagnosis of Adrenal Disorders. *Clin Chem*. 2017;63(12):1824–1835.

17. Chortis V, Bancos I, Nijman T, et al. Urine steroid metabolomics as a novel tool for detection of recurrent adrenocortical carcinoma. *J Clin Endocrinol Metab*. 2020;105(3).

18. Miller KC, Chintakuntlawar AV, Hilger C, et al. Salvage therapy with multikinase inhibitors and immunotherapy in advanced adrenal cortical carcinoma. *J Endocr Soc*. 2020;4(7):bvaa069.

Adrenal Cortical Carcinoma in a Patient With a History of Adrenal Incidentaloma

When a patient is incidentally discovered with an adrenal mass, two questions need to be answered: (1) Is the adrenal mass malignant? (2) Is the adrenal mass hormonally active?[1] Age, patient's history, tumor size, and imaging characteristics are useful in assessing the potential for adrenal malignancy.[2–4] Adrenal "incidentaloma" is frequently ignored by clinicians.[3] However, 3% of all adrenal incidentalomas are malignant. When imaging characteristics of the adrenal mass do not clearly exclude malignancy (i.e., malignancy is excluded if the unenhanced computed tomography [CT] attenuation is <10 Hounsfield units [HU]),[5,6] further action is needed and may include imaging monitoring, another imaging test, or adrenalectomy.

Case Report

The patient was a 29-year-old woman who presented for evaluation of a large adrenal mass. One year before referral, she discontinued oral contraceptive therapy in attempt to conceive. Six months before referral, she was evaluated by her gynecologist for secondary amenorrhea (she did not resume her menses since stopping oral contraceptive therapy). Workup at that time revealed elevated dehydroepiandrosterone sulfate (DHEA-S) and testosterone, and abdominal imaging was obtained and demonstrated a 7.3 × 5.8 × 7.0–cm left adrenal mass (unenhanced CT attenuation = 35 HU). The patient was then referred to our institution. Notably, the patient reported that more than 3 years prior, she had a CT scan for abdominal pain that

demonstrated an incidental adrenal nodule. She was advised that the adrenal incidentaloma was a benign finding that needed no further follow-up. She did not have workup for adrenal hormone excess at that time. On physical examination her body mass index was 33.6 kg/m² and blood pressure 145/104 mmHg. She was not cushingoid. Acne was present on her face, shoulders, and chest.

INVESTIGATIONS

Laboratory tests were obtained (Table 23.1). Marked hyperandrogenemia was noted with significantly elevated androstenedione and testosterone and mild elevation of DHEA-S. In addition, despite the absence of clinical features of Cushing syndrome, glucocorticoid autonomy was demonstrated with an

TABLE 23.1 Laboratory Tests

Biochemical Test	Result	Reference Range
Post–1-mg DST cortisol, mcg/dL	8.3	<1.8
ACTH, pg/mL	24	10–60
Aldosterone, ng/dL	<4	≤21
Plasma renin activity, ng/mL per hour	1.2	≤0.6–3
DHEA-S, mcg/dL	485	44–332
Total testosterone, ng/dL	256	8–60
Androstenedione, ng/dL	2010	30–200
Plasma metanephrine, nmol/L	<0.2	<0.5
Plasma normetanephrines, nmol/L	0.26	<0.9

ACTH, Corticotropin; *DHEA-S*, dehydroepiandrosterone sulfate; *DST*, dexamethasone suppression test.

abnormal dexamethasone suppression test. Workup for primary aldosteronism and catecholamine excess was negative.

Both current and abdominal CT scans from 3 years prior were reviewed. A 0.9 × 1.2 × 1.6–cm left adrenal mass (unenhanced CT attenuation = 23 HU) was visible on the first available imaging. On the abdominal CT scan 3 years later, the left adrenal mass demonstrated considerable enlargement measuring 7.5 × 5.2 × 6.8 cm (Fig. 23.1).

TREATMENT

The patient was advised that the most likely diagnosis of the adrenal mass was adrenal cortical carcinoma (ACC) as a result of a significant tumor growth over 3 years, current tumor size, indeterminate imaging characteristics, and a combined glucocorticoid and androgen excess. She underwent open resection of the left adrenal mass. On pathology, the mass weighed 145 g and measured 10.5 × 7.5 × 6.9 cm (Fig. 23.2). The tumor was hemorrhagic and necrotic, without

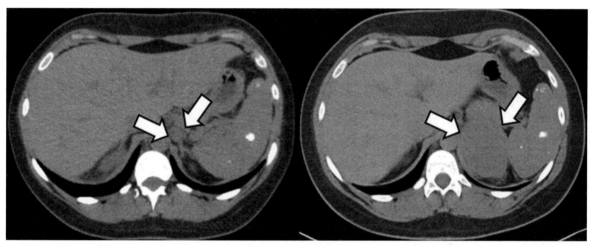

Fig. 23.1 Unenhanced axial computed tomography (CT) images 3 years apart (3 years ago, *left*, and current, *right*). A 0.9 × 1.2 × 1.6–cm left adrenal mass (unenhanced CT attenuation = 23 HU) was visible on the first available imaging (*left, arrows*). On the abdominal CT scan 3 years later, the left adrenal mass demonstrated a considerable enlargement measuring 7.5 × 5.2 × 6.8 cm and had an unenhanced CT attenuation of 35 Hounsfield units (*right, arrows*).

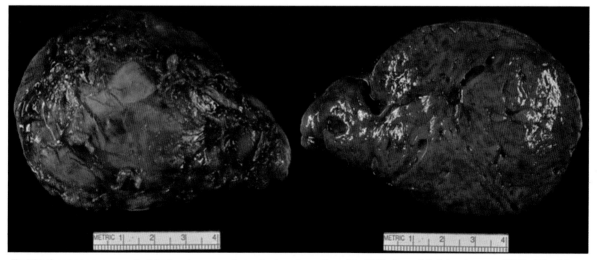

Fig. 23.2 On gross macroscopy, the left adrenal mass was hemorrhagic and necrotic, weighed 145 g (normal, 4–5 g) and measured 10.5 × 7.5 × 6.9 cm.

lymphovascular invasion. A tumor thrombus was identified in the left adrenal vein. ACC was diagnosed with a Ki-67 of 5%. She was discharged from the hospital on glucocorticoid therapy and opted to initiate postoperative treatment with mitotane 4 weeks later. Mitotane therapy was continued for 12 months and was stopped due to gastrointestinal side effects. Four years postoperatively the patient was doing very well and is in remission.

Discussion

Any patient with a newly discovered adrenal mass needs a conclusive evaluation for malignancy and hormone excess. Incidentally discovered adrenal tumors are less likely to be malignant or hormonally active when compared with patients presenting with symptoms, or with a history of malignancy. However, approximately 50% of all patients with ACC, pheochromocytomas, and overt hormone excess are discovered incidentally.[4] Our patient initially presented with a small adrenal mass (only 1.6 cm in the largest diameter) that demonstrated indeterminate imaging characteristics. Close monitoring, additional imaging, or adrenalectomy are the three options to consider in these situations.[7] Instead, the patient was falsely reassured, only to present 3 years later with a much larger adrenal mass and marked adrenal hormone excess.

Key Points

- Differential diagnosis of an indeterminate adrenal mass includes ACC, other malignant mass, pheochromocytoma, or lipid poor adenoma.
- Most patients with ACC are diagnosed with large adrenal tumors (>6 cm)[8] and have suboptimal prognosis with poor 5-year survival rates. In the case presented here, following the guidelines for detection of malignancy and hormone excess, ACC could have been diagnosed and treated at a very early stage, ensuring the best prognosis.

REFERENCES

1. Vaidya A, Hamrahian A, Bancos I, Fleseriu M, Ghayee HK. The evaluation of incidentally discovered adrenal masses. *Endocr Pract*. 2019;25(2):178–192.

2. Bancos I, Arlt W. Diagnosis of a malignant adrenal mass: the role of urinary steroid metabolite profiling. *Curr Opin Endocrinol Diabetes Obes*. 2017;24(3):200–207.

3. Ebbehoj A, Li D, Kaur RJ, et al. Epidemiology of adrenal tumours in Olmsted County, Minnesota, USA: a population-based cohort study. *Lancet Diabetes Endocrinol*. 2020;8(11):894–902.

4. Iniguez-Ariza NM, Kohlenberg JD, Delivanis DA, et al. Clinical, biochemical, and radiological characteristics of a single-center retrospective cohort of 705 large adrenal tumors. *Mayo Clin Proc Innov Qual Outcomes*. 2018;2(1):30–39.

5. Delivanis DA, Bancos I, Atwell TD, et al. Diagnostic performance of unenhanced computed tomography and (18) F-fluorodeoxyglucose positron emission tomography in indeterminate adrenal tumours. *Clin Endocrinol (Oxf)*. 2018;88(1):30–36.

6. Dinnes J, Bancos I, Ferrante di Ruffano L, et al. Management of endocrine disease: Imaging for the diagnosis of malignancy in incidentally discovered adrenal masses: a systematic review and meta-analysis. *Eur J Endocrinol*. 2016;175(2):R51–R64.

7. Fassnacht M, Arlt W, Bancos I, et al. Management of adrenal incidentalomas: European Society of Endocrinology Clinical Practice Guideline in collaboration with the European Network for the Study of Adrenal Tumors. *Eur J Endocrinol*. 2016;175(2):G1–G34.

8. Bancos I, Taylor AE, Chortis V, et al. Urine steroid metabolomics for the differential diagnosis of adrenal incidentalomas in the EURINE-ACT study: a prospective test validation study. *Lancet Diabetes Endocrinol*. 2020;8(9):773–781.

Unexpected Diagnosis of Adrenal Cortical Carcinoma: Role of Urinary Steroid Profiling

Adrenal "incidentaloma" is frequently ignored by clinicians.[1] However, approximately 50% of all patients with adrenocortical carcinomas (ACCs), pheochromocytomas, and overt hormone excess are discovered incidentally.[2] When imaging characteristics of the adrenal mass do not clearly exclude malignancy (i.e., malignancy is excluded if the unenhanced computed tomography [CT] attenuation is <10 Hounsfield units [HU]),[3,4] further action is needed, and may include imaging monitoring, another imaging test, or adrenalectomy. Urine steroid profiling was recently validated as an accurate diagnostic test for ACC.[5]

Case Report

The patient was a 21-year-old woman who 7 months prior presented to a local emergency department with symptoms of abdominal pain. CT of the abdomen demonstrated appendicitis, and she was treated with appendectomy. She recovered well, but on review of her hospital records noticed that the CT report also mentioned a 2.7 × 2.1 cm left adrenal mass. This discovery prompted her to perform internet research on adrenal tumors, and on reviewing the symptoms of Cushing syndrome, she requested her primary care physician to perform a hormonal workup and repeat the CT scan. Her symptoms included weight gain of 10 pounds over 3 months (unusual for her), exacerbation of anxiety and depression, and fatigue. She was a dancer, and despite intensifying her training, she noticed muscle weakness. In addition, she observed easy bruising and development of striae over her abdomen.

On physical examination her body mass index was 24.1 kg/m^2 and blood pressure was 110/80 mmHg. She presented clear cushingoid features, including facial rounding, dorsocervical and supraclavicular pads, facial plethora, and a few small striae.

INVESTIGATIONS

The patient's self-diagnosis of Cushing syndrome related to her adrenal mass (corticotropin [ACTH]-independent hypercortisolism) was completely accurate (Table 24.1). Both the abdominal CT scan obtained at the time of appendicitis (7 months prior) and the scan performed several weeks before referral were reviewed. On the contrast-enhanced CT scan from 7 months prior, a 2.2 × 2.9 × 2.7–cm left adrenal mass was demonstrated. Follow-up CT scan demonstrated an enlargement of the adrenal mass, measuring 2.5 × 3.6 × 3.2 cm; it had an unenhanced CT attenuation of 27 Hounsfield units (HU)

TABLE 24.1 Laboratory Tests

Biochemical Test	Result	Reference Range
AM cortisol, mcg/dL	9.2	7–25
PM cortisol, mcg/dL	8.7	2–14
Post–1-mg DST cortisol, mcg/dL	16	<1.8
ACTH, pg/mL	<5	10–60
DHEA-S, mcg/dL	77	44–332
24-Hour urine metanephrine, mcg/dL	52	30–180
24-Hour urine normetanephrines, mcg/dL	134	103–390

ACTH, Corticotropin; DHEA-S, dehydroepiandrosterone sulfate; DST, dexamethasone suppression test.

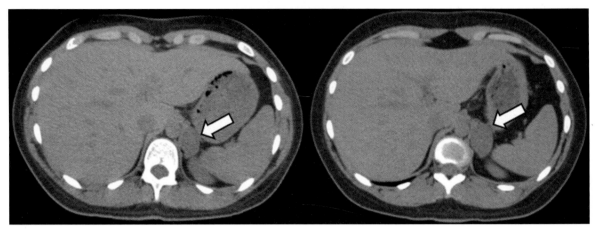

Fig. 24.1 Contrast-enhanced and unenhanced axial computed tomography (CT) images 7 months apart (7 months ago, *left*, and current, *right*). A 2.2 × 2.9 × 2.7–cm left adrenal mass was visible on the first available imaging (*left, arrow*). On the abdominal CT scan 7 months later, the left adrenal mass demonstrated an enlargement measuring 3.5 × 3.6 × 3.2 cm and had an unenhanced CT attenuation of 27 Hounsfield units (*right, arrow*).

and an absolute contrast washout of 74% at 10 minutes after contrast administration (Fig. 24.1). In addition, the patient provided a 24-hour urine sample for steroid profiling analysis: a research procedure at that time but now clinically available (http://www.mayocliniclabs.com/test-catalog/Overview/604986) (Table 24.2).

TREATMENT

The patient was advised that the tumor growth of 7 mm in 7 months, lipid-poor nature (>20 HU), and detectable serum dehydroepiandrosterone sulfate (DHEA-S) concentration in the setting of ACTH-independent hypercortisolism could be consistent with an ACC, whereas the contrast washout of >60% at 10 minutes was more suggestive of a benign adrenal mass. She underwent laparoscopic resection of the left adrenal mass. On pathology, the mass weighed 14.6 g (normal, 4–5 g) and measured 3.7 × 2.9 × 2.4 cm. Initially, the diagnosis of adrenal adenoma was given. She was discharged from the hospital on glucocorticoid therapy.

OUTCOME

The patient recovered well from surgery. Several weeks after adrenalectomy, the results of the urine steroid profiling were available and were strongly consistent with ACC: metabolites of 11-deoxycortisol (tetrahydrode-oxycortisol), 17-hydroxyprogesterone (pregnanetriol), and 17-hydroxypregnenolone (pregnanetriol) were

markedly elevated (see Table 24.2). Guided by these results, we asked for a rereview of pathology from adrenalectomy. Ki-67 immunostaining was performed and was elevated at 10%, reflecting the mitotic/proliferative activity. Because of clinical, biochemical, imaging, steroid profiling, and pathological findings, the patient was recommended for closer follow-up with repeat imaging at regular intervals. Five years since adrenalectomy, she remains in remission. She recovered from adrenal insufficiency and stopped hydrocortisone 8 months after adrenalectomy.

Discussion

A conclusive evaluation for malignancy and hormone excess is needed in any patient with a newly discovered adrenal mass. Features concerning for ACC in our patient included (1) rapid tumor growth, (2) unenhanced CT attenuation >20 HU, (3) young age, and (4) combined adrenal hormone excess (nonsuppressed DHEA-S in the setting of the ACTH-independent hypercortisolism). Notably, unlike unenhanced CT attenuation measurement, absolute contrast washout does not have sufficient evidence or accuracy in the diagnosis of ACC.[4] Urine steroid profiling has been recently validated as an accurate diagnostic test for ACC.[5] It is most useful in larger adrenal tumors with indeterminate imaging characteristics for diagnostic purposes, but also to establish an individual "steroid

TABLE 24.2   24-Hour Urine Steroid Profiling Results

Analyte	Full Name of Steroid	z Score
An	Androsterone	0.3
Etio	Etiocholanolone	2.2
DHEA	Dehydroepiandrosterone	−0.5
16a-DHEA	16α-Hydroxy-dehydroepiandrosterone	−0.8
5PT	Pregnenetriol	16
5PD	Pregnenediol	−0.2
THB	Tetrahydrocorticosterone	−1.7
THDOC	Tetrahydrodeoxycorticosterone	2.8
PD	Pregnanediol	−0.2
PT	Pregnanetriol	12
17HP	17α-Hydroxypregnenolone	1.8
PTONE	Pregnanetriolone	0.5
THS	Tetrahydrodeoxycortisol	284
Cortisol	Cortisol	0.2
Cortisone	Cortisone	0.6
6B-OH-Cortisol	6β-Hydroxycortisol	3.5
11B-OH-AN	11β-Hydroxyandrosterone	−0.5
11-OXO-ET	11-Oxoetiocholanolone	1.7
B-Cortol	β-Cortol	0.6
a-Cortolone	α-Cortolone	2.9
B-Cortolone	β-Cortolone	1.9
5a-THF	5α-Tetrahydrocortisol	0.9
THF	Tetrahydrocortisol	2.3
THE	Tetrahydrocortisone	2.6
11B-OH-ET	11β-Hydroxyetiocholanolone	1.1

z scores: standard deviations above normal. Normal: −2.5 to 2.5.

fingerprint" to monitor for recurrence after adrenalectomy.[6] In this case, urine steroid profiling was useful to diagnose a smaller ACC, prompting additional pathology rereview.

Key Points

- Differential diagnosis of an indeterminate adrenal mass includes ACC, other malignant mass, pheochromocytoma, or lipid poor adenoma.
- Most patients with ACC are diagnosed with large adrenal tumors (e.g., >6 cm)[5] and have suboptimal prognosis with poor 5-year survival rates. Early diagnosis of ACC is seldom outside cases such as the one illustrated here.
- Prompt workup of any adrenal mass ensures the best prognosis and is the responsibility of the medical team. In contrast, in the case presented here, it was the patient's careful review of her hospitalization records that led to further workup and treatment—possibly radically changing her prognosis outcome!

REFERENCES

1. Ebbehoj A, Li D, Kaur RJ, et al. Epidemiology of adrenal tumours in Olmsted County, Minnesota, USA: a population-based cohort study. *Lancet Diabetes Endocrinol.* 2020;8(11):894–902.
2. Iniguez-Ariza NM, Kohlenberg J, Delivanis DA, et al. Clinical, biochemical, and radiological characteristics of a single-center retrospective cohort of 705 large adrenal tumors. *Mayo Clin Proc Innov Qual Outcomes.* 2018;2(1):30–39.
3. Delivanis DA, Bancos I, Atwell TD, et al. Diagnostic performance of unenhanced computed tomography and (18) F-fluorodeoxyglucose positron emission tomography in indeterminate adrenal tumours. *Clin Endocrinol (Oxf).* 2018;88(1):30–36.
4. Dinnes J, Bancos I, Ferrante di Ruffano L, et al. Management of endocrine disease: Imaging for the diagnosis of malignancy in incidentally discovered adrenal masses: a systematic review and meta-analysis. *Eur J Endocrinol.* 2016;175(2):R51–R64.
5. Bancos I, Taylor AE, Chortis V, et al. Urine steroid metabolomics for the differential diagnosis of adrenal incidentalomas in the EURINE-ACT study: a prospective test validation study. *Lancet Diabetes Endocrinol.* 2020;8(9):773–781.
6. Chortis V, Bancos I, Nijman T, et al. Urine steroid metabolomics as a novel tool for detection of recurrent adrenocortical carcinoma. *J Clin Endocrinol Metab.* 2020;105(3):e307–e378.

Oncocytic Adrenocortical Carcinoma

The Weiss scoring system is the most popular system used in the histologic diagnosis of adrenocortical carcinoma (ACC) and includes assessment of diffuse architecture; clear cells; nuclear grade; mitotic rate; atypical mitotic figures; necrosis; and venous, sinusoidal, or capsular invasion.[1] However, it presents several limitations, including classification of borderline adrenal tumors (Weiss score of 3) or oncocytic and myxoid adrenal tumors. Oncocytic adrenocortical tumors demonstrate cells with eosinophilic cytoplasm, clear cells <25% of tumor volume, high-grade nuclear atypia, and diffuse architecture—all features diagnostic of ACC based on the Weiss scoring system and thus potentially misclassified. Oncocytic adrenocortical tumors are thus classified based on the Lin-Weiss-Bisceglia system that includes (1) major criteria (mitotic rate >5 mitoses/50 high-power fields, atypical mitoses, venous invasion) and (2) minor criteria (tumor size >10 cm or mass >200 g, necrosis, capsular invasion, sinusoidal invasion). The presence of any one major criterion is diagnostic of the oncocytic ACC, and the presence of at least one minor criterion indicates oncocytic neoplasm of uncertain malignant potential. The absence of any major or minor criteria is diagnostic of adrenocortical oncocytoma.[2,3] Here we present a case of oncocytic ACC.

Case Report

The patient was an 80-year-old woman incidentally discovered with a right adrenal mass during workup for acute abdominal pain, which was subsequently diagnosed as diverticulitis. Unenhanced computed tomography (CT) demonstrated a 8.2 × 7.1 × 6.3–cm right adrenal mass with an attenuation of 34 Hounsfield units (HU) (Fig. 25.1). Initial workup locally included a 1-mg dexamethasone suppression test, which was normal (cortisol <1.4 mcg/dL). The patient was referred to Mayo Clinic for further management of the adrenal mass.

On evaluation, she did not notice any symptoms suggestive of androgen, cortisol, aldosterone, or catecholamine excess. However, she did note an unusual sensation in her both breasts that she thought was very similar to what she felt when breastfeeding years ago. She had long-standing hypertension and prediabetes, both stable. Her blood pressure was 142/82 mmHg, heart rate was 81 beats per minute, and body mass index was 38.44 kg/m². Her only medication was losartan 75 mg daily.

INVESTIGATIONS

Laboratory evaluation showed normal levels of urinary metanephrines and normetanephrine; however, serum concentrations of progesterone and estradiol were higher than expected for the patient's postmenopausal status (Table 25.1). Positron emission tomography (PET) scan demonstrated intense F-18 fluorodeoxyglucose (FDG) uptake in the adrenal mass without any other foci of activity (see Fig. 25.1).

TREATMENT AND FOLLOW-UP

ACC was suspected because of the concerning imaging characteristics and the elevated progesterone and estradiol concentrations. The patient was treated with open right adrenalectomy. Final pathology demonstrated an oncocytic ACC that measured 9.5 × 7.5 × 7.0 cm and weighed 260 g (Fig. 25.2). The tumor displayed low mitotic activity, atypical mitoses, necrosis, and capsular invasion. The Ki-67 index was 17%. The patient declined mitotane therapy and was followed with periodic imaging. Two years postadrenalectomy she remains in remission.

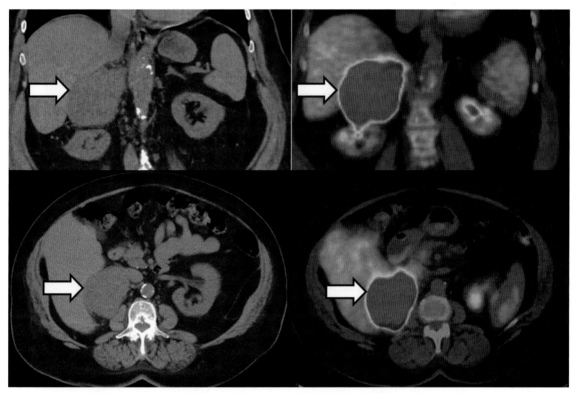

Fig. 25.1 Coronal and axial unenhanced computed tomography (CT) images (*left*) demonstrated a right adrenal mass (*arrows*) that measured 8.2 × 7.1 × 6.3 cm with a CT attenuation of 34 Hounsfield units. F-18 fluorodeoxyglucose positron emission tomography scan image (*right*) shows that the right adrenal mass (*arrows*) was markedly hypermetabolic, with maximum standard unit value (SUVmax) of 40.9.

TABLE 25.1 Laboratory Tests		
Biochemical Test	**Result**	**Reference Range**
Cortisol following overnight 1-mg DST, mcg/dL	1.4	<1.8
8 AM Cortisol, mcg/dL	12	7–21
ACTH, pg/mL	38	7.2–63
DHEA-S, mcg/dL	36	<15–157
Progesterone, ng/mL	0.72	<0.2
Estradiol, pg/mL	11	<10
Aldosterone, ng/dL	<4	<21
Plasma renin activity, ng/mL per hour	<0.6	≤0.6–3
24-Hour urine cortisol, mcg/24 h	29	<45
24-Hour urine metanephrines, mcg/24 h	57	<400
24-Hour urine normetanephrines, mcg/24 h	525	<900

ACTH, Corticotropin; *DHEA-S*, dehydroepiandrosterone sulfate; *DST*, dexamethasone suppression test.

Discussion

Our patient was diagnosed with a rare subtype of ACC—oncocytic ACC based on the Lin-Weiss-Bisceglia system. She had one major criterion (atypical mitoses) and several minor criteria (adrenal mass >200 g, necrosis, and capsular invasion). In addition, the Ki-67 index indicated a malignant tumor (17%). She had a R0 resection for her European Network for the Study of Adrenal Tumours (ENSAT) stage II disease, currently in remission. Accurate classification of adrenal neoplasms is key to ensure optimal management.

Key Points

- Oncocytic ACC is a rare subtype of ACC.
- Appropriate classification of adrenal neoplasms is important to ensure optimal management.
- The Ki-67 index can further clarify the malignancy potential in borderline adrenal tumors.

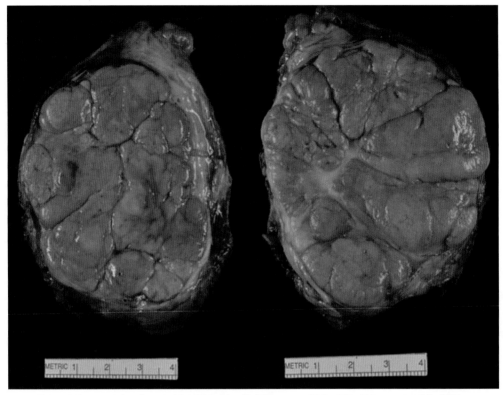

Fig. 25.2 Gross pathology image of the right oncocytic ACC measured 9.5 × 7.5 × 7.0 cm and weighed 260 g.

REFERENCES

1. Lau SK, Weiss LM. The Weiss system for evaluating adrenocortical neoplasms: 25 years later. *Hum Pathol.* 2009;40(6):757–768.

2. de Krijger RR, Papathomas TG. Adrenocortical neoplasia: evolving concepts in tumorigenesis with an emphasis on adrenal cortical carcinoma variants. *Virchows Arch.* 2012;460(1):9–18.

3. Erickson LA. Challenges in surgical pathology of adrenocortical tumours. *Histopathology.* 2018;72(1):82–96.

Mitotane Therapy in the ENSAT Stage II Adrenocortical Carcinoma

Adrenocortical carcinoma (ACC) can present with overt symptoms of hormone excess (usually androgen, cortisol, or combined hypersecretion) in 30%–40% of cases. Imaging characteristics include unenhanced attenuation >20 Hounsfield units (HU), heterogeneity, and positive F-18 fluorodeoxyglucose (FDG) uptake on positron emission tomography (PET). Prognosis depends on several factors, including the European Network for the Study of Adrenal Tumours (ENSAT) stage, R0 (complete) surgical resection by an expert surgeon, and Ki-67 index <10%. Adjuvant mitotane therapy is usually recommended for patients at high risk of recurrence. Recently, the results of the ADIUVO study that included patients with ENSAT stage I or II disease and Ki-67 index <10% did not support the routine use of mitotane therapy.

Case Report

The patient was a 23-year-old woman who initially presented for evaluation of acne and hirsutism of several months, duration, as well as development of irregular menses. Workup for androgen excess was performed. Because of significantly elevated serum androgen concentrations, computed tomography (CT) abdominal imaging was performed and demonstrated a heterogeneous right adrenal mass that measured 5.5 × 5.0 × 4.2 cm. The adrenal mass had an unenhanced CT attenuation of 31 HU and contained heterogeneity with areas of necrosis on contrast-enhanced CT. Subsequent FDG-PET scan demonstrated intense FDG uptake in the adrenal mass without any other foci of activity (Fig. 26.1). The patient was referred to Mayo Clinic for further management of the adrenal mass.

On evaluation, aside from acne and hirsutism, the patient denied any other symptoms and signs. She has not noticed cushingoid features or any changes in her

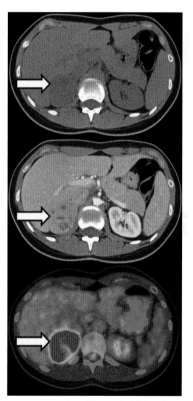

Fig. 26.1 Axial unenhanced (*top*) and contrast-enhanced (*middle*) computed tomography (CT) images and F-18 fluorodeoxyglucose positron emission tomography (FDG PET) scan image (*bottom*) show a heterogeneous right adrenal mass (*arrows*) measuring 5.5 × 5.0 × 4.2 cm. On unenhanced CT, the attenuation of adrenal mass was 31 Hounsfield units. On enhanced CT the adrenal mass demonstrated several areas of heterogeneity. On FDG PET scan, adrenal mass was FDG avid (maximum standard unit value [SUVmax] of 13.7).

blood pressure. On physical examination, her blood pressure was 124/68 mmHg and body mass index was 24.3 kg/m². She had facial acne and mild facial hirsutism. Her only medication was an oral contraceptive (drospirenone-ethinyl estradiol).

INVESTIGATIONS

Laboratory evaluation showed normal levels of urinary metanephrine and normetanephrine but was positive for significant androgen excess and possible glucocorticoid autonomy (abnormal dexamethasone suppression test while on oral contraceptive) (Table 26.1).

TREATMENT

ACC was suspected because of concerning imaging characteristics, severe hyperandrogenism of rapid onset, and possible combined glucocorticoid autonomy. The patient was treated with open right adrenalectomy. Final pathology demonstrated ACC that weighed 91 g and measured 6.4 × 6.2 × 4.2 cm. The yellow-brown soft heterogeneous mass did not extend beyond the adrenal gland (Fig. 26.2). Increased mitotic activity of 11 mitoses/50 high-power fields, atypical mitotic figure, and elevated Ki-67 proliferation index of 10% were noted. Capsular invasion was

not identified. A modified Weiss score of 5/7 was calculated.

The patient was treated with hydrocortisone after adrenalectomy. After discussion of mitotane therapy versus imaging follow-up without mitotane treatment for her ENSAT stage II disease, the patient elected to initiate mitotane therapy, which was started 4 weeks after surgery.

FOLLOW-UP

While the patient was on mitotane therapy, her hydrocortisone dosage was increased to a total daily dose of 40 mg in divided doses. Interval clinical, imaging, and biochemical monitoring was initiated. In addition to anticipated mitotane-induced adrenal insufficiency, she developed other side effects to mitotane. These included nausea, abdominal pain, diarrhea, and hypothyroidism. She was treated with levothyroxine for hypothyroidism. Imodium was tried for diarrhea, without success. As gastrointestinal symptoms were affecting the patient's quality of life, she decided to discontinue mitotane therapy 5 months after her operation. She continued to be in remission 5 years after adrenalectomy.

Discussion

Mitotane is an adrenolytic drug that is used in treatment of ACC. Until recently, all studies investigating mitotane to date have been retrospective.[1–3] These

TABLE 26.1   Laboratory Tests

Biochemical Test	Result	Reference Range
Cortisol after overnight 1-mg DST, mcg/dL	7.1	<1.8
Cortisol, mcg/dL	7.2	7–21
ACTH, pg/mL	7.5	7.2–63
DHEA-S, mcg/dL	1539	44–332
Androstenedione, ng/dL	430	30–200
Total testosterone, ng/dL	131	8–60
Aldosterone, ng/dL	21	<21
Plasma renin activity, ng/mL per hour	5.5	≤0.6–3
24-Hour urine cortisol, mcg/24 h	32	<45
24-Hour urine metanephrine, mcg/24 h	25	<400
24-Hour urine normetanephrine, mcg/24 h	144	<900

ACTH, Corticotropin; *DHEA-S,* dehydroepiandrosterone sulfate; *DST,* dexamethasone suppression test.

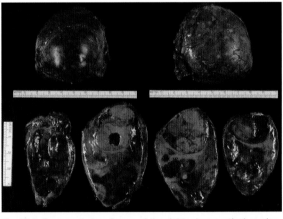

Fig. 26.2 Gross pathology image of the right adrenocortical carcinoma—a 6.4 × 6.2 × 4.2–cm yellow-brown soft heterogeneous mass that did not extend beyond the adrenal gland.

studies reported that mitotane therapy has been associated with a longer recurrence-free survival, a better 5-year survival, but not a better overall survival.[1–3] A recently completed trial (ADIUVO) aimed to assess the efficacy of adjuvant mitotane in patients with ENSAT stage I or II disease after a R0 resection and Ki-67 <10%. At the time of this chapter submission, the results of ADIUVO study are available only as an abstract. ADIUVO was a prospective observational study of 91 patients with ENSAT stage I–III and Ki-67 <10%. Overall, the recurrence-free survival was 75%, better than previously reported. No differences in the overall survival or the recurrence-free survival were noted between the mitotane versus observation arms. The decision on mitotane therapy in patients with ENSAT stage I–III and Ki-67 index <10% should be individualized.[4,5]

Mitotane-induced adrenal insufficiency should be anticipated and properly treated. Patients require increased dose of hydrocortisone while on mitotane therapy (30–60 mg daily in divided doses) as a result of the mitotane-induced increase in cortisol metabolism. Other common side effects include fatigue, nausea, diarrhea, gynecomastia, and, less commonly, confusion, dizziness, and ataxia. In addition to clinical evaluation for signs and symptoms of cortisol excess or deficiency and other side effects to mitotane, all patients require biochemical monitoring with serum electrolytes, liver function tests, thyroid function tests, lipid panel, and tests for mineralocorticoid deficiency.[4,5]

Key Points

- In retrospective studies, mitotane therapy was associated with a longer recurrence-free survival, a better 5-year survival, but not a better overall survival.
- In a prospective observational ADIUO study of 91 patients with ENSAT stage I–III disease and Ki-67 <10%, mitotane therapy was not found to be beneficial.
- Mitotane side effects include adrenal insufficiency, gastrointestinal side effects, fatigue, hypothyroidism, and several others.
- Clinical and biochemical monitoring every 3 months is required in any patient treated with mitotane.

REFERENCES

1. Calabrese A, Basile V, Puglisi S, et al. Adjuvant mitotane therapy is beneficial in non-metastatic adrenocortical carcinoma at high risk of recurrence. *Eur J Endocrinol*. 2019;180(6):387–396.
2. Puglisi S, Calabrese A, Basile V, et al. Mitotane concentrations influence the risk of recurrence in adrenocortical carcinoma patients on adjuvant treatment. *J Clin Med*. 2019;8(11).
3. Terzolo M, Angeli A, Fassnacht M, et al. Adjuvant mitotane treatment for adrenocortical carcinoma. *N Engl J Med*. 2007;356(23):2372–2380.
4. Kiseljak-Vassiliades K, Bancos I, Hamrahian A, et al. American Association of Clinical Endocrinology disease state clinical review on the evaluation and management of adrenocortical carcinoma in an adult: a practical approach. *Endocrine Practice*. 2020;26(11):1366–1383.
5. Fassnacht M, Dekkers OM, Else T, et al. European Society of Endocrinology Clinical Practice Guidelines on the management of adrenocortical carcinoma in adults, in collaboration with the European Network for the Study of Adrenal Tumors. *Eur J Endocrinol*. 2018;179(4):G1–G46.

Cortisol-Secreting Metastatic Adrenocortical Carcinoma: Role for Surgical Debulking of the Primary Tumor

When a patient presents with an acute onset of severe Cushing syndrome (CS) due to metastatic adrenocortical carcinoma (ACC), clinicians ask: "Should the primary tumor be resected?" This is a good question, and many times the best answer is uncertain. However, in general, if the primary ACC can be resected without too much operative-related morbidity, it makes sense to debulk the "cortisol-secreting factory." In this way, it provides the patient with a better quality of life while giving clinicians an opportunity to initiate treatment trials for the residual metastatic ACC.

Case Report

The patient was a 46-year-old woman who until recently had been quite healthy. Her only medication was losartan 50 mg daily for chronic hypertension. Two months previously she started developing signs and symptoms of CS, which included 30-pound weight gain; facial fullness; supraclavicular fat pads (Fig. 27.1); abrupt onset of acne affecting the face, neck, chest, and back; proximal muscle weakness; fatigue; accelerated hypertension; and ankle edema. On physical examination her body mass index was 42 kg/m^2 and blood pressure 150/104 mmHg. She was overtly cushingoid with a full, round, plethoric face. She had marked acne of the face, neck, upper back, and upper chest. There was hirsutism involving the

chin, sideburn areas, and upper lip. She had marked supraclavicular fat pads. There were no purple-red abdominal striae. She had 1+ ankle edema bilaterally.

INVESTIGATIONS

The baseline laboratory test results are shown in Table 27.1. Marked corticotropin (ACTH)-independent CS was clearly documented. In addition to cortisol, her adrenal tumor was hypersecreting adrenal androgens. There was associated hypokalemia and hyperglycemia.

An abdominal computed tomography (CT) scan showed a 13 × 7.3 × 9.6–cm right adrenal mass consistent with ACC (Fig. 27.2).[1] Chest CT showed two

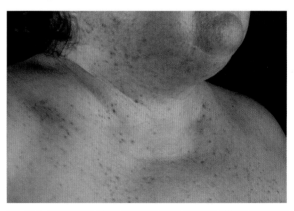

Fig. 27.1 Photograph of the patient's neck showing diffuse acne and supraclavicular fat pads.

TABLE 27.1 Laboratory Tests

Biochemical Test	Result	Reference Range
Sodium, mmol/L	143	135–145
Potassium, mmol/L	2.3	3.6–5.2
Fasting plasma glucose, mg/dL	231	70–100
Creatinine, mg/dL	0.9	0.6–1.1
8 AM serum cortisol, mcg/dL	57	7–25
4 PM serum cortisol, mcg/dL	51	2–14
ACTH, pg/mL	<5	10–60
Aldosterone, ng/dL	<4	≤21
Plasma renin activity, ng/mL per hour	<0.6	≤0.6–3
DHEA-S, mcg/dL	767	18–244
Total testosterone, ng/dL	152	8–60
24-Hour urine cortisol, mcg	462	3–45

ACTH, Corticotropin; *DHEA-S*, dehydroepiandrosterone sulfate.

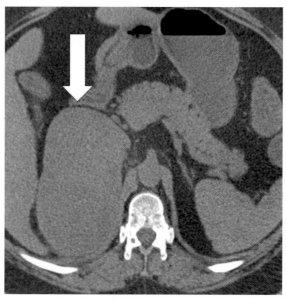

Fig. 27.2 Unenhanced axial computed tomography image shows a 13 × 7.3 × 9.6–cm right adrenal mass (*arrow*) with an attenuation of 28.1 Hounsfield units.

6-mm nodules in the left lung with imaging characteristics consistent with metastatic disease.

The patient was informed that she had severe CS caused by a right ACC, and that right adrenalectomy would likely cure the signs and symptoms of CS—the most urgent immediate problem.[2] She was also informed that she likely had metastatic ACC that would need to be addressed with systemic therapy after the adrenal surgery.

TREATMENT

The patient was treated with potassium chloride and spironolactone. *Pneumocystis jirovecii* pneumonia prophylaxis and deep venous thrombosis prophylaxis were initiated. Ten days after the initial endocrine consultation she underwent open resection of a right ACC; it weighed 465 g (normal adrenal gland weight, 4–5 g) and measured 18.5 × 18.0 × 5.2 cm. She declined postoperative treatment with mitotane. She was discharged from the hospital on prednisone 10 mg in the morning and 5 mg in the afternoon with a plan to taper to 5 mg every morning over 6 weeks and then transition to hydrocortisone.

OUTCOME AND FOLLOW-UP

Six months postoperatively the patient was doing very well. She had lost weight and her acne had improved dramatically. She felt completely back to normal. Blood pressure was controlled on monotherapy with a β-adrenergic blocker. Electrolyte levels were normal. Total and bioavailable testosterone levels were normal, and dehydroepiandrosterone sulfate was low-normal at 31.8 mcg/dL (normal, 18–244 mcg/dL). Her morning serum cortisol concentration was low-normal at 6.3 mcg/dL, indicating that her hypothalamic-pituitary-adrenal axis had not yet fully recovered. She was advised to continue her 10 mg morning dose of hydrocortisone. However, CT scan of chest, abdomen, and pelvis showed that the lung nodules had enlarged and that there was new adenopathy in the upper retroperitoneum between the aorta and inferior vena cava. Chemotherapy with etoposide, doxorubicin, and cisplatin (EDP) was initiated.[3] After three cycles there was partial tumor response; however, she discontinued treatment with EDP due to side effects. She sought alternative medicine approaches to her progressive metastatic ACC—during which time her ACC became widely metastatic. Unfortunately, 2 years after her adrenal surgery, signs and symptoms of severe CS recurred. She proceeded to develop a series of complications with pulmonary embolus, severe upper gastrointestinal bleeding, sepsis, and renal failure. She progressed to multiorgan system failure and death.

Key Points

- ACC is the most aggressive of all malignances seen by endocrinologists.
- ACC is associated with poor 5-year survival rates. The best survival rates are associated with stage I disease.[4]
- Stage IV ACC is not curable. However, life can be extended with debulking operations to provide short-term resolutions in life-threatening severe CS.

REFERENCES

1. Young WF Jr. Conventional imaging in adrenocortical carcinoma: update and perspectives. *Horm Cancer.* 2011;2(6):341–347.
2. Puglisi S, Perotti P, Pia A, Reimondo G, Terzolo M. Adrenocortical carcinoma with hypercortisolism. *Endocrinol Metab Clin North Am.* 2018;47(2):395–407.
3. Laganà M, Grisanti S, Cosentini D, et al. Efficacy of the EDP-M scheme plus adjunctive surgery in the management of patients with advanced adrenocortical carcinoma: the Brescia experience. *Cancers (Basel).* 2020;12(4):941.
4. Tella SH, Kommalapati A, Yaturu S, Kebebew E. Predictors of survival in adrenocortical carcinoma: an analysis from the National Cancer Database. *J Clin Endocrinol Metab.* 2018;103(9):3566–3573.

Adrenocortical Carcinoma and Severe Cushing Syndrome

Adrenocortical carcinoma (ACC) presents with overt symptoms of hormone excess (usually androgen, cortisol, or combined hypersecretion) in 30%–40% of cases.[1] Notably, even patients with incidentally discovered ACC or those presenting with symptoms of mass effect may have undiagnosed adrenal hormone excess. Uncontrolled or unrecognized overt Cushing syndrome (CS) carries additional morbidity and is a negative prognostic factor in patients with ACC. These patients are at high risk for deep venous thrombosis and pulmonary embolism, as well as infections. Surgical resection is the best therapy for ACC-related CS. However, when surgery is not possible, aggressive medical therapy for hypercortisolism should be initiated. Here, we present a case of metastatic ACC with severe CS of rapid onset.

Case Report

The patient was a 57-year-old man who was referred for evaluation of a newly found large adrenal mass. This was initially found on the ultrasound that was ordered to evaluate abdominal discomfort. In addition to abdominal pain, he reported other new symptoms for around 6 months. The symptoms included fatigue, mood changes, weight loss of around 10 pounds but with development of abdominal obesity, upper and lower extremity weakness, facial rounding and erythema, skin fragility and bruising, and curling hair. In addition, he developed uncontrolled hypertension and hypokalemia.

On physical examination, blood pressure was 152/86 mmHg, heart rate was 76 beats per minute, and body mass index was 25.1 kg/m^2.

Physical examination was positive for facial rounding and erythema, supraclavicular pads, abdominal obesity, multiple bruises over extremities and abdomen, and several skin tears. No significant myopathy was noticed on examination. He had bilateral 1+ lower extremity edema.

INVESTIGATIONS

Clinical presentation was highly suspicious for ACC and severe CS. Computed tomography (CT) of the abdomen, pelvis, and chest was performed for a better characterization of the adrenal mass and staging. A left lobulated heterogeneous adrenal mass measuring 18 × 14 × 15 cm was demonstrated (Fig. 28.1). In addition, several hepatic lesions measuring up to 12 cm were consistent with metastases. Other possible metastases included a vertebral T11 lesion of 1.2 cm and several indeterminate lung nodules measuring 3–5 mm.

Because of clinical findings of lower extremity edema and suspected severe hypercortisolism, the patient was considered at high risk for deep venous thrombosis. A lower extremity ultrasound was obtained and revealed an acute deep venous thrombosis through the right lower extremity (mid-low femoral vein, extending throughout the popliteal, posterior tibial, peroneal, soleal, and gastrocnemius veins).

Laboratory evaluation confirmed severe adrenal-dependent hypercortisolism, as well as androgen, estrogen, progesterone, and glucocorticoid and androgen precursor excess (Table 28.1).

Fine-needle aspiration of the liver metastasis was performed and confirmed metastatic ACC. Immunoperoxidase stains demonstrated neoplastic cells positive for Melan-A, SF1, inhibin, synaptophysin, and negative for pan-cytokeratin AE1/AE3, Sox10, arginase, and glypican-3.

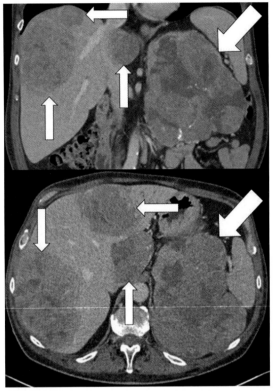

Fig. 28.1 Axial (*below*) and coronal (*above*) contrast-enhanced computed tomography images demonstrated a left lobulated heterogeneous adrenal mass (*large arrows*) measuring 18 × 14 × 15 cm and multiple large hepatic metastases (*small arrows*).

TABLE 28.1	Laboratory Tests	
Biochemical Test	Result	Reference Range
Cortisol, mcg/dL	27	7–21
ACTH, pg/mL	<5	7.2–63
DHEA-S, mcg/dL	3477	44–332
Androstenedione, ng/dL	1880	30–200
Total testosterone, ng/dL	181	240–950
Estradiol, pg/ml	83	10–40
Progesterone, ng/mL	2.5	<0.2
17-Hydroxypregnenolone, ng/dL	1140	55–455
Pregnenolone, ng/dL	371	33–248
17-Hydroxyprogesterone, ng/dL	207	<220
11-Deoxycortisol, ng/dL	832	10–79
Aldosterone, ng/dL	<4	<21
Plasma renin activity, ng/mL per hour	1.7	≤0.6–3
24-Hour urine cortisol, mcg/24 h	1723	<45
Plasma metanephrine, nmol/L	<0.2	<0.5
Plasma normetanephrine, nmol/L	0.24	<0.9

ACTH, Corticotropin; *DHEA-S*, dehydroepiandrosterone sulfate.

TREATMENT AND FOLLOW-UP

The patient was diagnosed with the ENSAT stage IV disease that was considered unresectable. Chemotherapy was discussed and planned with etoposide, doxorubicin, and cisplatin. Because of a high risk for opportunistic infections due to uncontrolled hypercortisolism, the patient was treated with one tablet of trimethoprim-sulfamethoxazole single strength daily. Anticoagulation was started to treat deep venous thrombosis. Spironolactone therapy was initiated to control hypercortisolism-related hypertension and hypokalemia. Mitotane therapy was initiated and quickly titrated to 5 g per day. As mitotane alone was not expected to be fully effective, osilodrostat was added at 5 mg twice per day. Subsequently, mitotane was decreased to 2 g per day due to poor tolerance, and osilodrostat was increased to 7 mg twice a day. The 24-hour urine cortisol excretion decreased to 70 mcg 2 months later, and then to 56 mcg 4 months later (normal <45 mcg/24 h). Monitoring with blood pressure and potassium measurements was performed periodically, and the potassium supplement dose was adjusted. At the last follow-up (6 months after initial diagnosis), an interval decrease of 2–4 cm in the size of left adrenal mass and hepatic metastases was noted.

Discussion

Mitotane is an adrenolytic drug that is used in treatment of ACC and rarely in CS.[2] Mitotane-induced adrenal insufficiency should be anticipated and properly treated. However, in patients with severe CS due to metastatic ACC, adrenal insufficiency is unlikely to develop with mitotane. Most patients require additional cortisol-lowering therapy to control hypercortisolism. Several medications can be used, including metyrapone and osilodrostat (11-β-hydroxylase inhibitors that block conversion of 11-deoxycortisol to cortisol), ketoconazole, and mifepristone.[3–7] Keto-conazole may cause hepatotoxicity and is contraindicated in patients with liver disease.[6,7] The choice of other medications depends on whether concomitant hyperglycemia is present (mifepristone) and insurance coverage.[8] In this case, osilodrostat was affordable and available quickly. A combination of mitotane and osilodrostat in this patient was effective in decreasing the 24-hour urinary cortisol excretion from 1721 mcg to 56 mcg. Side effects of osilodrostat include hypokalemia and hypertension due to accumulation of circulating aldosterone precursor levels.

Key Points

- Uncontrolled severe CS contributes to poor prognosis in patients with ACC.
- In patients with unresectable ACC and CS, aggressive medical therapy with cortisol-lowering agents should be urgently initiated with the goal of significant decrease or normalization of cortisol concentrations. This goal is usually achieved only with a combination of medications.
- Prophylaxis for opportunistic infections with trimethoprim-sulfamethoxazole and anticoagulation to prevent deep venous thrombosis should be considered in all patients with severe CS.

REFERENCES

1. Iniguez-Ariza NM, Kohlenberg JD, Delivanis DA, et al. Clinical, biochemical, and radiological characteristics of a single-center retrospective cohort of 705 large adrenal tumors. *Mayo Clin Proc Innov Qual Outcomes*. 2018;2(1):30–39.
2. Baudry C, Coste J, Bou Khalil R, et al. Efficiency and tolerance of mitotane in Cushing's disease in 76 patients from a single center. *Eur J Endocrinol*. 2012;167(4):473–481.
3. Fleseriu M, Molitch ME, Gross C, Schteingart DE, Vaughan TB, 3rd, Biller BM. A new therapeutic approach in the medical treatment of Cushing's syndrome: glucocorticoid receptor blockade with mifepristone. *Endocr Pract*. 2013;19(2):313–326.
4. Daniel E, Aylwin S, Mustafa O, et al. Effectiveness of metyrapone in treating cushing's syndrome: a retrospective multicenter study in 195 patients. *J Clin Endocrinol Metab*. 2015;100(11):4146–4154.
5. Duggan S. Osilodrostat: first approval. *Drugs*. 2020;80(5):495–500.
6. Newell-Price J. Ketoconazole as an adrenal steroidogenesis inhibitor: effectiveness and risks in the treatment of Cushing's disease. *J Clin Endocrinol Metab*. 2014;99(5):1586–1588.
7. Castinetti F, Guignat L, Giraud P, et al. Ketoconazole in Cushing's disease: is it worth a try? *J Clin Endocrinol Metab*. 2014;99(5):1623–1630.
8. Feelders RA, Newell-Price J, Pivonello R, Nieman LK, Hofland LJ, Lacroix A. Advances in the medical treatment of Cushing's syndrome. *Lancet Diabetes Endocrinol*. 2019;7(4):300–312.

Pure Aldosterone-Secreting Adrenocortical Carcinoma

Approximately 50% of adrenocortical carcinomas (ACCs) hypersecrete adrenal steroids. When secretory, ACCs are typically plurihormonal—most commonly glucocorticoids and adrenal androgens. Rarely ACCs secrete a single steroid in excess. The case presented herein is an example of a patient with a pure aldosterone-producing ACC, a subtype of ACC that may be associated with a more indolent clinical course.

Case Report

In the year 2000, this 51-year-old woman came to Mayo Clinic for refractory hypertension and hypokalemia. She had been diagnosed with hypertension and hypokalemia 23 years previously when her blood pressure was 170/115 mmHg. Body computed tomography (CT) was available at only a few medical centers in the United States in 1977.[1] She lived outside of the United States and, instead of CT-based imaging, she underwent adrenal venography, which demonstrated asymmetric adrenal size and led to left adrenalectomy. The pathology report indicated the adrenal gland was in two pieces and weighed 3.3 g and no tumor was seen. Hypertension and hypokalemia persisted following the operation, and she was treated with a mineralocorticoid receptor antagonist (spironolactone 100 mg daily) and a β-adrenergic blocker (propranolol 80 mg daily). In 1995, her blood pressure was 230/110 mmHg and serum potassium was 2.0 mEq/L on the same two medications. Plasma aldosterone concentration (PAC) was markedly elevated and plasma renin activity (PRA) was suppressed. An abdominal CT scan showed a 4-cm left adrenal mass and she underwent her second surgery, which was an open left adrenalectomy removing a 4.5 × 4.0 × 4.0–cm

tumor that weighed 31 g. Postoperatively her blood pressure and serum potassium level were normal for 3 years. In 1998, she had recurrent primary aldosteronism (PA) and she was treated with spironolactone. In 2000, due to progressive hypertension and hypokalemia despite 300 mg of spironolactone daily she underwent right adrenalectomy and a 9.2-g adrenal gland without an adenoma was found. Two months later, in April 2000, at 51 years of age she came to Mayo Clinic for the first time.

She had refractory hypertension and hypokalemia. Her medications included propranolol 160 mg daily, spironolactone 200 mg daily, fosinopril 40 mg daily, cortisone acetate 25 mg twice daily, and potassium chloride 80 mEq daily. Except for the hypertension and symptoms related to hypokalemia, she felt reasonably well. There were no signs or symptoms of glucocorticoid or androgen excess.

INVESTIGATIONS

Laboratory studies completed in April 2000 are shown in Table 29.1. Her blood pressure averaged 160/100 mmHg on a 6-hour ambulatory blood pressure monitor. She had positive case detection testing for PA with a plasma aldosterone concentration (PAC) >10 ng/dL and the plasma renin activity (PRA) was <1.0 ng/mL per hour.[2] In addition, PA was confirmed because when a patient has spontaneous hypokalemia and the PAC >20 ng/dL, there are no other differential diagnostic possibilities beyond PA.[2,3] Thus formal confirmatory testing with oral sodium loading or a saline infusion test was not needed for this patient. The 24-hour urine for 17-ketosteroids was normal and indicated that the patient was not producing excess adrenal androgens (see Table 29.1). In addition, the 24-hour urine for ketogenic steroids and cortisol was normal. Thus the patient had a pure aldosterone-secreting neoplasm.

TABLE 29.1 Laboratory Tests		
Biochemical Test	Result	Reference Range
Sodium, mmol/L	143	135–145
Potassium, mmol/L	3.4	3.6–5.2
Creatinine, mg/dL	1.3	0.8–1.3
Aldosterone, ng/dL	116	≤21 ng/dL
Plasma renin activity ng/mL per hour	<0.6	≤0.6–3
24-Hour urine 17-ketosteroids, mg	2.3	4–17
24-Hour urine ketogenic steroids, mg	7	2–12
24-Hour urine free cortisol, mcg	61.8	<108

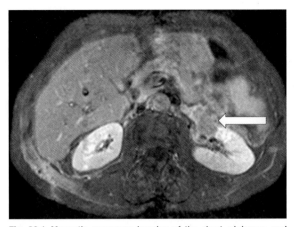

Fig. 29.1 Magnetic resonance imaging of the chest, abdomen, and pelvis. Axial T2-weighted image shows a 3-cm lobulated mass (*arrow*) between the anterior aspect of the left renal hilum and the tail of the pancreas.

Magnetic resonance imaging (MRI) of the chest, abdomen, and pelvis detected a 3-cm lobulated mass between the anterior aspect of the left renal hilum and the tail of the pancreas (Fig. 29.1).

TREATMENT

The patient underwent open laparotomy—her fourth abdominal operation. There was a firm lobulated mass that was adherent to the renal parenchyma and extended around the renal hilar vessels. A left nephrectomy was necessary to remove the mass in its entirety. Pathologic examination showed recurrent ACC forming a mass measuring 4.3 × 3.5 × 2.6 cm and there were two ACC implants present on the surface of the kidney measuring 0.5 and 1.2 cm.

OUTCOME AND FOLLOW-UP

Three days after surgery the PAC was undetectable (<1 ng/dL). Treatment with spironolactone and potassium chloride was discontinued. Treatment with fludrocortisone was initiated. Three months after surgery, PAC remained undetectable and blood pressure was normal without the aid of antihypertensive medications. Three years after surgery, except for a tiny posterior left lower lobe lung nodule (Fig. 29.2), there was no imaging or biochemical evidence of recurrent disease. However, the patient returned to Mayo Clinic 13 years later (2013) with an enlarging left lower lung nodule (see Fig. 29.2) that had a high signal on 18F-fluorodeoxyglucose (FDG)

positron emission tomography (PET) CT. She had developed hypertension that was well controlled on amlodipine 5 mg daily and atenolol 25 mg daily. Laboratory studies showed no biochemical evidence of recurrent aldosterone-secreting ACC: PAC <4 ng/dL, PRA <0.6 ng/mL per hour, and, DHEA-S <15 mcg/dL (normal, 15–157). She underwent left lower lobe wedge resection for metastatic ACC forming a 3.2 × 2.3 × 1.5–cm subpleural circumscribed mass. Thus the pulmonary metastasis was not hypersecreting aldosterone. Subsequently, PAC remained undetectable and there was no anatomic evidence of recurrent disease based on CT scans of chest, abdomen, and pelvis every 6 months. Her last follow-up was in April 2020, and she had no laboratory or imaging evidence of recurrent disease—43 years after her initial diagnosis of primary aldosteronism, 20 years after resection of the primary ACC and local metastatic disease, and 7 years after resection of a pulmonary metastasis.

In 2002, we published a series of 10 patients (including the patient reported herein) with pure aldosterone-secreting ACC out of 141 with ACC who had been evaluated at Mayo Clinic Rochester from 1957 to 2000.[4] Disease recurred in seven patients (70%) with a median interval of 17 months. Five-year survival was 52%. Patients with aldosterone-secreting ACC had an increased risk of perioperative mortality, yet they had an overall median survival of 63 months compared to 19 months for patients with non–aldosterone-secreting

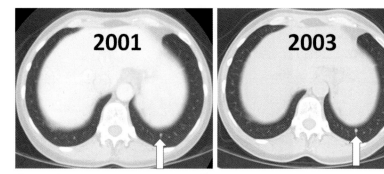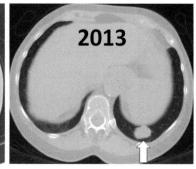

Fig. 29.2 Serial chest computed tomography (CT) scans showed a <5-mm posterior left lower lobe nodule (*arrows*) in 2001 and 2003. However, in 2013, this nodule measured 2.3 × 2.7 cm (*arrow*) and was fluorodeoxyglucose-avid on F-18 flurodeoxyglucose positron emission tomography-CT and proved to be metastatic adrenocortical carcinoma.

ACC.[4] The patient reported herein is especially unique with a 43-year course of her disease. In most patients with ACC, if not cured with the initial resection, it is a progressive malignancy with 15%–30% 5-year survival rates. Aldosterone-secreting ACC appears to be a unique and indolent subtype even in the setting of distant metastatic disease.

Key Points

- Pure aldosterone-secreting ACC is a rare subtype of ACC and may be associated with better survival compared to other forms of ACC.
- Due to the high risk of delayed recurrent metastatic disease, patients with "cured" ACC should be followed for life.

REFERENCES

1. Young WF Jr. Conventional imaging in adrenocortical carcinoma: update and perspectives. *Horm Cancer*. 2011;2(6):341–347.
2. Young WF Jr. Diagnosis and treatment of primary aldosteronism: practical clinical perspectives. *J Intern Med*. 2019;285(2):126–148.
3. Funder JW, Carey RM, Mantero F, et al. The management of primary aldosteronism: case detection, diagnosis, and treatment: an Endocrine Society Clinical Practice Guideline. *J Clin Endocrinol Metab*. 2016;101(5):1889–1916.
4. Kendrick ML, Curlee K, Lloyd R, et al. Aldosterone-secreting adrenocortical carcinomas are associated with unique operative risks and outcomes. *Surgery*. 2002;132(6):1008–1011; discussion 1012.

Long-Standing Primary Aldosteronism in a Patient Diagnosed With Metastatic Adrenocortical Carcinoma

Most cases of primary aldosteronism (PA) are the results of either an aldosterone-producing adenoma or bilateral hyperplasia.[1] Adrenocortical carcinoma (ACC) is a very rare cause of PA, accounting for <1% of all cases.

Case Report

A 49-year-old man was referred to our clinic for management of metastatic ACC. As highlighted in the text that follows, he had a remarkable history leading to current evaluation.

26 YEARS BEFORE CURRENT EVALUATION

He developed hypertension and had an evaluation for secondary causes of hypertension at our institution. At the time of initial evaluation, his blood pressure was 156/108 mmHg. His medications included metoprolol, hydrochlorothiazide, amlodipine, and Accupril. In addition, because of hypokalemia, he was taking 20 mEq of potassium chloride daily. Workup for PA was performed with a positive case detection and confirmatory testing (Table 30.1). He was advised to proceed with abdominal imaging and consider adrenal venous sampling if interested in a potential surgical cure. At that time, he declined and elected therapy with spironolactone. He continued his care locally. Imaging was not performed.

1 YEAR BEFORE CURRENT EVALUATION

Because of worsening hypertension, reevaluation for PA was performed locally. Computed tomography (CT) abdominal imaging was performed and demonstrated a right adrenal mass measuring $5.8 \times 5.0 \times 4.7$ cm with an unenhanced CT attenuation of 29 Hounsfield units (HU) and a left adrenal mass measuring $2.0 \times 1.9 \times 1.8$ cm with an unenhanced CT attenuation of 2 HU (Fig. 30.1). The patient was referred for adrenal venous sampling, which reportedly demonstrated a right-sided aldosterone secretion (results are not available), and he was recommended to proceed with a laparoscopic right adrenalectomy. Surgery was performed elsewhere. Pathology revealed a 5.7-cm ACC with tumor necrosis, increased mitotic activity of 20 mitoses per 50 high-power fields, and a Ki-67 proliferative index of 10%. He was advised to be followed with serial imaging but no other therapy. Follow-up imaging 5 months after the right adrenalectomy demonstrated bilateral indeterminate lung and mediastinal nodules. Biopsy confirmed metastatic ACC. The patient was referred to our institution for further care.

CURRENT EVALUATION

On evaluation, the patient reported fatigue and shortness of breath. He did not have weight gain, abdominal striae, and supraclavicular or dorsocervical pads. On physical examination, his blood pressure was 154/94 mmHg, and on chest examination, decreased breath sounds were noted on the left side. He had mild bilateral edema. Medications included amlodipine, lisinopril, metoprolol, and eplerenone. He was also taking potassium supplements at 40 mEq daily. On imaging, metastatic

TABLE 30.1   Laboratory Tests

Biochemical Test	Age 23 Result	Age 49 Result	Reference Range
Cortisol, mcg/dL		19	7–21
ACTH, pg/mL		37	7.2–63
DHEA-S, mcg/dL		29	32–395
Pregnenolone, ng/dL		304	33–248
17-Hydroxypregnenolone, ng/dL		33	55–455
17-Hydroxyprogesterone, ng/dL		47	<220
11-Deoxycortisol, ng/dL		109	10–79
11-Deoxycorticosterone, ng/dL		447	<10
Total testosterone, ng/dL		388	240–950
Aldosterone, ng/dL	11	87	<21
Plasma renin activity, ng/mL per hour	<0.6	<0.6	≤0.6–3
24-Hour urine cortisol, mcg/24 h		62	<45
24-Hour urine aldosterone, mcg/24 h	19	264	<10
24-Hour urine sodium, mmol/24 h	267	375	41–227

ACTH, Corticotropin; *DHEA-S*, dehydroepiandrosterone sulfate.

implants were noted in right suprarenal space, lung, mediastinum, and appendix (Fig. 30.2).

TREATMENT AND FOLLOW-UP

The patient was treated with multiple regimens, including etoposide, doxorubicin, and cisplatin, pembrolizumab, mitotane, gemcitabine, and docetaxel. Hypertension and hypokalemia related to aldosterone excess were difficult to control, requiring high doses of a mineralocorticoid receptor antagonist (600 mg spironolactone per day), potassium supplements of 80–140 mEq per day, metoprolol, doxazosin, nifedipine, and lisinopril. Despite multiple therapies, his disease progressed over the 12 months after evaluation at our institution. Because of progressive symptomatic decline, hospice was recommended.

Discussion

ACC is a very rare cause of PA.[1–4] Once the diagnosis of PA is made, abdominal imaging is recommended even if patient elects medical therapy with mineralocorticoid receptor blockade.[1] In this case, the patient had a well-controlled hypertension and PA for more than 20 years before the imaging that demonstrated a suspicious adrenal mass. It is unclear whether the adrenal mass was present at the time of the initial diagnosis. Cases of small adrenal tumors that are stable in size for years later to develop into ACC have been described.[5]

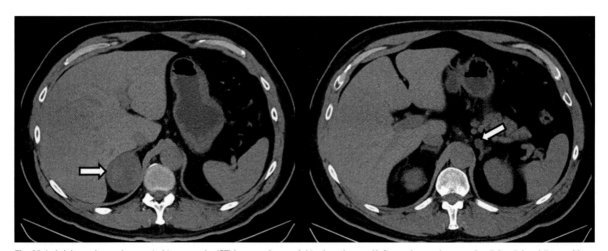

Fig. 30.1 Axial unenhanced computed tomography (CT) images show a right adrenal mass (*left panel, arrow*) measuring 5.8 × 5.0 × 4.7 cm with an unenhanced CT attenuation of 29 Hounsfield units (HU) and a left adrenal mass measuring 2.0 × 1.9 × 1.8 cm with an unenhanced CT attenuation of 2 HU (*right panel, arrow*).

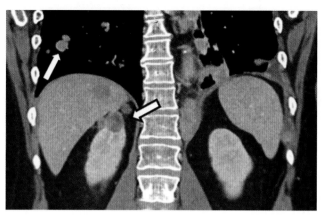

Fig. 30.2 Coronal contrast enhanced computed tomography (CT) image of abdomen shows multiple metastases in the right suprarenal space and chest (*arrows*).

In a setting of clear diagnosis of PA and a suspicious adrenal mass likely to be ACC (as in this case), adrenal venous sampling is unnecessary. Surgical decision is based on the imaging characteristics with the main goal of resecting a potentially malignant mass. Open adrenalectomy is recommended for ACC to ensure a complete resection.[2,6]

Key Points

- A minority of ACCs present with PA.
- ACC is a very rare cause of PA.
- In a patient with PA and a suspicious adrenal mass, adrenalectomy should be based on imaging characteristics and adrenal venous sampling is unnecessary.
- Open adrenalectomy is the treatment of choice in patients with ACC.

REFERENCES

1. Young WF Jr. Diagnosis and treatment of primary aldosteronism: practical clinical perspectives. *J Intern Med*. 2019;285(2):126–148.
2. Fassnacht M, Dekkers OM, Else T, et al. European Society of Endocrinology Clinical Practice Guidelines on the management of adrenocortical carcinoma in adults, in collaboration with the European Network for the Study of Adrenal Tumors. *Eur J Endocrinol*. 2018;179(4):G1–G46.
3. Iniguez-Ariza NM, Kohlenberg JD, Delivanis DA, et al. Clinical, biochemical, and radiological characteristics of a single-center retrospective cohort of 705 large adrenal tumors. *Mayo Clin Proc Innov Qual Outcomes*. 2018;2(1):30–39.
4. Kiseljak-Vassiliades K, Bancos I, Hamrahian A, et al. American Association of Clinical Endocrinology Disease state clinical review on the evaluation and management of adrenocortical carcinoma in an adult: a practical approach. *Endocrine Practice*. 2020;26(11):1366–1383.
5. Gagnon N, Boily P, Alguire C, et al. Small adrenal incidentaloma becoming an aggressive adrenocortical carcinoma in a patient carrying a germline APC variant. *Endocrine*. 2020;68(1):203–209.
6. Fassnacht M, Arlt W, Bancos I, et al. Management of adrenal incidentalomas: European Society of Endocrinology Clinical Practice Guideline in collaboration with the European Network for the Study of Adrenal Tumors. *Eur J Endocrinol*. 2016;175(2):G1–G34.

Adrenocortical Carcinoma Associated With Lynch Syndrome

Most cases of adrenocortical carcinoma (ACC) are sporadic; however, some occur as a part of a hereditary syndrome, such as Li-Fraumeni syndrome, multiple endocrine neoplasia type 1, familial adenomatous polyposis, neurofibromatosis type 1, Beckwith-Wiedemann syndrome, or Lynch syndrome. Here we present an incidentally discovered ACC in a patient with undiagnosed Lynch syndrome.

Case Report

This 65-year-old woman was initially evaluated for postmenopausal vaginal bleeding. Transvaginal ultrasound showed endometrial thickening and several uterine fibroids, and subsequent histology demonstrated benign endometrial hyperplasia. Incidentally, on the initial ultrasound, a large right adrenal mass was noted. Subsequent computed tomography (CT) scan revealed a heterogeneous right adrenal mass, measuring 7.8 × 6.0 × 5.1 cm (Fig. 31.1). The patient was referred to Mayo Clinic for further management of the adrenal mass.

On evaluation, the patient reported fatigue and a weight loss of 3 pounds over several weeks. On physical examination, her blood pressure was 135/83 mmHg and body mass index was 24.7 kg/m^2. She did not have any signs of androgen, cortisol, or aldosterone excess.

Recently, her sister was diagnosed with Lynch syndrome. Subsequently, our patient was also tested and found positive for a familial pathogenic variant in *MutS homolog 6 (MSH6)*. Colonoscopy, performed several months previously, was normal.

INVESTIGATIONS

Laboratory evaluation showed normal levels of 24-hour urinary metanephrine and normetanephrine but was positive for androgen precursor and androgen excess, hypercortisolism, and estrogen excess (Table 31.1).

TREATMENT

ACC was suspected because of concerning imaging characteristics and the adrenal plurihormonal excess. The patient was treated with open right adrenalectomy. Final pathology demonstrated an adrenal oncocytic

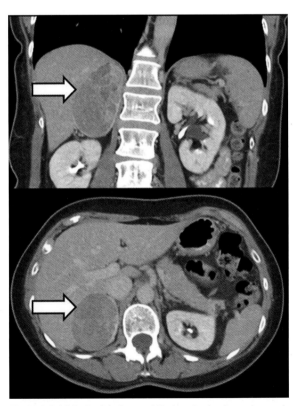

Fig. 31.1 Axial (*bottom*) and coronal (*top*) contrast-enhanced computed tomography images showed a heterogeneous right adrenal mass (*arrows*) measuring 4.8 × 5.7 × 7.9 cm.

TABLE 31.1 Laboratory Tests

Biochemical Test	Result	Reference Range
Cortisol after overnight 1-mg DST, mcg/dL	13	<1.8
Cortisol, mcg/dL	14	7–21
ACTH, pg/mL	<5	7.2–63
DHEA-S, mcg/dL	403	<15–157
Androstenedione, ng/dL	151	30–200
17-Hydroxyprogesterone, ng/dL	167	<51
17-Hydroxypregnenolone, ng/dL	888	31–455
Total testosterone, ng/dL	30	8–60
Estradiol, pg/mL	113	<10 (postmenopausal)
Aldosterone, ng/dL	20	<21
Plasma renin activity, ng/mL per hour	2	≤0.6–3
24-Hour urine cortisol, mcg/24 h	68	<45
24-Hour urine metanephrine, mcg/24 h	68	<400
24-Hour urine normetanephrine, mcg/24 h	340	<900

ACTH, Corticotropin; *DHEA-S,* dehydroepiandrosterone sulfate; *DST,* dexamethasone suppression test.

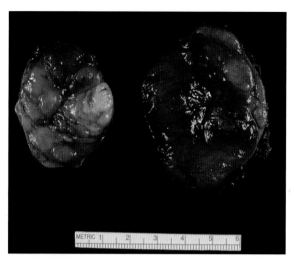

Fig. 31.2 Gross pathology image of the right oncocytic adrenal cortical carcinoma measuring 9.2 × 5.9 × 4.8 cm.

carcinoma with extracapsular extension into periadrenal adipose tissue, mitotic count of 40 mitoses/50 high-power fields, and Ki-67 index of 15% (Fig. 31.2). Surgical margins were negative for the tumor.

Peri- and postoperatively, the patient was treated with hydrocortisone for adrenal insufficiency. As the patient was considered high risk for recurrent disease (European Network for the Study of Adrenal Tumours [ENSAT] stage III disease, Ki-67 of 15%), mitotane therapy was initiated 6 weeks after surgery but stopped 12 months later because of a personal preference.

OUTCOME AND FOLLOW-UP

The patient was in remission for more than 3 years but later developed hepatic metastases at 40 months after adrenalectomy. She underwent resection of the liver metastases and currently is in remission 10 months later.

Discussion

Lynch syndrome[1] is an autosomal dominant disorder caused by a germline pathogenic variant in the DNA mismatch repair genes, including *MutL homolog 1 (MLH1)*, *MutS homolog 2 (MSH2)*, *MutS homolog 6 (MSH6)*, and *postmeiotic segregation 2 (PMS2)*. Our patient was found to have a germline pathogenic variant in *MSH6*, which is located on chromosome 2p16.3.[2] Patients with Lynch syndrome are at higher risk for colorectal cancer, other gastrointestinal cancers, endometrial cancer, genitourinary cancer, gliomas, and other cancers. ACC is a rare manifestation of Lynch syndrome, with only a handful of cases reported (including the one presented here).[2,3] In a study of 114 patients with ACC, the prevalence of Lynch syndrome was 3.2%.[3]

Key Points

- Patients with Lynch syndrome are at increased risk for colorectal and endometrial cancer but also other malignancies.
- Prevalence of Lynch syndrome in patients with ACC is 3.2%.
- Careful clinical examination for ACC should be performed in patients with known Lynch syndrome.
- In a patient with Lynch syndrome and an incidentally discovered adrenal mass, prompt workup and management should be pursued.

REFERENCES

1. Lynch HT, de la Chapelle A. Hereditary colorectal cancer. *N Engl J Med*. 2003;348(10):919–932.

2. Kaur RJ, Pichurin PN, Hines JM, Singh RJ, Grebe SK, Bancos I. Adrenal cortical carcinoma associated with lynch syndrome: a case report and review of literature. *J Endocr Soc*. 2019;3(4):784–790.

3. Raymond VM, Everett JN, Furtado LV, et al. Adrenocortical carcinoma is a lynch syndrome-associated cancer. *J Clin Oncol*. 2013;31(24):3012–3018.

Adrenocortical Carcinoma Associated With Multiple Endocrine Neoplasia Type 1

Although adrenocortical nodularity is fairly common in patients with multiple endocrine neoplasia type 1 (MEN-1), adrenocortical carcinoma (ACC) is rare. The case presented herein is a cautionary notice for clinicians who have patients with small lipid-poor adrenal masses that are thought to be benign adrenal adenomas.

Case Report

This 51-year-old man came to Mayo Clinic for treatment of recurrent left adrenal ACC. He had been diagnosed with MEN-1 21 years previously when he presented with a duodenal gastrinoma and primary hyperparathyroidism—both of which were treated effectively surgically. Subsequently, he was diagnosed with a pituitary prolactinoma, facial angiofibromas, left hip lipoma, and left adrenal "adenoma." His mother and maternal grandmother had previously been diagnosed with MEN-1. Germline genetic testing was not performed.

The left adrenal tumor was first detected on a computed tomography (CT) scan 11 years previously (Fig. 32.1). At that time, it was 1.6 cm in diameter with an unenhanced CT attenuation of 39.1 Hounsfield units (HU). Enhanced CT imaging completed at 4 and 5 years after the initial discovery showed the left adrenal mass to be slightly larger at 1.8 cm (see Fig. 32.1). Laboratory evaluation showed normal levels of plasma fractionated metanephrines, serum cortisol, 24-hour urinary free cortisol, and dehydroepiandrosterone sulfate (DHEA-S). Two years before coming to Mayo Clinic

he underwent left adrenalectomy after the left adrenal mass had markedly enlarged. However, details of the operation, preoperative imaging, and pathologic examination were not available for our review.

INVESTIGATIONS

The image labeled "11 yrs" in Fig. 32.1 was obtained after his adrenal surgery and 3 months before his Mayo Clinic consultation. Magnetic resonance imaging (MRI) at Mayo Clinic showed numerous nodular deposits of locally recurrent tumor in the splenectomy and distal pancreatectomy bed with extension into the renal hilum and renal cortex and more than five bilobar hepatic metastases; the largest lesion in hepatic segment VIII measured 2.7 cm in maximal diameter (Fig. 32.2). All adrenocortical function testing was normal.

TREATMENT

Because of the recurrent tumor, the patient underwent en bloc resection that included distal pancreatectomy, left hemicolectomy, and left nephrectomy (Fig. 32.3). In addition, intraoperative radiofrequency ablation was used to destroy six deep-seated hepatic metastases. At pathology, metastatic ACC formed a 7.5 × 3.5 × 2.0–cm mass with additional multiple tumor deposits ranging between 1.0 and 2.5 cm. Immunohistochemistry showed that the tumor cells were positive for synaptophysin, inhibin, and Melan-A and negative for keratin and chromogranin, thus supporting the diagnosis of ACC.

OUTCOME AND FOLLOW-UP

The patient recovered well from surgery. After hospital dismissal, treatment was initiated with mitotane and

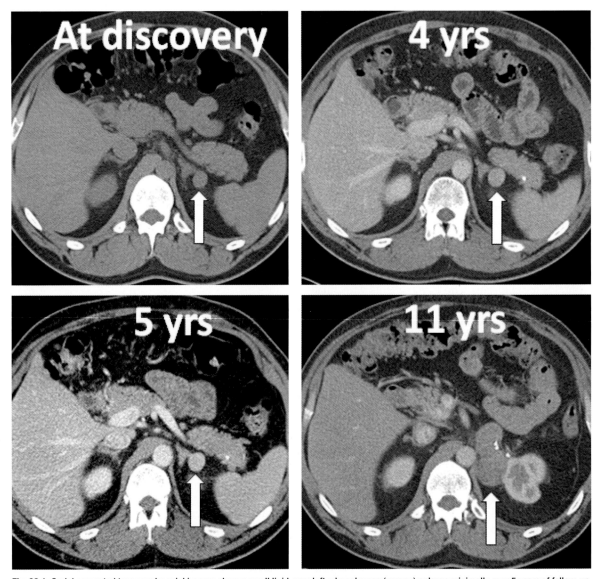

Fig. 32.1 Serial computed tomography axial images show a small lipid-poor left adrenal mass (*arrows*) enlarge minimally over 5 years of follow-up. The "11-yrs" image shows 3.6 × 4.4 cm recurrent adrenocortical carcinoma after surgery performed elsewhere.

hydrocortisone. There was no further follow-up information after he returned home.

Discussion

Although unusual, the occurrence ACC in the setting of MEN-1 has been previously reported.[1,2] In a report on 715 patients with MEN-1 from a multicenter database collected between 1956 and 2008, adrenal enlargement was reported in 20.4% (146/715) of patients.[2] Compared with an adrenal incidentaloma cohort, MEN-1–related tumors showed a decreased prevalence of pheochromocytoma and an increased prevalence primary aldosteronism and ACC. They

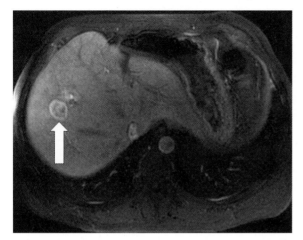

Fig. 32.2 Abdominal magnetic resonance imaging axial diffusion weighted image shows the largest (2.7 cm) metastasis (*arrow*) in hepatic segment VIII.

reported 10 ACCs in 8 patients (8 of 715; 1.4%). Interestingly, just as the case reported herein, ACCs occurred after several years of follow-up of small adrenal tumors in two of the eight patients. They found no genotype-phenotype correlations for the occurrence of adrenal lesions or ACC.[2]

Key Points

- The major life-shortening risk for patients with MEN-1 is metastatic pancreatic neuroendocrine tumor. However, there are rare MEN-1–associated neoplasms such as ACC and thymic carcinoid that may supersede the pancreatic tumor risk.
- Lipid-poor adrenal masses labeled as stable "adenomas" by radiologists should either be resected or followed closely in all patients (also see Case 6).

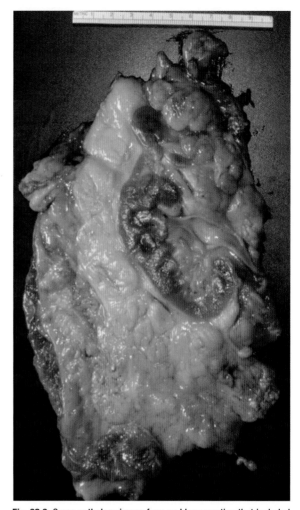

Fig. 32.3 Gross pathology image from en bloc resection that included distal pancreatectomy, left hemicolectomy, and left nephrectomy. Metastatic adrenocortical carcinoma formed a 7.5 × 3.5 × 2.0–cm mass with additional multiple tumor deposits ranging between 1.0 and 2.5 cm in diameter.

REFERENCES

1. Ventura M, Melo M, Carrilho F. Outcome and long-term follow-up of adrenal lesions in multiple endocrine neoplasia type 1. *Arch Endocrinol Metab*. 2019;63(5):516–523.

2. Gatta-Cherifi B, Chabre O, Murat A, et al. Adrenal involvement in MEN1. Analysis of 715 cases from the Groupe d'etude des Tumeurs Endocrines database. *Eur J Endocrinol*. 2012;166(2):269–279.

Adrenocortical Carcinoma Presenting With Inferior Vena Cava Thrombus

The prognosis of patients with adrenocortical carcinoma (ACC) depends on several factors, including the European Network for the Study of Adrenal Tumours (ENSAT) stage, R0 (complete) surgical resection by an expert surgeon, and Ki-67 index.[1,2] ACC can present with the inferior vena cava (IVC), renal vein, or adrenal vein tumor thrombus in up to 25% of cases.[3–5] Patients with the IVC thrombus are considered to have ENSAT stage III disease and are at high risk of recurrence. Here we present a patient with a locally advanced ACC and a large IVC tumor thrombus.

Case Report

The patient was a 60-year-old woman who initially presented for evaluation of abdominal pain. Computed tomography (CT) abdominal imaging was performed and demonstrated a heterogeneous right adrenal mass that measured 11.0 × 10.5 × 10.0 cm (Fig. 33.1). Subsequent F-18 fluorodeoxyglucose (FDG) positron emission tomography (PET) scan demonstrated intense FDG uptake in the adrenal mass without any other foci of activity. On evaluation, the patient noted a 40-pound weight gain over 2 years, facial fullness, but no hirsutism or acne. Her review of system was otherwise negative. On physical examination, her blood pressure was 149/90 mmHg and body mass index was 28.9 kg/m². She had mild facial hirsutism and facial fullness without erythema. She had mild supraclavicular pads but no dorsocervical pad. She had no signs of proximal myopathy, no striae, and no edema. She was not taking any medications.

INVESTIGATIONS

Laboratory evaluation showed normal levels of urinary metanephrine and normetanephrine but was positive for increased excretion of cortisol, androgens, estrogen, progesterone, and steroid precursors (11-deoxycortisol, pregnenolone, 17-hydroxypregnenolone) (Table 33.1).

TREATMENT

ACC was suspected because of concerning imaging characteristics and adrenal hormonal excess.

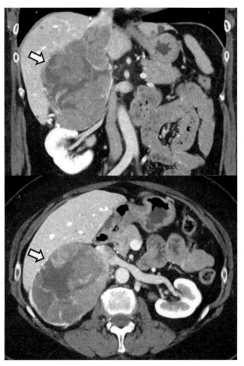

Fig. 33.1 Axial (*bottom*) and coronal (*top*) contrast-enhanced computed tomography images showed a heterogeneous right adrenal mass (*arrows*) measuring 11.0 × 10.5 × 10.0 cm. Extension of the adrenal mass into the inferior vena cava was noted. The adrenocortical carcinoma caused mass effect on the inferior posterior right hepatic lobe, displaced the right kidney, and abutted the posterior medial right hemidiaphragm.

TABLE 33.1 Laboratory Tests		
Biochemical Test	**Result**	**Reference Range**
Cortisol, mcg/dL	17.8	7–21
ACTH, pg/mL	<5	7.2–63
DHEA-S, mcg/dL	685, 931	<15–157
Androstenedione, ng/dL	87	30–200
Total testosterone, ng/dL	18	8–60
Estradiol, pg/mL	28, 36	<10
Progesterone, ng/mL	0.81	<0.20
17-Hydroxyprogesterone, ng/dL	70	<51
Pregnenolone, ng/dL	260	33–248
17-Hydroxypregnenolone, ng/dL	597	31–455
11-Deoxycortisol, ng/dL	176	10–79
Aldosterone, ng/dL	<4	<21
Plasma renin activity, ng/mL per hour	1.9	≤0.6–3
24-Hour urine cortisol, mcg/24 h	270, 189	<45
24-Hour urine metanephrine, mcg/24 h	20	<400
24-Hour urine normetanephrine, mcg/24 h	182	<900

ACTH, Corticotropin; *DHEA-S*, dehydroepiandrosterone sulfate.

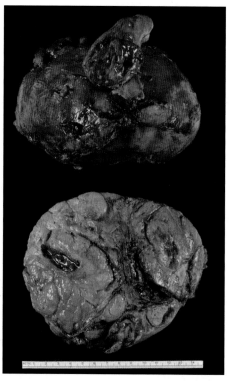

Fig. 33.2 Gross pathology image of the right adrenocortical carcinoma—a 16.8 × 11.4 × 8.2–cm heterogeneous adrenal mass with intravenous portion containing a 7.5 × 5.6 × 2.5–cm tumor thrombus.

Resection was anticipated to be difficult and included a multispecialty surgical team: adrenal surgeon, liver surgeon, vascular surgeon, and a cardiovascular surgeon. The patient was treated with open right adrenalectomy, IVC tumor extraction, vena cava thrombectomy, repair of retrohepatic and infrahepatic IVC with bovine pericardial patch angioplasty, tumor removal from the right atrium, and closure of patent foramen ovale. The patient was hospitalized for 1 week after the surgery.

Final pathology demonstrated an ACC that weighed 790 g and measured 16.8 × 11.4 × 8.2 cm. In addition, a 7.5 × 5.6 × 2.5–cm intravenous thrombus was noted. The adrenal mass extended beyond the adrenal gland. The surgical margins were free of tumor. The Ki-67 proliferation index was 40%. Both lymphovascular and capsular invasion were noted (Fig. 33.2).

FOLLOW-UP

The patient was treated with hydrocortisone after adrenalectomy. One week after hospital discharge, her postoperative course was complicated by a pulmonary embolism without significant hypoxia or hemodynamic instability. Another week later, she developed a pericardial effusion that necessitated pericardiocentesis. After these two complications necessitating therapy and hospitalizations, she recovered well. At the 6-week postoperative visit, mitotane therapy was initiated and titrated up to 3 g daily without significant side effects. Seven months after surgery, lung and liver metastases were detected. At that time, it was decided to stop mitotane and to start cisplatin, doxorubicin, and etoposide (EDP). With 5 months of EDP she had near-complete response in several metastases and had stable disease at 18 months after initial diagnosis. At that time, she was treated with radiation therapy of 50 Gy to left lower lobe metastases. She is now 3 years after adrenalectomy and continues to have nearly stable metastatic disease in the lungs without any additional therapy.

Discussion

Extension of ACC into the IVC, renal vein, or adrenal vein can occur in up to 25% of cases.[3–5] In a retrospective study of 65 patients with locally advanced ACC who underwent resection, overall survival was lower in patients with IVC thrombus.[6] The overall 3-year survival was reported to be 25% when venous resection is performed in patients with locally advanced disease.[4] Tumor invasion into adjacent organs or venous tumor thrombus in IVC is considered a T4 disease, ENSAT stage III, and these patients are at high risk of recurrence.[2] In addition to a complete resection, these patients may benefit from additional cytotoxic therapy.[2] Published evidence on the benefit of cytotoxic therapy in this setting is very limited, and as such, management of patients with IVC thrombus should be individualized.

In this case, the course of disease was remarkable for a better than expected prognosis.

Key Points

- ACC with IVC tumor thrombus is T4 disease, ENSAT stage III, and these patients are at high risk of recurrence.

- Complete resection of ACC and thrombectomy are associated with an improved prognosis.
- Management of these patients should be individualized and it may include cytotoxic chemotherapy.

REFERENCES

1. Kiseljak-Vassiliades K, Bancos I, Hamrahian A, et al. American Association of Clinical Endocrinology Disease state clinical review on the evaluation and management of adrenocortical carcinoma in an adult: a practical approach. *Endocrine Practice*. 2020;26(11):1366–1383.

2. Fassnacht M, Dekkers OM, Else T, et al. European Society of Endocrinology Clinical Practice Guidelines on the management of adrenocortical carcinoma in adults, in collaboration with the European Network for the Study of Adrenal Tumors. *Eur J Endocrinol*. 2018;179(4):G1–G46.

3. Chiche L, Dousset B, Kieffer E, Chapuis Y. Adrenocortical carcinoma extending into the inferior vena cava: presentation of a 15-patient series and review of the literature. *Surgery*. 2006;139(1):15–27.

4. Mihai R, Iacobone M, Makay O, et al. Outcome of operation in patients with adrenocortical cancer invading the inferior vena cava—a European Society of Endocrine Surgeons (ESES) survey. *Langenbecks Arch Surg*. 2012;397(2):225–231.

5. Turbendian HK, Strong VE, Hsu M, Ghossein RA, Fahey TJ 3rd. Adrenocortical carcinoma: the influence of large vessel extension. *Surgery*. 2010;148(6):1057–1064, discussion 1064.

6. Laan DV, Thiels CA, Glasgow A, et al. Adrenocortical carcinoma with inferior vena cava tumor thrombus. *Surgery*. 2017;161(1):240–248.

Management of Mitotane Therapy in Adrenocortical Carcinoma

The prognosis of adrenocortical carcinoma (ACC) depends on several factors, including the European Network for the Study of Adrenal Tumours (ENSAT) stage, R0 (complete) surgical resection by an expert surgeon, and Ki-67 index.[1,2] Therapy with adjuvant mitotane, an adrenolytic agent, is usually recommended for patients at high risk of recurrence, such as ENSAT stage III disease.[1,2] Careful discussion of mitotane-associated side effects and monitoring should be performed before initiation of therapy.

Case Report

The patient was a 29-year-old man who developed an acute-onset severe abdominal pain in the right upper quadrant during jogging. He presented to a local emergency department where a computed tomography (CT) scan was obtained, and a right large adrenal mass was found. He was referred to our institution for further evaluation and management.

History was positive for nocturnal night sweats for several month but no other symptoms. His weight was stable. On physical examination, his blood pressure was 136/97 mmHg and body mass index was 22 kg/m². There was no evidence of any features of Cushing syndrome. He did not take any medications.

INVESTIGATIONS

A large heterogeneous right adrenal mass measuring 14.6 × 14.0 × 17.0 cm with areas of internal calcification and central necrosis was demonstrated on CT scan (Fig. 34.1, upper panel). The mass caused inferior displacement of the right kidney, superior displacement of the liver, and compression of the inferior vena cava. Subsequent F-18 fluorodeoxyglucose (FDG) positron emission tomography (PET) scan demonstrated intense FDG uptake in the adrenal mass (maximum standardized uptake value = 9.9) without any other foci of activity (see Fig. 34.1, lower panel).

Laboratory evaluation documented corticotropin (ACTH)-independent hypercortisolism and a 100-fold elevation in 11-deoxycortisol (Table 34.1).

TREATMENT

ACC was suspected because of concerning imaging characteristics, associated ACTH-independent hypercortisolism, and elevated 11-deoxycortisol. The patient was treated with open right adrenalectomy and segment 6 liver resection. The adrenal mass weighed 1865 g and measured 19.7 × 14.7 × 12.5 cm. The Ki-67 proliferation index was 15% (Fig. 34.2). Although lymphovascular invasion was not identified, the tumor did invade through the adrenal capsule. Surgical margins were free of tumor. The patient was diagnosed with the ENSAT stage III disease. Postoperatively, 11-deoxycortisol decreased from 7270 ng/dL to 12 ng/dL (normal range, 10–79 ng/dL). He was initiated on hydrocortisone (20 mg daily in divided doses) treatment for anticipated adrenal insufficiency.

FOLLOW-UP

Mitotane therapy was started 4 weeks after adrenalectomy, at which point hydrocortisone therapy was increased to a total daily dose of 50 mg in divided doses. The initial dose of mitotane was 500 mg daily, which was titrated up to 3 g daily after 2 weeks. The blood mitotane concentration at that time was 2 mcg/mL. The approach of using mitotane based on tolerance versus based on mitotane levels was discussed. After an attempt to increase mitotane to 4 g daily, side effects of nausea and dizziness developed, and resolved when the dose was decreased to 3.5 g daily. The patient was

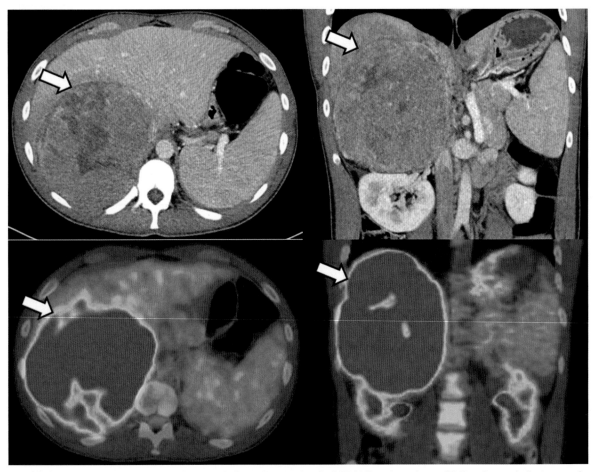

Fig. 34.1 Axial contrast-enhanced computed tomography image (*top panel*) and axial F-18 fluorodeoxyglucose (FDG) positron emission tomography (PET) scan image (*bottom panel*) showed a heterogeneous 14.6 × 14.0 × 17.0–cm right adrenal mass (*arrows*) with areas of internal calcification and central necrosis. The adrenal mass was FDG avid with a maximum standard unit value (SUVmax) of 9.9.

able to tolerate this dose and it was continued. His blood mitotane concentrations while on 3.5 g daily varied between 5 and 8.3 mcg/mL. Based on patient tolerance, it was decided to not increase the mitotane dosage above 3.5 g per day. Thus monitoring of blood mitotane levels was considered unnecessary and was discontinued.

Several months after initiating mitotane therapy, mild abnormalities in thyroid function tests and dyslipidemia were noted. Dyslipidemia was mild with elevation of low-density lipoprotein cholesterol (175 mg/dL). It was decided not to treat with statin therapy. The abnormality in thyroid function resolved when the mitotane dosage was decreased from 4 g to

3.5 g daily. The patient developed unilateral gynecomastia 8 months into mitotane therapy. There were no symptoms of hypogonadism. At that time total testosterone was 1670 ng/dL (normal range, 240–950 ng/dL) and bioavailable testosterone was 184 ng/dL (normal range, 72–235 ng/dL). Gynecomastia improved without any intervention 3 months later.

The patient continued supplemental therapy with hydrocortisone, 30 mg on waking and 20 mg at noon. He had no symptoms or signs of under- or overreplacement with glucocorticoids. In addition, symptoms of potential mineralocorticoid deficiency were periodically evaluated, and the patient did not develop hypotension, orthostasis, or salt craving. In addition, renin

TABLE 34.1	**Laboratory Tests**		
Biochemical Test		**Result**	**Reference Range**
Cortisol after overnight 1-mg DST, mcg/dL		11	<1.8
Cortisol, mcg/dL		11	7–21
ACTH, pg/mL		<5	7.2–63
DHEA-S, mcg/dL		548	105–728
Pregnenolone, ng/dL		243	33–248
17-Hydroxypregnenolone, ng/dL		178	55–455
17-Hydroxyprogesterone, ng/dL		157	<220
11-Deoxycortisol, ng/dL		7270	10–79
Aldosterone, ng/dL		<4	<21
Plasma renin activity, ng/mL per hour		<0.6	≤0.6–3
24-Hour urine cortisol, mcg/24 h		97	<45
Plasma metanephrine, nmol/L		<0.20	<0.50
Plasma normetanephrine, nmol/L		0.24	<0.90

ACTH, Corticotropin; *DHEA-S,* dehydroepiandrosterone-sulfate; *DST,* dexamethasone suppression test.

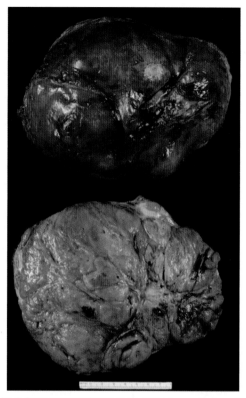

Fig. 34-2 Gross pathology image of the right adrenocortical carcinoma. The adrenal mass weighed 1865 g and measured 19.7 × 14.7 × 12.5 cm. Sectioning showed areas of tan, soft, friable tissue with hemorrhage, necrosis, and calcifications. The residual normal adrenal gland could not be identified.

plasma activity was also monitored every 3 months while the patient was on mitotane therapy and was within the normal range. The patient's last follow-up was 20 months after adrenalectomy; imaging was stable with indeterminate lung nodules.

Discussion

Mitotane is an adrenolytic drug that is used in treatment of ACC. Mitotane therapy has been associated with a longer recurrence-free survival, a better 5-year survival, but not a better overall survival.[3–5] Approaches to mitotane therapy dosing vary. One approach is to use mitotane at a lower dose of 1–3 g daily—a dose that is associated with fewer side effects and higher tolerance. In a study of 177 patients with ACC, adjuvant mitotane therapy at this dose was associated with a higher recurrence-free survival.[5] Notably, 13% of patients required a temporary dose reduction.[5] Another approach to mitotane dosing is based on achieving therapeutic mitotane serum levels of 14–20 mcg/mL. With this approach, mitotane is usually titrated to doses of up to 3–6 g a day and is accompanied by measurement of mitotane levels every 2–4 weeks.

Several studies suggested that therapeutic benefit is higher when mitotane levels are within 14–20 mcg/mL.[6–8] A third and more practical approach is to slowly titrate the dosage of mitotane to the high dosage that the patient tolerates; in this way the highest tolerated blood concentrations of mitotane are achieved without the need to measure blood mitotane levels. Careful discussion of mitotane-associated side effects and monitoring should be performed before initiation of therapy (Table 34.2). Mitotane-induced adrenal insufficiency should be anticipated and properly treated. Patients require an increased dose of hydrocortisone while on mitotane therapy (30–60 mg daily in divided doses) as a result of mitotane-induced increase in cortisol metabolism. Other common side effects include fatigue, nausea, diarrhea, gynecomastia, and, less commonly, confusion, dizziness, and ataxia. In addition to

TABLE 34.2	Mitotane Therapy: Dosing, Monitoring, and Side Effects			
	Therapy	**Clinical Monitoring**	**Biochemical Monitoring**	**Comments**
Adrenal insufficiency	Start glucocorticoid therapy at the time or several weeks after mitotane therapy initiation (hydrocortisone at 30–60 mg daily) or prednisone (10 mg daily). Provide patient education on sick day rules.	Monitor for symptoms of adrenal insufficiency or cortisol excess (history, physical examination).	Plasma ACTH may be helpful to determine the appropriateness of glucocorticoid dose. Serum electrolytes and plasma renin activity are helpful to determine whether mineralocorticoid deficiency is present.	Adrenal insufficiency may persist for months after stopping mitotane. Permanent primary adrenal insufficiency is possible.
Gastrointestinal side effects (nausea, vomiting, diarrhea, anorexia)	Consider suboptimal glucocorticoid replacement as a cause (i.e., adrenal insufficiency). Metoclopramide, ondansetron, and Imodium If severe: hold or decrease mitotane.	Monitor for symptoms.	—	—
Neurologic (lethargy, sedation, confusion, sedation, ataxia, and dizziness)	Consider suboptimal glucocorticoid replacement as a cause (i.e., adrenal insufficiency).	Monitor for symptoms.	—	Severe neurologic side effects (e.g., ataxia) usually occur at mitotane levels >30 mcg/mL.
Dyslipidemia	If mild: no therapy is needed. Consider pravastatin or rosuvastatin.	—	Lipid profile every 3–6 months	Mitotane stimulates the rate-limiting enzyme in cholesterol synthesis resulting in increased blood levels of LDL cholesterol.
Hypothyroidism	Levothyroxine	Monitor for symptoms of hypothyroidism.	Thyroid function tests every 3–6 months	Mitotane increases concentration of thyroid hormone binding globulin → decrease in free thyroxine. Mitotane directly inhibits TSH secretion.
Hepatic toxicity	Decrease or stop mitotane.		Liver function tests every 3 months	
Male hypogonadism	Testosterone replacement therapy	Monitor for symptoms; physical examination: gynecomastia.	Total and free testosterone concentrations if symptoms of hypogonadism or gynecomastia	Mitotane increases concentrations of binding globulins, including cortisol and sex binding globulin. Mitotane inhibits 5-α-reductase activity.

ACTH, Corticotropin; *LDL,* low-density lipoprotein; *TSH,* thyroid-stimulating hormone.

clinical evaluation for signs and symptoms of cortisol excess or deficiency and other side effects to mitotane, all patients require biochemical monitoring with serum electrolytes, liver function tests, thyroid function tests, serum cholesterol, and tests for mineralocorticoid deficiency.[1,2]

Key Points

- Dosing of mitotane is mainly based on tolerance.
- Mitotane concentrations of 14–20 mcg/mL have been reported to be associated with a higher therapeutic benefit.
- Mitotane side effects include adrenal insufficiency, nausea, diarrhea, fatigue, hypothyroidism, confusion, lethargy, sedation, dizziness, and ataxia.
- Clinical and biochemical monitoring every 3 months is required in any patient treated with mitotane.

REFERENCES

1. Kiseljak-Vassiliades K, Bancos I, Hamrahian A, et al. American Association of Clinical Endocrinology Disease state clinical review on the evaluation and management of adrenocortical carcinoma in an adult: a practical approach. *Endocrine Practice.* 2020;26(11):1366–1383.

2. Fassnacht M, Dekkers OM, Else T, et al. European Society of Endocrinology Clinical Practice Guidelines on the management of adrenocortical carcinoma in adults, in collaboration with the European Network for the Study of Adrenal Tumors. *Eur J Endocrinol.* 2018;179(4):G1–G46.

3. Calabrese A, Basile V, Puglisi S, et al. Adjuvant mitotane therapy is beneficial in non-metastatic adrenocortical carcinoma at high risk of recurrence. *Eur J Endocrinol.* 2019;180(6):387–396.

4. Puglisi S, Calabrese A, Basile V, et al. Mitotane Concentrations influence the risk of recurrence in adrenocortical carcinoma patients on adjuvant treatment. *J Clin Med.* 2019;8(11):1850.

5. Terzolo M, Angeli A, Fassnacht M, et al. Adjuvant mitotane treatment for adrenocortical carcinoma. *N Engl J Med.* 2007;356(23):2372–2380.

6. Haak HR, Hermans J, van de Velde CJ, et al. Optimal treatment of adrenocortical carcinoma with mitotane: results in a consecutive series of 96 patients. *Br J Cancer.* 1994;69(5):947–951.

7. van Slooten H, Moolenaar AJ, van Seters AP, Smeenk D. The treatment of adrenocortical carcinoma with o,p'-DDD: prognostic implications of serum level monitoring. *Eur J Cancer Clin Oncol.* 1984;20(1):47–53.

8. Hermsen IG, Fassnacht M, Terzolo M, et al. Plasma concentrations of o,p'DDD, o,p'DDA, and o,p'DDE as predictors of tumor response to mitotane in adrenocortical carcinoma: results of a retrospective ENSAT multicenter study. *J Clin Endocrinol Metab.* 2011;96(6):1844–1851.

Pheochromocytoma and Paraganglioma

Catecholamine-secreting tumors that arise from the chromaffin cells in the adrenal medulla and the sympathetic ganglia are referred to as *pheochromocytoma* (PHEO) and *catecholamine-secreting paraganglioma* (PGL), respectively.[1,2] Because they have similar clinical presentations and are treated with similar approaches, many clinicians use the term *pheochromocytoma* to refer to both adrenal PHEO and extraadrenal catecholamine-secreting PGLs. However, the distinction between PHEO and PGL (PPGL) is important because of the implications for associated neoplasms and syndromes are different and the risk for metastatic disease is higher in patients with PGL.[1] Catecholamine-secreting PPGL should be suspected in patients who have one or more of the following: an incidentally discovered adrenal mass with imaging characteristics consistent with PHEO (e.g., lipid poor, hypervascular, and partially cystic) (see Cases 35, 36, and 37); a familial syndrome that predisposes to catecholamine-secreting PPGLs (e.g., multiple endocrine neoplasia type 2 [see Cases 40 and 46], neurofibromatosis type 1 [see Case 39], von Hippel-Lindau disease [see Case 41]); a family history of PPGL; pressor response during anesthesia, surgery, or angiography; hyperadrenergic spells (e.g., self-limited episodes of nonexertional forceful palpitations, diaphoresis, headache, tremor, or pallor)[3]; treatment-resistant hypertension; onset of hypertension at a young age; and idiopathic dilated cardiomyopathy. The symptoms, listed in Table E.1, are caused by the pharmacologic effects of excess concentrations of circulating catecholamines.[4] However, when a PPGL is diagnosed in the presymptomatic stage, it is common for these patients to have normal blood pressure.[5] In approximately 60% of patients with adrenal PHEO the tumors are discovered incidentally on imaging performed for other reasons.[5] In addition, small PPGLs may not be large enough to be biochemically detectable (see Case 36).

Most people tested for catecholamine-secreting PPGL do not have these rare neoplasms.[3] Levels of fractionated catecholamines and metanephrines may be elevated in several clinical scenarios, including any acute illness (e.g., subarachnoid hemorrhage, migraine headache, preeclampsia, or illness requiring intensive care unit hospitalization), withdrawal from medications or drugs (e.g., clonidine, alcohol), and administration of many drugs and medications (Table E.2). Tricyclic antidepressants is the drug class that interferes most frequently with the interpretation of fractionated metanephrines and catecholamines. To effectively screen for catecholamine-secreting tumors, treatment with tricyclic antidepressants and other psychoactive agents listed in Table E.2 should be tapered and discontinued at least 2 weeks before any hormonal assessments. In some clinical situations it is contraindicated to discontinue certain medications (e.g., antipsychotics), and if case-detection testing is positive, then CT or MRI of the abdomen and pelvis would be needed to exclude a catecholamine-secreting tumor. A normal computed tomography CT or MRI of the abdomen and pelvis makes a symptomatic PPGL extremely unlikely because (1) 95% of catecholamine-secreting tumors are found between the diaphragm and pubis; and (2) the average size of a symptomatic PPGL is 4.5 cm.

TABLE E.1 Signs and Symptoms Associated With Catecholamine-Secreting Tumors

Paroxysm-Related Signs and Symptoms

Anxiety and fear of impending death

Diaphoresis

Dyspnea

Epigastric or chest pain

Headache

Hypertension

Nausea and vomiting

Pallor

Palpitation (forceful heartbeat)

Tremor

Chronic Signs and Symptoms

Cold hands and feet

Congestive heart failure—dilated or hypertrophic cardiomyopathy

Constipation that may progress to obstipation

Dyspnea

Ectopic hormone secretion–dependent symptoms (e.g., CRH/ACTH, GHRH, PTHrP, VIP)

Epigastric or chest pain

Fatigue

Fever

General increase in sweating

Grade II to IV hypertensive retinopathy

Headache

Hyperglycemia and secondary diabetes mellitus

Hypertension

Nausea and vomiting

Orthostatic hypotension

Painless hematuria (associated with urinary bladder paraganglioma)

Pallor

Palpitation (forceful heartbeat)

Paroxysms precipitated by micturition (associated with urinary bladder paraganglioma)

Tremor

Weight loss

Not Typical of Pheochromocytoma

Flushing

ACTH, Corticotropin; *CRH*, corticotropin–releasing hormone; *GHRH*, growth hormone–releasing hormone; *PTHrP*, parathyroid hormone–related peptide; *VIP*, vasoactive intestinal polypeptide.
Adapted from Young WF Jr. Pheochromocytoma, 1926–1993. *Trends Endocrinol Metab.* 1993;4:122–127.

TABLE E.2 Medications That May Increase Measured Levels of Norepinephrine, Normetanephrine, and Dopamine

Tricyclic antidepressants (including cyclobenzaprine): up to 10-fold elevations in NE and Normet

Levodopa: up to 20-fold elevations in DA and 4-fold in NE and Normet

Antipsychotic agents and buspirone: up to 10-fold elevations in NE and Normet

Serotonin-norepinephrine reuptake inhibitor: up to 5-fold elevations in NE and Normet

Selective serotonin reuptake inhibitors: up to 2-fold elevations in NE and Normet

Prochlorperazine: up to 5-fold elevations in NE and Normet

Reserpine: up to 10-fold elevations in NE and Normet

Drugs containing adrenergic receptor agonists (e.g., decongestants): up to 5-fold elevations in NE and Normet

Amphetamines: up to 10-fold elevations in NE and Normet

Withdrawal from clonidine and other drugs: up to 10-fold elevations in NE and Normet

Illicit drugs (e.g., cocaine, heroin): up to 10-fold elevations in NE and Normet

Ethanol: up to 5-fold elevations in NE and Normet

DA, Dopamine; *NE,* norepinephrine; *Normet,* normetanephrine.

Genetic testing should be considered in all patients with PPGL.[1,2] When bilateral PHEO or multiple PGLs are found, there is always has a genetic cause (see Cases 40, 41, 42, 45, and 46). The probability of finding a pathogenic variant in a PPGL susceptibility gene is inversely correlated with age—germline pathogenic variants are found in approximately 85% of those with a PPGL detected in the first decade of life and 25% when PPGL is diagnosed in the sixth decade of life.[1] Pathogenic variants in PPGL susceptibility genes have three general transcription signatures: (1) cluster 1, genes encoding proteins that function in the cellular response to hypoxia; (2) cluster 2, genes encoding proteins that activate kinase signaling; and (3) cluster 3, Wnt signaling pathway genes (Table E.3).

When the results of abdominal and pelvic cross-sectional imaging are negative in patients with biochemically confirmed catecholamine-secreting PPGL or in patients with metastatic PPGL, additional localization

TABLE E.3 Pheochromocytoma and Paraganglioma Susceptibility Genes

Syndrome/Name	Gene	Typical Tumor Location and Other Associations
Hypoxic Pathway: Cluster 1[a]		
SDHD pathogenic variant	*SDHD*	Primarily skull base and neck; occasionally adrenal medulla, mediastinum, abdomen, pelvis; GIST; possible pituitary adenoma
SDHAF2 pathogenic variant[b]	*SDHAF2*	Primarily skull base and neck; occasionally abdomen and pelvis
SDHC pathogenic variant	*SDHC*	Primarily skull base and neck; occasionally abdomen, pelvis, or chest; GIST; possible pituitary adenoma
SDHB pathogenic variant	*SDHB*	Abdomen, pelvis, and mediastinum; rarely adrenal medulla, skull base, and neck; GIST; renal cell carcinoma; possible pituitary adenoma
SDHA pathogenic variant	*SDHA*	Primarily skull base and neck; occasionally abdomen and pelvis; GIST; possible pituitary adenoma
von Hippel-Lindau (VHL) disease	*VHL*	Adrenal medulla, frequently bilateral; occasionally paraganglioma that may be localized from skull base to pelvis; VHL-associated findings, including retinal angiomas, cerebellar hemangioblastomas, spinal hemangioblastomas, renal cell carcinoma, pancreatic neuroendocrine tumors, and endolymphatic sac tumor
Hereditary leiomyomatosis and renal cell carcinoma (Reed syndrome)—*fumarate hydratase* pathogenic variant	*FH*	Multifocal and metastatic paraganglioma; associated with hereditary leiomyomatosis, uterine fibroids, and renal cell carcinoma
Endothelial PAS	*EPAS1*	Paraganglioma, polycythemia, and rarely somatostatinomas
Familial erythrocytosis associated with pathogenic variant in *prolyl hydroxylase isoform 1 (PDH1)*	*EGLN2* (Egl-9 family)	Polycythemia associated with pheochromocytoma and paraganglioma
Familial erythrocytosis associated with pathogenic variant in *prolyl hydroxylase isoform 2 (PDH2)*	*EGLN1* (Egl-9 family)	Polycythemia associated with pheochromocytoma and paraganglioma
Kinesin family member 1B	*KIF1B*	Paraganglioma, ganglioneuroma, leiomyosarcoma, lung adenocarcinoma, neuroblastoma, ganglioneuroma
Malate dehydrogenase 2	*MDH2*	Pheochromocytoma and paraganglioma—penetrance and associated conditions not yet characterized
Solute carrier family 25 Member 11	*SLC25A11*	Pheochromocytoma and paraganglioma—penetrance and associated conditions not yet characterized
DNA methyltransferase 3 α	*DNMT3A*	Pheochromocytoma and paraganglioma—penetrance unknown; acute myeloid leukemia
Isocitrate dehydrogenase [NADP(+)] 1	*IDH1*	Pheochromocytoma and paraganglioma—penetrance and associated conditions not yet characterized
Dihydrolipoamide S-succinyltransferase	*DLST*	Pheochromocytoma and paraganglioma—penetrance and associated conditions not yet characterized
Glutamic-oxaloacetic transaminase 2	*GOT2*	Pheochromocytoma and paraganglioma—penetrance and associated conditions not yet characterized

Continued

TABLE E.3 Pheochromocytoma and Paraganglioma Susceptibility Genes—cont'd		
Syndrome/Name	Gene	Typical Tumor Location and Other Associations
Kinase Signaling Pathway: Cluster 2[c]		
MEN2A	*RET*	Pheochromocytoma in 50% (frequently bilateral); medullary thyroid carcinoma in 100%, primary hyperparathyroidism in 20%, and cutaneous lichen amyloidosis in 5%
MEN2B	*RET*	Pheochromocytoma in 50% (frequently bilateral); medullary thyroid carcinoma in 100%; mucocutaneous neuromas in most (typically involving the tongue, lips, and eyelids); skeletal deformities (kyphoscoliosis or lordosis) in most; joint laxity in most; myelinated corneal nerves in many; and intestinal ganglioneuromas (Hirschsprung disease) in most
Neurofibromatosis type 1 (NF1)	*NF1*	Pheochromocytoma or periadrenal paraganglioma in 3%; café au lait spots; subcutaneous or plexiform neurofibromas; axillary or inguinal freckling; optic glioma; iris hamartomas (Lisch nodules); and osseous lesions (e.g., sphenoid dysplasia)
MYC associated factor X[b]	*MAX*	Adrenal medulla
Transmembrane protein 127	*TMEM127*	Adrenal medulla; possible renal cell carcinoma
Wnt Signaling Pathway: Cluster 3[d]		
Cold shock domain containing E1	*CSDE1*	Pheochromocytoma and paraganglioma—penetrance and associated conditions not yet characterized
Mastermind like transcriptional coactivator 3	*MAML3*	Pheochromocytoma and paraganglioma—penetrance and associated conditions not yet characterized

[a]Cluster 1 tumors are mostly extraadrenal paragangliomas (except in VHL where most tumors are localized to the adrenal) and nearly all have a noradrenergic biochemical phenotype.
[b]Associated with maternal imprinting.
[c]Cluster 2 tumors are usually adrenal pheochromocytomas with an adrenergic biochemical phenotype.
[d]Cluster 3 tumors are adrenal or extraadrenal in location with variable biochemical phenotype.
GIST, Gastrointestinal stromal tumor; *MEN,* multiple endocrine neoplasia; *SDH,* succinate dehydrogenase.

imaging is indicated with either gallium 68 (Ga-68) 1,4,7,10-tetraazacyclododecane-1,4,7,10-tetraacetic acid (DOTA)-octreotate (DOTATATE) positron emission tomography (PET) (Ga-68 DOTATATE PET) or scintigraphy with iodine-123 (I-123) metaiodobenzylguanidine (I-123 MIBG) (see Cases 47 and 48).

The treatment of choice for PPGL is complete surgical resection. Most catecholamine-secreting tumors are benign and can be totally excised. The most common complications are intraoperative blood pressure lability and postoperative hypotension.[6] Careful preoperative pharmacologic preparation is crucial for successful treatment. Some form of preoperative pharmacologic preparation is indicated for all patients with catecholamine-secreting neoplasms, including those who are asymptomatic and normotensive.[6] Combined

α- and β-adrenergic blockade is one approach to control blood pressure and prevent intraoperative hypertensive crises. α-Adrenergic blockade with either doxazosin or phenoxybenzamine should be started at least 7–10 days preoperatively to normalize blood pressure and expand the contracted blood volume. When compared to doxazosin, use of phenoxybenzamine is more effective in preventing intraoperative hemodynamic instability.[7]

Because all PPGLs have malignant potential, all patients should have annual biochemical follow-up with measurement of fractionated metanephrines. With the exception of multiple endocrine neoplasia type 2 and neurofibromatosis type 1 (where the PPGL is always adrenal or periadrenal), periodic imaging from skull base to pelvis is indicated to detect nonfunctioning PGLs in patients with pathogenic variants in PPGL susceptibility genes. There is no cure for metastatic PPGL.[8] However, most patients with metastatic PPGL have an indolent course and a median disease-specific survival of 33 years.[9] The aggressiveness of the treatment approach should match the pace of progression of the metastatic PPGL. Treatment options include observation (see Case 52), ablative therapies[10] (see Case 51), chemotherapy[11] (see Case 50), or radiation therapy[12] (see Case 53).

REFERENCES

1. Neumann HPH, Young WF, Jr., Eng C. Pheochromocytoma and paraganglioma. *N Engl J Med*. 2019;381(6):552–565.

2. Lenders JW, Duh QY, Eisenhofer G, et al. Pheochromocytoma and paraganglioma: an Endocrine Society clinical practice guideline. *J Clin Endocrinol Metab*. 2014;99(6):1915–1942.

3. Young WF, Jr., Maddox DE. Spells: in search of a cause. *Mayo Clin Proc*. 1995;70(8):757–765.

4. Young WF, Jr., Pheochromocytoma: 1926–1993. *Trends Endocrinol Metab*. 1993;4(4):122–127.

5. Gruber LM, Hartman RP, Thompson GB, et al. Pheochromocytoma characteristics and behavior differ depending on method of discovery. *J Clin Endocrinol Metab*. 2019;104:1386–1393.

6. Weingarten TN, Welch TL, Moore TL, et al. Preoperative levels of catecholamines and metanephrines and intraoperative hemodynamics of patients undergoing pheochromocytoma and paraganglioma resection. *Urology*. 2017;100:131–138.

7. Buitenwerf E, Osinga TE, Timmers H, Lenders JWM, Feelders RA, Eekhoff EMW, et al. Efficacy of alpha-blockers on hemodynamic control during pheochromocytoma resection: a randomized controlled trial. *J Clin Endocrinol Metab*. 2020;105(7):2381–2391.

8. Young WF. Metastatic pheochromocytoma: in search of a cure. *Endocrinology*. 2020;161(3):bqz019.

9. Hamidi O, Young WF, Jr. Iñiguez-Ariza NM, et al. Malignant pheochromocytoma and paraganglioma: 272 patients over 55 years. *J Clin Endocrinol Metab*. 2017;102(9):3296–3305.

10. Kohlenberg J, Welch B, Hamidi O, et al. Efficacy and safety of ablative therapy in the treatment of patients with metastatic pheochromocytoma and paraganglioma. *Cancers (Basel)*. 2019;11(2):195.

11. Huang H, Abraham J, Hung E, et al. Treatment of malignant pheochromocytoma/paraganglioma with cyclophosphamide, vincristine, and dacarbazine: recommendation from a 22-year follow-up of 18 patients. *Cancer*. 2008;113(8):2020–2028.

12. Breen W, Bancos I, Young WF, Jr. Bible KC, Laack NN, Foote RL, Hallemeier CL. External beam radiation therapy for advanced/unresectable malignant paraganglioma and pheochromocytoma. *Adv Radiat Oncol*. 2017;3(1):25–29.

Most Pheochromocytomas Grow Slowly

The clinical presentation of pheochromocytoma has changed dramatically since Dr. Charlie Mayo successfully resected the first pheochromocytoma in North America in 1926.[1] In the early days nearly all patients presented with hypertension and signs and symptoms of catecholamine excess. However, at Mayo Clinic since 2005, in most patients with pheochromocytoma their tumor was discovered incidentally on imaging performed for other reasons. We have also learned over the past two decades that although all pheochromocytomas have malignant potential, they grow slowly over time—by approximately 3–5 mm in diameter per year. Herein we share such a case.

Case Report

The patient was a 71-year-old man referred for evaluation of an incidentally discovered right adrenal mass. The initial computed tomography (CT) scan was obtained 5 years previously to evaluate left lower quadrant abdominal pain and incidentally detected a 1.8-cm right adrenal mass that was lipid poor (40.6 Hounsfield units [HU]) on unenhanced images (Fig. 35.1). Subsequent CT scans demonstrated that the right adrenal mass was enlarging by an average of 4 mm in diameter per year and at the time of referral to endocrinology measured 3.8 × 3.3 cm (see Fig. 35.1). The patient was asymptomatic. His hypertension of 5 years duration was effectively treated with a calcium channel blocker (diltiazem 240 mg daily), an angiotensin receptor blocker (losartan 50 mg daily), and a β-adrenergic receptor blocker (metoprolol 25 mg daily). His diabetes of 2 years duration was treated with metformin (1000 mg twice daily) and rosiglitazone (4 mg twice daily).

The patient had no signs or symptoms of adrenocortical or medullary dysfunction. He did have a history of prostate cancer treated with radiation therapy 3 years previously. His body mass index was 22.7 kg/m², blood pressure was 120/70 mmHg, and heart rate 56 beats per minute.

INVESTIGATIONS

The laboratory studies were remarkable for marked elevation of normetanephrine in the blood and marked elevations of norepinephrine and normetanephrine the 24-hour urine collection (Table 35.1). The patient was taking no medications that would cause false-positive elevations in norepinephrine or normetanephrine.

TREATMENT

The findings on biochemical testing were diagnostic for a catecholamine-secreting tumor. In preparation for surgery, phenoxybenzamine was added to his list of medications and losartan was discontinued. The phenoxybenzamine was titrated for a target low-normal systolic blood pressure. The patient underwent laparoscopic right adrenalectomy. The adrenal gland weighed 19.8 g (normal, 4–5 g) and the pheochromocytoma measured 2.5 × 1.5 × 1.5 cm. Phenoxybenzamine was discontinued postoperatively, and the patient was discharged from the hospital the day after surgery.

OUTCOME AND FOLLOW-UP

Five days after surgery the patient's blood glucose was normal without pharmacologic treatment. In addition, blood pressure was normal on his low-dose β-adrenergic blocker alone. One year later his plasma fractionated metanephrines were normal and his glycosylated hemoglobin was normal without the aid of

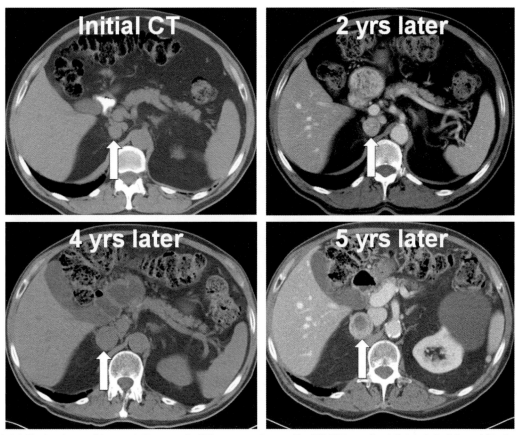

Fig. 35.1 Axial images from serial computed tomography (CT) scans over 5 years. The initial CT scan (*top left*) detected a 1.8-cm right adrenal mass (*arrow*) with an unenhanced CT attenuation of 40.6 Hounsfield units (HU). Two years later on a contrast-enhanced CT scan the right adrenal mass (*arrow*) measured 2.6 × 2.4 cm (*top right*). Four years after the initial CT scan the adrenal mass (*arrow*) measured 3.2 × 2.9 cm and the unenhanced CT attenuation was 38.7 HU (*bottom left*). Five years after the initial CT scan and at the time of referral to endocrinology, the adrenal mass (*arrow*) was cystic and vascular and measured 3.8 × 3.3 cm. The unenhanced CT attenuation of the solid component was 40.6 HU (*bottom right*).

TABLE 35.1 Laboratory Tests		
Biochemical Test	**Result**	**Reference Range**
Sodium, mmol/L	139	135–145
Potassium, mmol/L	5.4	3.6–5.2
Creatinine, mg/dL	1.0	0.8–1.3
Glycosylated hemoglobin, %	5.8	4–6
AM serum cortisol, mcg/dL	17	7–25
PM serum cortisol, mcg/dL	7.6	2–14
Plasma metanephrine, nmol/L	0.34	<0.5
Plasma normetanephrine, nmol/L	8.59	<0.9
Aldosterone, ng/dL	8	≤21 ng/dL

TABLE 35.1 Laboratory Tests—cont'd		
Biochemical Test	**Result**	**Reference Range**
Plasma renin activity ng/mL per hour	14	≤0.6–3
24-Hour urine:		
Metanephrine, mcg	173	<400
Normetanephrine, mcg	3147	<900
Norepinephrine, mcg	455	<80
Epinephrine, mcg	7.2	<20
Dopamine, mcg	160	<400
Cortisol, mcg	19	3.5–45

medications. His blood pressure continued to be well controlled on monotherapy. Fourteen years after surgery the patient continued to do well with no evidence for recurrent pheochromocytoma or diabetes mellitus.

Key Points

- As a result of the widespread use of computed abdominal imaging, most patients with pheochromocytoma are discovered incidentally on imaging performed for other reasons.[2]
- Lipid-poor adrenal masses should be considered pheochromocytoma until proven otherwise.
- Although patients may not have the classic paroxysms associated with catecholamine hypersecretion, pheochromocytoma can result in sustained hypertension and may be responsible for diabetes mellitus.[3]

- Approximately 25% of patients with pheochromocytoma have diabetes mellitus, and it resolves in about 75% of patients after tumor resection.[3]
- Although all pheochromocytomas have malignant potential, they grow slowly over time—by approximately 3–5 mm in diameter per year.

REFERENCES

1. Mayo CH. Paroxysmal hypertension with tumor of the retroperitoneal nerve: report of a case. *JAMA*. 1927;89(13):1047–1050.

2. Gruber LM, Hartman RP, Thompson GB, et al. Pheochromocytoma characteristics and behavior differ depending on method of discovery. *J Clin Endocrinol Metab*. 2019;104(5):1386–1393.

3. Beninato T, Kluijfhout WP, Drake FT, et al. Resection of pheochromocytoma improves diabetes mellitus in the majority of patients. *Ann Surg Oncol*. 2017;24(5):1208–1213.

The "Prebiochemical" Pheochromocytoma

All pheochromocytomas are biochemically undetectable when small—they require a sizable "factory" to become biochemically detectable. Thus publications that report that a laboratory test is 98% or 100% sensitive in detecting pheochromocytomas is simply wrong—just not possible! Computed abdominal imaging is being performed for a never-ending list of reasons. We are finding "baby" pheochromocytomas before they become symptomatic or biochemically detectable. Herein is such a case.

Case Report

The patient was a healthy 49-year-old man who had been troubled by intermittent right upper quadrant pain, which was thought to be related to gallbladder dysfunction. Abdominal computed tomography (CT) incidentally discovered a 1.6-cm lipid-poor and vascular left adrenal mass (Fig. 36.1). He had no signs or symptoms of adrenal cortical or medullary dysfunction. He took no regular medications. His blood pressure was 128/78 mmHg, heart rate 74 beats per minute, and body mass index 26.51 kg/m^2.

INVESTIGATIONS

All adrenal-related laboratory studies normal (Table 36.1).

TREATMENT

The patient was informed that he had a dense and vascular adrenal mass that could be a prebiochemical pheochromocytoma or a very small adrenocortical carcinoma. He was advised to either have a laparoscopic left adrenalectomy or close imaging follow-up. The patient elected to proceed with surgery. He was prepared with the α-adrenergic blocker doxazosin, which was titrated for low-normal systolic blood pressure for age. The patient underwent laparoscopic left adrenalectomy. The adrenal gland weighed 8 g (normal, 4–5 g), and the pheochromocytoma measured 2.1 × 1.7 × 1.3 cm (Fig. 36.2). The patient was discharged from the hospital the day after surgery.

OUTCOME AND FOLLOW-UP

The patient recovered from surgery over the subsequent 7 days and he returned to work. One year later his plasma fractionated metanephrines were normal. Abdominal computed tomography (CT) was performed for other reasons and his right adrenal gland appeared normal and there was no sign of a paraganglioma. The patient declined germline genetic testing.

Discussion

We are frequently asked about whether preoperative adrenergic blockade should be administered to patients with pheochromocytoma or paraganglioma who have normal levels of fractionated catecholamines and metanephrines. In our review of 258 patients who underwent resection of a pheochromocytoma or paraganglioma, intraoperative hemodynamic variability was greater with higher preoperative levels of fractionated catecholamines and metanephrines (P < .001).[1] However, substantial hemodynamic variability was observed even when preoperative fractionated catecholamines and metanephrines were within the normal range.[1]

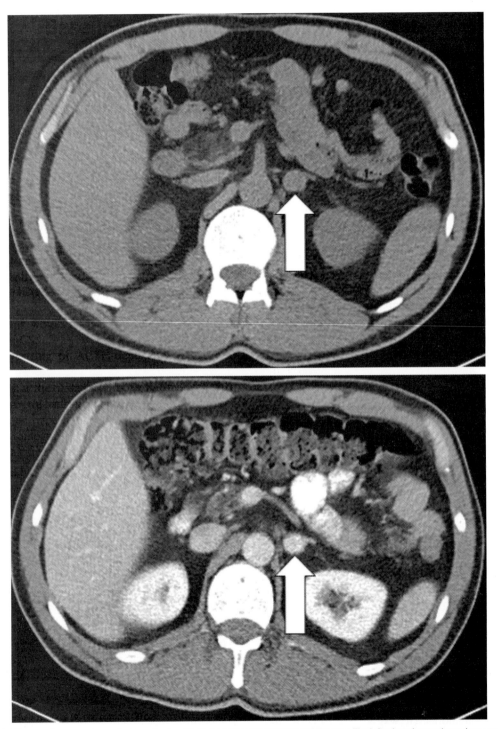

Fig. 36.1 Axial images from unenhanced and contrast-enhanced computed tomography (CT) scans. The left adrenal mass (*arrow*) measured 1.6 cm in maximal diameter. The unenhanced CT attenuation was 41.4 Hounsfield units (*upper panel*). The adrenal mass enhanced markedly with contrast administration (*lower panel*).

TABLE 36.1 Laboratory Tests

Biochemical Test	Result	Reference Range
Sodium, mmol/L	142	135–145
Potassium, mmol/L	4.2	3.6–5.2
Creatinine, mg/dL	1.15	0.74–1.35
AM serum cortisol, mcg/dL	16	7–25
ACTH, pg/mL	44	10–60
Plasma metanephrine, nmol/L	<0.2	<0.5
Plasma normetanephrine, nmol/L	0.55	<0.9
Aldosterone, ng/dL	5.3	≤21 ng/dL
Plasma renin activity ng/mL per hour	2	≤0.6–3
24-Hour urine:		
Metanephrine, mcg	151	<400
Normetanephrine, mcg	447	<900
Norepinephrine, mcg	61	<80
Epinephrine, mcg	7.6	<20
Dopamine, mcg	201	<400

ACTH, Corticotropin.

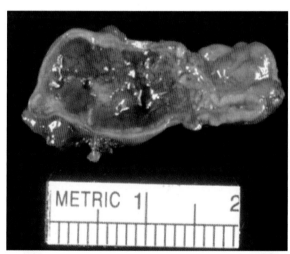

Fig. 36.2 Gross pathology image of the left adrenal gland containing a 2.1 × 1.7 × 1.3–cm pheochromocytoma.

Key Points

- With the advent of widespread use of computed abdominal imaging, most patients with pheochromocytoma are discovered incidentally on imaging performed for other reasons.[2]
- Lipid-poor adrenal masses should be considered pheochromocytoma until proven otherwise.
- All pheochromocytomas are "prebiochemical" when small. There is no biochemical test that carries 100% sensitivity.
- Patients with pheochromocytoma or paraganglioma that is associated with normal levels of fractionated catecholamines and metanephrines should be prepared for surgery with adrenergic blockade.

REFERENCES

1. Weingarten TN, Welch TL, Moore TL, et al. Preoperative levels of catecholamines and metanephrines and intraoperative hemodynamics of patients undergoing pheochromocytoma and paraganglioma resection. *Urology.* 2017;100:131–138.
2. Gruber LM, Hartman RP, Thompson GB, et al. Pheochromocytoma characteristics and behavior differ depending on method of discovery. *J Clin Endocrinol Metab.* 2019;104(5):1386–1393.

Huge Catecholamine-Secreting Tumor

The average size of a symptomatic catecholamine-secreting tumor is 4.5 cm. Some of the very large pheochromocytomas or paragangliomas (PPGLs) (e.g., >10 cm in diameter) are biochemically non-functioning. However, there is a unique subset of patients with PPGL who are asymptomatic despite large tumors and massive catecholamine hypersecretion. We describe one such case here.

Case Report

The patient was a 47-year-old man who was incidentally discovered to have a large right adrenal pheochromocytoma during an elective partial sigmoidectomy to remove large benign colon polyps. There was no problem with blood pressure lability intraoperatively. After his partial sigmoidectomy, abdominal magnetic resonance imaging showed a massive right retroperitoneal tumor (20 × 10 × 12 cm) (Fig. 37.1). He always had normal blood pressure and denied paroxysms, palpitations, headaches, or sweating. There is no family history of pheochromocytoma. On physical examination his body mass index was 25.9 kg/m², blood pressure 108/65 mmHg, and heart rate 87 beats per minute.

INVESTIGATIONS

Blood and 24-hour urine studies provided unequivocal proof that this was a catecholamine-secreting tumor (Table 37.1). The 24-hour urinary excretion of dopamine, normetanephrine, and metanephrine was increased 124-fold, 7-fold, and 5-fold above the upper limits of the respective reference ranges.

Scintigraphy with 123-I metaiodobenzylguanidine found no extraadrenal paragangliomas or sites of metastatic disease.

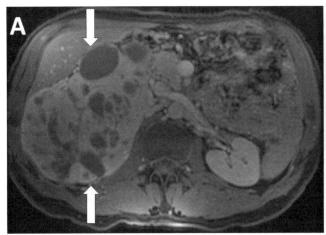
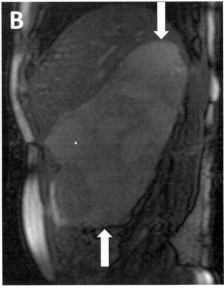

Fig. 37.1 Axial (A) and sagittal (B) images from abdominal magnetic resonance imaging revealed huge pheochromocytoma measuring 20 × 10 × 12 cm (longitudinal, transverse, and AP diameters, respectively). The tumor had numerous cystic and necrotic areas throughout and displaced the right kidney inferiorly and anteriorly.

TABLE 37.1 Laboratory Tests		
Biochemical Test	Result	Reference Range
Sodium, mmol/L	143	135–145
Potassium, mmol/L	4.4	3.6–5.2
Creatinine, mg/dL	1.0	0.6–1.1
Plasma metanephrine, nmol/L	1.9	<0.5
Plasma normetanephrine, nmol/L	15.0	<0.9
24-Hour urine:		
Metanephrine, mcg	2155	<400
Normetanephrine, mcg	6361	<900
Norepinephrine, mcg	374	<80
Epinephrine, mcg	1.7	<20
Dopamine, mcg	49,662	<400

TREATMENT

Treatment with phenoxybenzamine was started at 10 mg per day and titrated for a low-normal systolic blood pressure. Simultaneous with starting phenoxybenzamine, the patient was placed on a high-sodium diet. The dosage of phenoxybenzamine was increased to 10 mg twice daily. Propranolol extended release 60 mg daily was added 3 days before surgery. The patient underwent an open laparotomy, and the pheochromocytoma was resected intact with great care to avoid tumor capsule rupture. The tumor measured 23 × 16 × 8.5 cm (Fig. 37.2).

OUTCOME AND FOLLOW-UP

The 24-hour urine collected on the fourth postoperative day showed normalization of the 24-hour urine

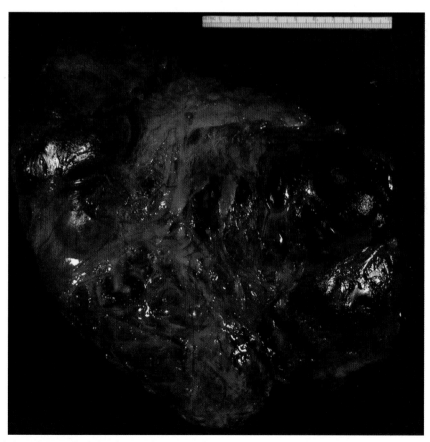

Fig. 37.2 Gross pathology photograph of pheochromocytoma measuring 23 × 16 × 8.5 cm. The tumor was well circumscribed, nearly black, and had no areas of necrosis. On immunohistochemistry the tumor cells were positive for synaptophysin and chromogranin and negative for S-100 and Melan-A.

fractionated metanephrines and catecholamines. For example, the 24-hour urinary dopamine excretion was 204 mcg (normal <400 mcg; preoperatively it was 49,662 mcg). The patient recovered well from the operation and was dismissed from the hospital on the fifth postoperative day. Germline genetic testing did not detect a pathogenic variant in any of the genes known to be associated with PPGL. He was followed with annual measurement of 24-hour urine fractionated metanephrines and catecholamines—these remained normal at last follow-up, which was 12 years after his surgery.

Key Points

- There is a unique subset of patients with PPGL who are asymptomatic despite large tumors and massive catecholamine hypersecretion.[1,2] In this setting clinicians frequently assume that there must be a laboratory error. Although it is unclear why these patients lack symptoms, it may be as a result of the slow growth of the PPGL over decades and catecholamine receptor downregulation.
- Although the laparoscopic approach to adrenalectomy is the procedure of choice for patients with pheochromocytoma, when the pheochromocytomas is large (e.g., >8 cm), the priority is a complete and safe resection without tumor capsule rupture[3]; many times this will require an open laparotomy.

REFERENCES

1. Machairas N, Papaconstantinou D, Papala A, Ioannidis A, Patapis P, Misiakos EP. A huge asymptomatic pheochromocytoma. *Clin Case Rep*. 2018;6(7):1366–1367.
2. Afaneh A, Yang M, Hamza A, Schervish E, Berri R. Surgical management of a giant pheochromocytoma. *In Vivo*. 201;32(3):703–706.
3. Rafat C, Zinzindohoue F, Hernigou A, et al. Peritoneal implantation of pheochromocytoma following tumor capsule rupture during surgery. *J Clin Endocrinol Metab*. 2014;99(12):E2681–E2685.

Metyrosine Use in a Patient With Metastatic Pheochromocytoma

The treatment of choice for pheochromocytoma is complete surgical resection. The success of surgery depends on the experience and expertise of a multidisciplinary team that includes an endocrinologist, endocrine surgeon, and anesthesiologist team. Careful preoperative pharmacologic preparation is crucial for successful treatment and is usually accomplished with combined α- and β-adrenergic blockade to prevent intraoperative hypertensive crises. In certain situations, metyrosine therapy can be used in addition to or instead of α-adrenergic blockade. We describe one such case here.

Case Report

The patient was a 21-year-old man with no significant medical history until the development of acute symptoms that occurred in the setting of physical activity several days before evaluation. While running, he developed a lower extremity pain with muscle cramping. By the time he completed his run, his pain progressed to the abdomen and left lower back, and he vomited. He was transported to the emergency department, where his blood pressure was found to be elevated at 203/117 mmHg, thought to be the result of severe pain. To further evaluate the abdominal pain, computed tomography (CT) of abdomen was performed and revealed a heterogeneous 7-cm left adrenal mass, along with a possible lymphadenopathy and several bony lesions (Fig. 38.1). In retrospect, he recalled progressive symptoms of diaphoresis over several years, without palpitations or headaches. Review of systems was otherwise negative. Family history was negative for any genetic syndromes or pheochromocytomas. The patient was not taking any medications.

On physical examination his body mass index was 26.3 kg/m^2, blood pressure was 130/97 mmHg, and heart rate was 97 beats per minute. He had mild tremor in outstretched fingers. Physical examination was otherwise unrevealing.

INVESTIGATIONS

The laboratory tests confirmed catecholamine excess with a noradrenergic biochemical phenotype (Table 38.1). A 68-gallium DOTATATE positron emission tomography scan was obtained (Fig. 38.2) and revealed heterogeneous

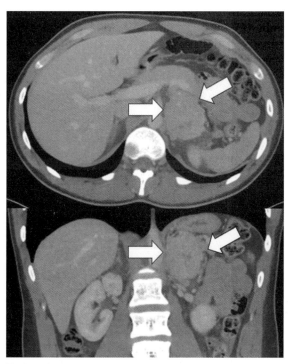

Fig. 38.1 Coronal (*below*) and axial (*above*) images from the contrast-enhanced computed tomography scan demonstrated a heterogeneous left adrenal mass, measuring 7.5 × 6.0 × 6.0–cm mass (*arrows*).

radiotracer uptake in the left adrenal mass (SUVmax of 16.3); a large left retroperitoneal lymph node; and multiple radiotracer avid lytic skeletal metastases in C1, C6, T3, T9, T10, T12 vertebral bodies, sacrum, and right posterior acetabulum.

TABLE 38.1 Laboratory Tests

Biochemical Test	Baseline Result	1 Month After Adrenalectomy Result	Reference Range
Plasma metanephrine, nmol/L	<0.2	<0.2	<0.5
Plasma normetanephrine, nmol/L	15	1.3	<0.9
24-Hour urine:			
Metanephrine, mcg	149	84	<400
Normetanephrine, mcg	9644	1421	<900
Norepinephrine, mcg	1093	125	<80
Epinephrine, mcg	9.2	2.8	<20
Dopamine, mcg	342	332	<400

TREATMENT

Open adrenalectomy was recommended, and α-adrenergic blockade therapy with doxazosin was initiated. However, despite optimal hydration and salt intake, the patient could not tolerate even a small (e.g., 1 mg) dose of doxazosin, developing severe orthostatic symptoms and tachycardia. Metyrosine therapy was initiated with the following protocol: 250 mg every 6 hours on day 1, 500 mg every 6 hours on day 2, 750 mg every 6 hours on day 3, 1000 mg every 6 hours on day 4, with the last dose of 1000 mg on the morning of the surgery.[1] The patient tolerated metyrosine well, with side effects of mild somnolence on the fourth day of therapy. He was treated with open left adrenalectomy and resection of nearby lesions thought to be lymph nodes. Pathology revealed a 7.1 × 6.1 × 5.9–cm pink-tan soft mass located in the medulla, extending beyond the adrenal gland to invade the perirenal fat (Fig. 38.3). Two additional paragangliomas measuring 2.4 cm and 2.5 cm were demonstrated. Immunostains were positive for chromogranin and synaptophysin, and succinate dehydrogenase (SDH) B loss was demonstrated.

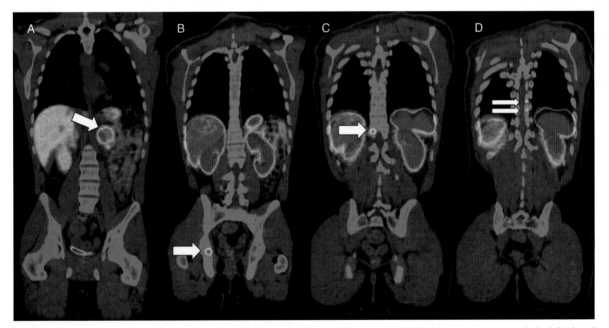

Fig. 38.2 68-Gallium DOTATATE positron emission tomography scan demonstrated a large 7.5-cm lobulated heterogenous mass in the left adrenal (A), with a maximum standard unit value (SUVmax) of 16.3, Krenning score 3 (A–D). Adjacent to left adrenal, lesions (paragangliomas versus lymph nodes) measuring around 2 cm demonstrated poor radiotracer uptake (Krenning score 1); not shown. Multiple radiotracer avid lytic skeletal metastases were noted in C1, C6, T3, T9, T10, T12, sacrum, and right posterior acetabulum (B–D).

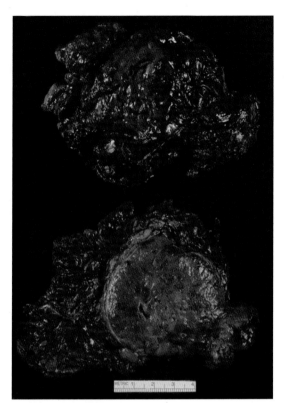

Fig. 38.3 Gross pathology revealed a 7.1 × 6.1 × 5.9–cm pink-tan soft mass located in the medulla, weighing 190 g.

OUTCOME AND FOLLOW-UP

After adrenalectomy, catecholamine excess significantly improved (Table 38.1). Genetic testing revealed a heterozygous variant in *SDHAF2*, c.*12C>T (g.61213555), which was first characterized as variant of uncertain significance and later reclassified as likely benign. He was later treated with cryoablation of vertebral lesions and was initiated on therapy with zoledronic acid 4 mg infused intravenously every 3 months.[2] Stable metastatic disease was demonstrated during subsequent monitoring over 18 months.

Discussion

Resection of the primary tumor is associated with a better prognosis in patients with metastatic pheochromocytoma.[3] Preoperative pharmacologic preparation with α- and β-adrenergic blockade therapy is key to ensuring a successful surgery. Metyrosine is a tyrosine hydroxylase inhibitor, a key enzyme in catecholamine synthesis, that can be considered in patients at high risk for a procedure-related excessive catecholamine release. At our institution, metyrosine was commonly used in patients with anticipated difficult resection (44%), inability to achieve an adequate α-adrenergic blockade (28%), in patients planned to have an ablative procedure of a metastasis (20%), or other indications (<10%).[1] Two-thirds of patients treated with metyrosine report side effects, with most being mild. Drowsiness and fatigue are the most common side effects (19%–94%).[1] Occasionally, extrapyramidal side effects can be seen. Other side effects include anxiety, depression, diarrhea, and weight gain (with longer-term use).[1]

Key Points

- Preoperative pharmacologic preparation with α- and β-adrenergic blockade therapy is key to ensure successful surgery.
- Metyrosine is a tyrosine hydroxylase inhibitor, a key enzyme in catecholamine synthesis.
- Metyrosine is indicated for patients undergoing procedures with anticipated excessive catecholamine release, or when α-adrenergic blockade is inadequate.
- Drowsiness and fatigue are the most common side effects of metyrosine, with more rare side effects including extrapyramidal manifestations and depression.

REFERENCES

1. Gruber LM, Jasim S, Ducharme-Smith A, Weingarten T, Young WF, Bancos I. The role for metyrosine in the treatment of patients with pheochromocytoma and paraganglioma. *J Clin Endocrinol Metab.* 2021;106(6): e2393–e2401.
2. Jeon HL, Oh IS, Baek YH, et al. Zoledronic acid and skeletal-related events in patients with bone metastatic cancer or multiple myeloma. *J Bone Miner Metab.* 2020;38(2):254–263.
3. Hamidi O, Young WF Jr, Iniguez-Ariza NM, et al. Malignant pheochromocytoma and paraganglioma: 272 patients over 55 years. *J Clin Endocrinol Metab.* 2017;102(9):3296–3305.

Case 39

Pheochromocytoma in a Patient With Neurofibromatosis Type 1

Neurofibromatosis type 1 (NF1) is an autosomal dominant disease caused by mutations in the *NF1* gene located on chromosome 17q11.2. Approximately 50% of patients with NF1 present with de novo germline mutations. Clinical diagnosis is based on at least two of the following features: six or more café au lait spots, two or more neurofibromas or one plexiform neurofibroma, freckling in axillae or inguinal areas, optic glioma, two or more Lisch nodules, bony lesions, or a first-degree relative with NF1. Pheochromocytomas can occur in 3% of patients with NF1.[1,2]

Case Report

The patient was a 21-year-old man who presented for evaluation of an 8-cm left adrenal mass. He was diagnosed with NF1 at 6 months of age when café-au-lait spots and neurofibromas were detected on physical examination. He described progressive symptoms of palpitations, anxiety, and headaches for the 9 years prior. Over the last year these symptoms were precipitated by straining, and he also developed abdominal pain. Computed tomography (CT) of the abdomen was obtained to investigate the origin of the abdominal pain and led to the incidental discovery of the adrenal mass. The patient's medical history was positive for attention deficit disorder, and he was not taking any medications. He had no family history of NF1. On physical examination, his blood pressure was 143/92 mmHg, heart rate 80 beats per minute, and body mass index 24.1 kg/m². Café-au lait spots and axillary freckling were visible on examination (Fig. 39.1).

INVESTIGATIONS

Abdominal CT revealed a heterogeneous left adrenal mass of 6.7 × 7.7 × 7.8 cm causing inferior displacement of the left kidney (Fig. 39.2). The right adrenal gland appeared normal. Subsequent I-123 metaiodobenzylguanidine scintigraphy demonstrated increased radiotracer uptake in the left adrenal mass without any additional abnormal radiotracer uptake in the abdomen and pelvis (Fig. 39.3). Preoperative laboratory studies are shown in Table 39.1. The levels of metanephrine in the blood and urine were diagnostic of an adrenergic pheochromocytoma.

TREATMENT

The patient was prepared with the α-adrenergic blocker phenoxybenzamine (30 mg three times daily) and the β-adrenergic blocker propranolol (20 mg three times daily). Left laparoscopic adrenalectomy was performed without complications. The left adrenal gland weighed 275 g (normal, 4–5 g) and contained a 9.5 × 7.5 × 7.0–cm pheochromocytoma (Fig. 39.4). Postoperatively, the adrenergic blockade was discontinued and he was discharged from the hospital. The patient recovered well from surgery. He was recommended to have yearly monitoring for recurrent pheochromocytoma with a 24-hour urine for fractionated catecholamines and metanephrines.

Discussion

The prevalence of pheochromocytoma in patients with NF1 is 3%, and most are discovered incidentally on imaging performed for another reason.[3,4] Bilateral disease can occur in 15%–20% of patients and metastatic or recurrent disease in 7%.[4] Patients demonstrate an adrenergic biochemical profile (predominant elevations in epinephrine and metanephrine).[5] All patients

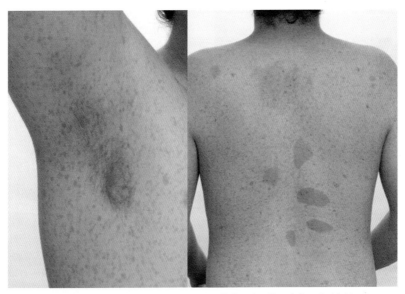

Fig. 39.1 Photographs of axillary freckling (*left*) and café-au-lait spots (*right*).

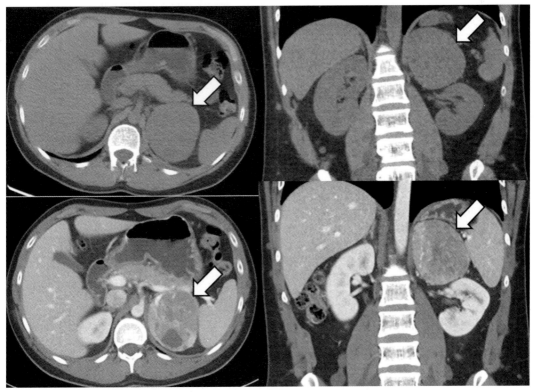

Fig. 39.2 Axial (*left*) and coronal (*right*) unenhanced (*top*) and contrast-enhanced (*bottom*) abdominal computed tomography (CT) scan images showed a left 6.7 × 7.7 × 7.8–cm adrenal mass (*arrows*) causing inferior displacement of the left kidney. The adrenal mass was lipid poor (42 Hounsfield units) on unenhanced CT and heterogeneous on contrast-enhanced CT.

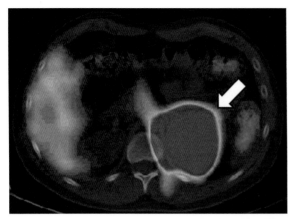

Fig. 39.3 Axial image from fused I-123 metaiodobenzylguanidine (MIBG) computed tomography scan demonstrated intense I-123 MIBG uptake in the left adrenal mass (*arrow*) without additional foci of abnormal radiotracer uptake.

TABLE 39.1 Laboratory Tests		
Biochemical Test	**Result**	**Reference Range**
Plasma metanephrine, nmol/L	12	<0.5
Plasma normetanephrine, nmol/L	31	<0.9
24-Hour urine:		
Metanephrine, mcg	13,532	<400
Normetanephrine, mcg	13,881	<900

with NF1 should undergo biochemical case detection testing for pheochromocytoma every 3 years, before elective surgical procedures, and before pregnancy. Patients with a history of pheochromocytoma should be monitored yearly for recurrence.[4]

Key Points

- Patients with NF1 should undergo biochemical case detection testing for pheochromocytoma every 3 years.
- Bilateral pheochromocytomas can occur in 15%–20% and metastatic or recurrent disease in 7% of patients with NF1.

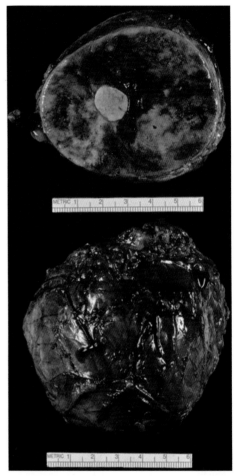

Fig. 39.4 Gross pathology photographs of the left adrenal gland (intact *below* and cut section *above*). The left adrenal gland weighed 275 g (normal, 4–5 g) and contained a 9.5 × 7.5 × 7.0–cm pheochromocytoma. The medullary adrenal mass was heterogeneous, tan-to-mahogany in color, firm, focally cystic, and hemorrhagic; it did not extending beyond the adrenal gland. A region of tumor necrosis was present.

REFERENCES

1. Bausch B, Borozdin W, Neumann HP. European-American Pheochromocytoma Study G. Clinical and genetic characteristics of patients with neurofibromatosis type 1 and pheochromocytoma. *N Engl J Med*. 2006;354(25):2729–2731.

2. National Institutes of Health Consensus Development Conference Statement: neurofibromatosis. Bethesda, MD, USA, July 13-15, 1987. *Neurofibromatosis*. 1988;1(3):172–178.

3. Gruber LM, Hartman RP, Thompson GB, et al. Pheochromocytoma characteristics and behavior differ depending on method of discovery. *J Clin Endocrinol Metab*. 2019;104(5):1386–1393.

4. Gruber LM, Erickson D, Babovic-Vuksanovic D, Thompson GB, Young WF Jr. Bancos I. Pheochromocytoma and paraganglioma in patients with neurofibromatosis type 1. *Clin Endocrinol (Oxf)*. 2017;86(1):141–149.

5. Yan Q, Bancos I, Gruber LM, et al. When biochemical phenotype predicts genotype: pheochromocytoma and paraganglioma. *Am J Med*. 2018;131(5):506–509.

New Diagnosis of Multiple Endocrine Neoplasia Type 2A in a Patient With Bilateral Pheochromocytomas

Multiple endocrine neoplasia type 2A (MEN2A) is an autosomal dominant disorder caused by the mutations in the rearranged during transfection (RET) protein. Patients with MEN2A present with medullary thyroid carcinoma, pheochromocytomas, and primary hyperparathyroidism as a result of parathyroid hyperplasia.

Case Report

The patient was a 39-year-old man who presented with a 2-year history of spells, manifested by a headache, palpitations, and paroxysmal hypertension (as high as 240/120 mmHg). Occasionally these episodes were accompanied by tremor, nausea, and diaphoresis. The spells lasted 10–15 minutes, occurring one to four times a day. Over time, the spells became more intense and more frequent—ultimately leading to his presentation to his primary care physician. Pheochromocytoma was suspected, and workup confirmed catecholamine excess (Table 40.1). He was initiated on lisinopril and amlodipine for hypertension and referred to our institution for further evaluation. He had no family history of pheochromocytoma, thyroid neoplasm, or hypercalcemia. On physical examination, his blood pressure was 148/95 mmHg, heart rate 73 beats per minute, and body mass index 23.3 kg/m^2. His physical examination was normal.

INVESTIGATIONS

Abdominal computed tomography (CT) revealed bilateral adrenal tumors: a 3.9 × 4.2 × 5.2–cm left adrenal mass and a 2.4 × 2.9 × 2.4–cm right adrenal mass (Fig. 40.1). Additional CT findings included bilateral renal cysts and a 5-mm obstructive stone in the left ureter. Review of outside records demonstrated a history of hypercalcemia. Additional laboratory studies were obtained (see Table 40.1). The levels of metanephrines in the blood and urine were diagnostic of adrenergic pheochromocytomas. In addition, calcitonin concentrations were elevated, and workup confirmed primary hyperparathyroidism. Thyroid ultrasound demonstrated a 0.9 × 0.6 × 0.7–cm solid hypoechoic irregular nodule with punctate echogenic foci, with high suspicion for malignancy. Genetic testing confirmed a pathogenic variant in the *RET* gene (c.19OOT>C; p.Cys634Arg).

TREATMENT AND OUTCOME

The patient was advised that his initial surgery should be bilateral adrenalectomy. He was prepared with the α-adrenergic blocker doxazosin (14 mg twice daily)

TABLE 40.1 Laboratory Tests

Biochemical Test	Result	Reference Range
Plasma metanephrine, nmol/L	9	<0.5
Plasma normetanephrine, nmol/L	15	<0.9
Calcitonin, pg/mL	52	<14.3
Parathyroid hormone, pg/mL	179	15–65
Calcium, mg/dL	11.4	8.6–10
24-Hour urine:		
Calcium, mg	410	<250
Metanephrine, mcg	7729	<400
Normetanephrine, mcg	6011	<900

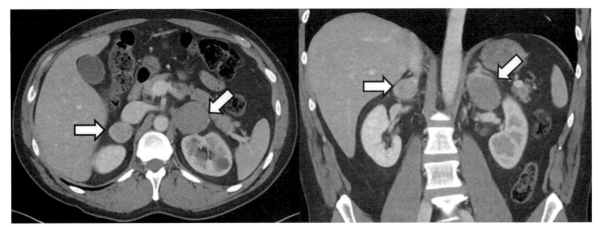

Fig. 40.1 Axial (*left*) and coronal (*right*) contrast-enhanced abdominal computed tomography scan images showed a left 3.9 × 4.2 × 5.2–cm adrenal mass and a right 2.4 × 2.9 × 2.4–cm adrenal mass (*arrows*).

and amlodipine (2.5 mg daily). Initially, cortical sparing adrenalectomy was planned, but given the anatomy, this was not possible, and a complete bilateral laparoscopic adrenalectomy was performed without complications. Pathology confirmed bilateral pheochromocytomas (Fig. 40.2). Postoperatively, therapy with hydrocortisone and fludrocortisone was initiated and the adrenergic blockade was discontinued. Two months later, the patient underwent total thyroidectomy, central lymph node dissection, and a subtotal parathyroidectomy (left superior, left inferior, right inferior parathyroid glands). Medullary thyroid carcinoma (MTC) was present in the right thyroid lobe (0.9 × 0.5 cm), with surgical margins being negative for tumor. A single (1 of 15) lymph node was involved by MTC. Levothyroxine was initiated for treatment of primary iatrogenic hypothyroidism. Postoperatively, the hypercalcemia resolved and the serum calcitonin concentration was undetectable. Monitoring was implemented. After the diagnosis of MEN2A, family members were tested and the patient's 10-year-old daughter was also found to have the same genetic predisposition. She was treated with prophylactic thyroidectomy.

Discussion

MTC is the main cause of morbidity and mortality among the patients with MEN2A.[1,2] Prophylactic total thyroidectomy is recommended in all patients

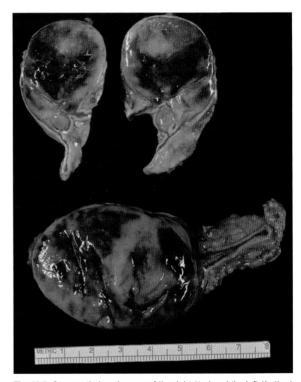

Fig. 40.2 Gross pathology images of the right (*top*) and the left (*bottom*) adrenal glands. The right adrenal gland weighed 16.5 g (normal, 4–5 g) and contained a 3.6 × 2.8 × 2.2–cm pheochromocytoma. The right adrenal mass was red-brown, firm, and located in the medulla. The left adrenal gland weighed 61.6 g and contained a 6.0 × 4.3 × 3.3–cm pheochromocytoma. The left adrenal mass was yellow-brown, necrotic, hemorrhagic, soft mass, and located in the medulla.

early in life.[3] Around half of the patients with MEN2A develop pheochromocytomas. Pheochromocytomas are often multifocal and bilateral, though metastatic pheochromocytoma is extremely unlikely.[4–7] Pheochromocytomas present with an adrenergic biochemical phenotype.[8] Primary hyperparathyroidism occurs in up to 25% of patients with MEN2A and is usually the result of parathyroid hyperplasia. Case detection testing for pheochromocytoma should be performed yearly, as well as before an elective surgical procedure or pregnancy.

Key Points

- Pheochromocytoma in the setting of MEN2A is frequently bilateral.
- All patients with MEN2A need lifelong monitoring for manifestations of MEN2A.

REFERENCES

1. Rohmer V, Vidal-Trecan G, Bourdelot A, et al. Prognostic factors of disease-free survival after thyroidectomy in 170 young patients with a RET germline mutation: a multicenter study of the Groupe Francais d'Etude des Tumeurs Endocrines. *J Clin Endocrinol Metab*. 2011;96(3):E509–E518.

2. Cupisti K, Wolf A, Raffel A, et al. Long-term clinical and biochemical follow-up in medullary thyroid carcinoma: a single institution's experience over 20 years. *Ann Surg*. 2007;246(5):815–821.

3. Wells SA Jr., Asa SL, Dralle H, et al. Revised American Thyroid Association guidelines for the management of medullary thyroid carcinoma. *Thyroid*. 2015;25(6):567–610.

4. Castinetti F, Maia AL, Peczkowska M, et al. The penetrance of MEN2 pheochromocytoma is not only determined by RET mutations. *Endocr Relat Cancer*. 2017;24(8):L63–LL7.

5. Bausch B, Boedeker CC, Berlis A, et al. Genetic and clinical investigation of pheochromocytoma: a 22-year experience, from Freiburg, Germany to international effort. *Ann N Y Acad Sci*. 2006;1073:122–137.

6. Gruber LM, Hartman RP, Thompson GB, et al. Pheochromocytoma characteristics and behavior differ depending on method of discovery. *J Clin Endocrinol Metab*. 2019;104(5):1386–1393.

7. Neumann HPH, Young WF Jr., Eng C. Pheochromocytoma and paraganglioma. *N Engl J Med*. 2019;381(6):552–565.

8. Yan Q, Bancos I, Gruber LM, et al. When biochemical phenotype predicts genotype: pheochromocytoma and paraganglioma. *Am J Med*. 2018;131(5):506–509.

Pheochromocytoma in a Patient With von Hippel-Lindau Disease

Pheochromocytoma and paraganglioma (PPGL) are associated with a genetic predisposition in at least 40% of patients. Von Hippel-Lindau (VHL) disease is an autosomal dominant syndrome that manifests by the retinal, brain, and spine hemangioblastomas; renal cell carcinomas; pheochromocytomas; endolymphatic sac tumors of the middle ear; pancreatic serous cystadenomas; and neuroendocrine tumors of the pancreas. Patients with VHL develop PPGL in up to 18% of cases.[1]

Case Report

The patient was a 20-year-old woman who presented for evaluation of multifocal PPGL. She reported that at 6 years of age, she initially presented with a hypertension-induced seizure secondary to the renal artery stenosis. At 10 years of age, she again presented with hypertension, and at that time was diagnosed with a right adrenal pheochromocytoma that was treated with laparoscopic adrenalectomy. She was symptom free until several months before referral to our institution, when she developed hypertension associated with lightheadedness, diaphoresis, blurry vision, and headaches. Because of her history of pheochromocytoma, a 24-hour urine collection was analyzed for fractionated catecholamines and metanephrines and confirmed noradrenergic-type catecholamine excess (Table 41.1). Computed tomography (CT) of abdomen was performed and demonstrated three arterially enhancing retroperitoneal masses: a 2.7-cm left adrenal mass, a 2.6-cm left paraadrenal mass anterior to the left renal pelvis, and a 2.3-cm right retroperitoneal mass posterior to the inferior vena cava and adjacent to the right renal artery (Fig. 41.1). Her blood pressure was 133/81 mmHg, heart rate 93 beats per minute, and body mass index 34.1 kg/m^2. Family history was positive for a pheochromocytoma in the patient's mother and maternal grandfather.

INVESTIGATIONS

Preoperative laboratory studies are shown in Table 41.1. The levels of normetanephrine in the blood and urine were diagnostic of a noradrenergic catecholamine-secreting tumor(s). In addition to the abdominal CT scan (see Fig. 41.1), outside images from the I-123 metaiodobenzylguanidine (MIBG) scintigraphy were reviewed, demonstrating I-123 MIBG uptake in three regions: (1) a left abdominal lesion possibly arising from the left adrenal gland; (2) a lesion of increased uptake in the left side of the abdomen just inferior to the mass abutting the left adrenal gland and adjacent to the aorta and between the left renal artery and vein; and (3) a region of uptake in the right side of the abdomen (Fig. 41.2). Genetic analysis revealed a pathogenic variant in the exon 1 of the *VHL* gene (c.202 T>C), consistent with VHL disease.

TREATMENT

The patient was prepared with the α-adrenergic blocker doxazosin (total daily dose of 8 mg) and the

TABLE 41.1 Laboratory Tests

Biochemical Test	Result	Reference Range
Plasma metanephrine, nmol/L	<0.2	<0.5
Plasma normetanephrine, nmol/L	7.9	<0.9
24-Hour urine:		
Epinephrine, mcg	1.1	<21
Norepinephrine, mcg	313	15–80
Dopamine, mcg	191	65–400
Metanephrine, mcg	48	<400
Normetanephrine, mcg	4340	<900

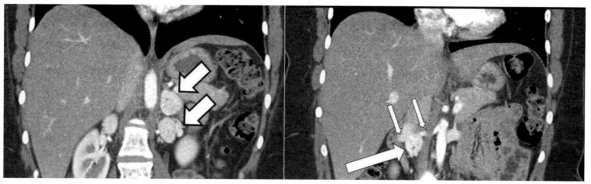

Fig. 41.1 Coronal contrast-enhanced abdominal computed tomography (CT) scan images showed three arterially enhancing retroperitoneal masses: two lesions on the left (a 2.7 × 2.3 × 2.5–cm pheochromocytoma and a 2.1 × 2.6 × 2.5–cm paraganglioma) and one lesion on the right: a 2.3 × 1.2 × 2.1–cm paracaval paraganglioma just inferior to the right renal artery.

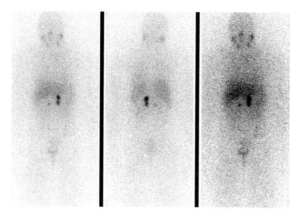

Fig. 41.2 I-123 metaiodobenzylguanidine (MIBG) scintigraphy demonstrated three regions of focal increased MIBG uptake, correlating with computed tomography findings.

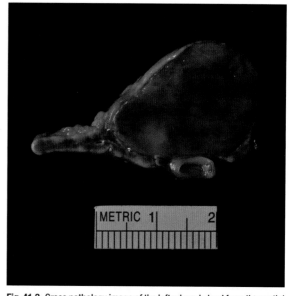

Fig. 41.3 Gross pathology image of the left adrenal gland from the partial left adrenalectomy demonstrated a 2.9 × 2.4 × 2.0–cm pheochromocytoma. Not shown are the 3.2 × 3.0 × 1.7–cm left paraaortic paraganglioma and a 3.0 × 2.5 × 1.5–cm right paracaval paraganglioma.

β-adrenergic blocker propranolol (total daily dose of 40 mg). Open abdominal exploration was performed with a subtotal cortical sparing left adrenalectomy (Fig. 41.3), resection of left paraaortic paraganglioma, and resection of right paracaval paraganglioma. Postoperatively the adrenergic blockade was discontinued, and the patient was dismissed from the hospital on glucocorticoid replacement.

OUTCOME AND FOLLOW-UP

The patient recovered well from surgery. On reassessment of adrenal function, cortisol was excellent at 22 mcg/dL (normal, 7–25 mcg/day), corticotropin (ACTH) was 26 pg/mL (normal, 10–60 pg/mL), and dehydroepiandrosterone sulfate was mid-normal at 148 mcg/dL (normal, 44–332 mcg/dL). Hydrocortisone therapy was discontinued. Postoperative plasma fractionated metanephrines were normal. The patient was advised about the risk for hemangioblastomas of the retina, cerebellum, and spinal cord, pancreatic lesions, renal cancer, and additional PPGLs. Lifelong monitoring for VHL-associated conditions was recommended.

Key Points

- Patients with VHL should be advised on life-long surveillance to ensure an early detection and treatment of VHL-associated manifestations.
- VHL-associated PPGL can be biochemically silent or demonstrate noradrenergic catecholamine excess.[2]
- Prevalence of PPGL in VHL is approximately 18%, with high likelihood of bilateral adrenal or multifocal disease.[1,2]
- Cortical sparing adrenalectomy in patients with VHL can be attempted when technically feasible. In a study that included patients with bilateral pheochromocytomas resulting from VHL disease and multiple endocrine neoplasia type 2, 13% of those treated with cortical sparing adrenalectomy developed another pheochromocytoma within the remnant adrenal after a median of 8 years.[3]
- Success of the cortical sparing adrenalectomy in preserving adrenocortical function is approximately 75%.[3]

REFERENCES

1. Baghai M, Thompson GB, Young WF Jr., Grant CS, Michels VV, van Heerden JA. Pheochromocytomas and paragangliomas in von Hippel-Lindau disease: a role for laparoscopic and cortical-sparing surgery. *Arch Surg.* 2002;137(6):682–688; discussion 8-9.

2. Yan Q, Bancos I, Gruber LM, et al. When biochemical phenotype predicts genotype: pheochromocytoma and paraganglioma. *Am J Med.* 2018;131(5):506–509.

3. Neumann HPH, Tsoy U, Bancos I, et al. Comparison of pheochromocytoma-specific morbidity and mortality among adults with bilateral pheochromocytomas undergoing total adrenalectomy vs cortical-sparing adrenalectomy. *JAMA Netw Open.* 2019;2(8):e198898.

Bilateral Pheochromocytoma in a Patient With MYC-Associated Protein X (*MAX*) Genetic Predisposition

Pheochromocytoma and paraganglioma (PPGL) are associated with a genetic predisposition in at least 40% of patients and likely 100% when presenting with bilateral or multifocal PPGL. Most patients with bilateral pheochromocytomas will prove to have neurofibromatosis type 1, multiple endocrine neoplasia type 2, or von Hippel-Lindau disease.[1] Bilateral pheochromocytoma associated with the loss of function in the *MAX* (MYC-associated factor X) gene represents 1.7% of cases.[1–3]

Case Report

The patient was a 56-year-old man who presented for evaluation of incidentally discovered bilateral adrenal tumors during computed tomography (CT) of chest performed for lung cancer screening. Subsequent abdominal CT demonstrated a 2.8-cm left adrenal mass with an unenhanced CT attenuation of 38 Hounsfield units (HU) and a 3.5-cm right adrenal mass with an unenhanced CT attenuation of 27 HU (Fig. 42.1). Hormonal workup demonstrated catecholamine excess (Table 42.1). Medical history included diabetes mellitus type 2 and hypertension of 5 years, duration. His medication regimen included six antihypertensive medications (amlodipine, benazepril, carvedilol, clonidine, hydrochlorothiazide, and doxazosin) and glyburide and metformin for diabetes mellitus. His blood pressure was 126/83 mmHg, heart rate 72 beats per minute, and body mass index 30.9 kg/m². Family history

was positive for a metastatic pheochromocytoma in his sister, who died of complications from PPGL. His sister did undergo germline mutation testing, which was unrevealing.

INVESTIGATIONS

Preoperative laboratory studies are shown in Table 42.1. The levels of normetanephrine in the blood and urine were diagnostic of noradrenergic pheochromocytoma. An abdominal CT scan showed bilateral adrenal nodules

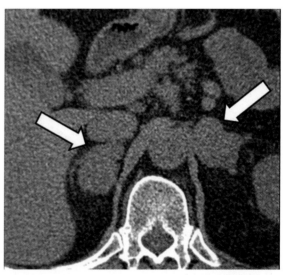

Fig. 42.1 Axial unenhanced adrenal computed tomography (CT) scan image showed a lipid-poor (38 Hounsfield units [HU]) 2.8-cm left adrenal mass (*arrow*) and a lipid-poor (27 HU) 3.5-cm right adrenal mass (*arrow*).

(2.8-cm left adrenal mass and a 3.5-cm right adrenal mass) (Fig. 42.2). I-123 metaiodobenzylguanidine (MIBG) scintigraphy demonstrated intense I-123 MIBG uptake in the bilateral adrenal nodules, without additional foci of abnormal radiotracer uptake. Genetic analysis revealed a pathogenic variant in *MAX* (c.97C>T; p.Arg33*).

TREATMENT

The patient was prepared with the α-adrenergic blocker doxazosin 30 mg daily (dosage titrated up from 2 mg daily) and the β-adrenergic blocker carvedilol (12.5 mg twice daily). Bilateral laparoscopic adrenalectomy was planned: cortical sparing on the right and complete on the left. The right adrenal gland weighed 26 g (normal, 4–5 g) and contained a 4.1 × 2.6 × 2.2–cm brown soft pheochromocytoma. The left adrenal gland

weighed 39 g and contained two distinct nodules, one 3.9 × 3.7 × 2.7–cm solid red-brown soft mass in central medulla, and a 3.0 × 2.7 × 2.7 cm cystic red-brown mass at the periphery: both left adrenal nodules were pheochromocytomas (Fig. 42.3). Postoperatively the adrenergic blockade was discontinued and the patient was dismissed from the hospital on glucocorticoid replacement.

OUTCOME AND FOLLOW-UP

The patient recovered well from surgery. On reassessment of adrenal function, he continued to demonstrate glucocorticoid deficiency but not mineralocorticoid deficiency. He continued with hydrocortisone therapy and stopped fludrocortisone. He had not developed additional PPGLs when last seen 3 years after surgery.

Discussion

PPGL can occur in patients with loss of function in the *MAX* (MYC-associated factor X) gene, representing approximately 1% of all cases and 1.7% of patients with bilateral pheochromocytoma.[1–3] The *MAX* gene is located on chromosome 14q23.3 and encodes *MAX* protein that acts as tumor suppressor. Patients usually present with pheochromocytomas that could be bilateral or multifocal in 50%–60% of cases and malignant in up to 25%.[2] Lifelong monitoring is required.

TABLE 42.1 Laboratory Tests		
Biochemical Test	**Result**	**Reference Range**
Plasma metanephrine, nmol/L	0.3	<0.5
Plasma normetanephrine, nmol/L	17	<0.9
24-Hour urine:		
Metanephrine, mcg	259	<400
Normetanephrine, mcg	4882	<900

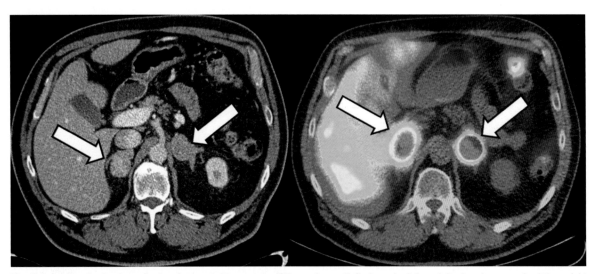

Fig. 42.2 Axial contrast-enhanced adrenal computed tomography (CT) scan image (*left*) showed a 2.8-cm left adrenal mass and a 3.5-cm right adrenal mass (*left*). I-123 metaiodobenzylguanidine (MIBG) scintigraphy demonstrated intense I-123 MIBG uptake in bilateral adrenal nodules (*right*), without additional foci of abnormal radiotracer uptake.

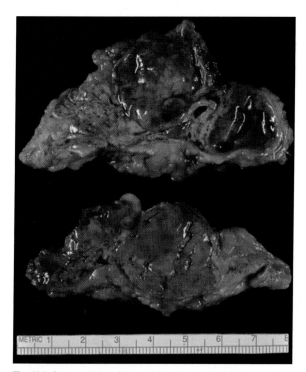

Fig. 42.3 Gross pathology image of the left adrenal gland (*above*) and the right adrenal gland (*below*). The left adrenal gland weighed 39 g (normal, 4–5 g) and contained two distinct nodules: a 3.9 × 3.7 × 2.7–cm solid red-brown soft pheochromocytoma in the central medulla and a 3.0 × 2.7 × 2.7–cm cystic red-brown pheochromocytoma at the periphery. The right adrenal gland weighed 26 g and contained a 4.1 × 2.6 × 2.2–cm brown soft pheochromocytoma.

Key Points

- Pheochromocytoma in the setting of *MAX* can be bilateral or multifocal in 50%–60% of cases.
- Cortical sparing adrenalectomy in patients with *MAX* can be attempted when technically feasible. The data on long-term outcomes of patients with *MAX* are not available; however, in a study that included patients with bilateral pheochromocytomas resulting from von Hippel-Lindau disease and multiple endocrine neoplasia type 2, 13% of those treated with cortical sparing adrenalectomy developed another pheochromocytoma within the remnant adrenal after a median of 8 years.[1]
- The success of the cortical sparing adrenalectomy in preserving adrenocortical function is approximately 75%.[1]

REFERENCES

1. Neumann HPH, Tsoy U, Bancos I, et al. Comparison of pheochromocytoma-specific morbidity and mortality among adults with bilateral pheochromocytomas undergoing total adrenalectomy vs cortical-sparing adrenalectomy. *JAMA Netw Open.* 2019;2(8):e198898.
2. Comino-Mendez I, Gracia-Aznarez FJ, Schiavi F, et al. Exome sequencing identifies *MAX* mutations as a cause of hereditary pheochromocytoma. *Nat Genet.* 2011;43(7):663–667.
3. Brito JP, Asi N, Bancos I, et al. Testing for germline mutations in sporadic pheochromocytoma/paraganglioma: a systematic review. *Clin Endocrinol (Oxf).* 2015;82(3):338–345.

The Cystic Pheochromocytoma

As pheochromocytomas enlarge, they develop areas of hemorrhagic necrosis. Most pheochromocytomas >4 cm in diameter have some cystic component that is evident on computed cross-sectional imaging. Some pheochromocytomas become progressively cystic to the point that the radiologist interprets them as adrenal cysts. Such a case is reported herein.

Case Report

The patient was a 50-year-old woman who presented with persistent and recurrent emesis that led to abdominal computed tomography (CT). Incidentally discovered on the CT scan was a 7 × 8.3–cm cystic right adrenal mass (Fig. 43.1). The patient was morbidly obese (body mass index 51.6 kg/m^2). She had well-controlled hypertension of 7 years, duration that was treated with a β-adrenergic blocker (atenolol 100 mg daily) and an angiotensin receptor antagonist (valsartan 80 mg daily). She also had type 2 diabetes mellitus diagnosed 5 years previously and treated with metformin 500 mg once daily. Her blood pressure was 136/76 mmHg and heart rate was 76 beats per minute.

INVESTIGATIONS

The plasma fractionated metanephrines and 24-hour urine for fractionated metanephrines and catecholamines unequivocally confirmed the diagnosis of pheochromocytoma (Table 43.1).

TREATMENT

Treatment with valsartan was discontinued, and phenoxybenzamine was started at 10 mg per day and titrated for a low normal systolic blood pressure. The atenolol was continued at the same dosage. The patient was started on a high-sodium diet for volume expansion and to prevent orthostasis. Blood pressure was monitored daily in the outpatient setting, and 8 days later she went to surgery with open approach for right adrenalectomy (Fig. 43.2). An open surgical approach was favored over the laparoscopic approach to avoid intraoperative rupture of the cystic pheochromocytoma. Tumor rupture during surgical resection can be a fatal

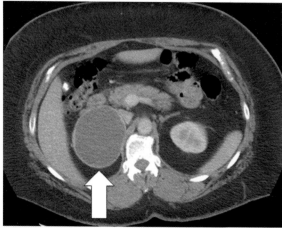

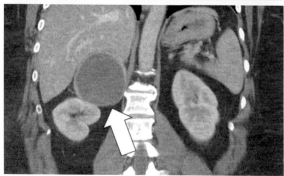

Fig. 43.1 Axial image (*upper*) and coronal image (*lower*) from a contrast-enhanced computed tomography scan. The cystic right adrenal mass (*arrows*) measured 7.0 × 8.3 cm.

TABLE 43.1 Laboratory Tests

Biochemical Test	Result	Reference Range
Sodium, mmol/L	141	135–145
Potassium, mmol/L	4.0	3.6–5.2
Creatinine, mg/dL	0.8	0.6–1.04
Glycosylated hemoglobin, %	7.0	4.2–5.6
Plasma metanephrine, nmol/L	1.1	<0.5
Plasma normetanephrine, nmol/L	14.0	<0.9
Aldosterone, ng/dL	10	≤21 ng/dL
Plasma renin activity ng/mL per hour	14	≤0.6–3
24-Hour urine:		
Metanephrine, mcg	1022	<400
Normetanephrine, mcg	6761	<900
Norepinephrine, mcg	239	<80
Epinephrine, mcg	9.1	<20
Dopamine, mcg	219	<400

complication—there is peritoneal and retroperitoneal dissemination leading to peritoneal carcinomatosis and metastatic disease.[1] Phenoxybenzamine was stopped the day after surgery. The patient was discharged from the hospital on the fourth postoperative day. She declined to pursue germline genetic testing.

OUTCOME AND FOLLOW-UP

One week after surgery the plasma fractionated metanephrines were normal with a metanephrine of <0.2 nmol/L (normal, <0.5) and normetanephrine 0.86 nmol/L. Three months after surgery her blood pressure was under excellent control on monotherapy (atenolol 50 mg daily). She continued on low-dose metformin (500 mg once daily), and her glycosylated hemoglobin was improved (6.4%). Plasma fractionated metanephrines remained normal when checked annually. She died from metastatic endometrial cancer 8 years after her adrenalectomy.

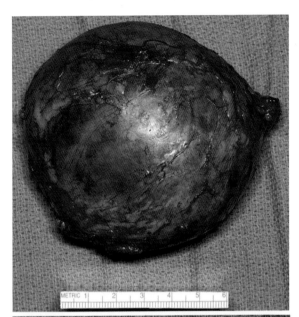

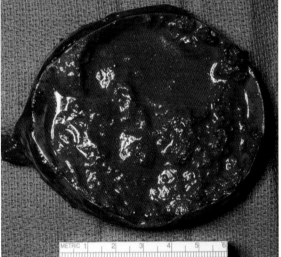

Fig. 43.2 Gross pathology image of right adrenal gland containing a pheochromocytoma forming a cystic adrenal mass measuring 9.4 × 8.2 × 6.6 cm with extensive hemorrhagic necrosis. Intact surgical specimen is shown in the upper panel and bisected pheochromocytoma showing hemorrhagic necrosis is shown in the lower panel.

Key Points

- Most pheochromocytomas >4 cm in diameter have some cystic component resulting from hemorrhage necrosis.
- Beware of the adrenal cyst! Large pheochromocytomas can be nearly totally cystic.[2–5] All patients with adrenal cysts should have biochemical testing for pheochromocytoma.
- If a patient is on a β-adrenergic blocker when diagnosed with pheochromocytoma, don't stop it—simply add α-adrenergic blockade with a target low-normal systolic blood pressure for age.

REFERENCES

1. Rafat C, Zinzindohoue F, Hernigou A, et al. Peritoneal implantation of pheochromocytoma following tumor capsule rupture during surgery. *J Clin Endocrinol Metab.* 2014;99(12):E2681–E2685.

2. Cajipe KM, Gonzalez G, Kaushik D. Giant cystic pheochromocytoma. *BMJ Case Rep.* 2017;2017:bcr2017222264.

3. Kumar S, Parmar KM, Aggarwal D, Jhangra K. Simple adrenal cyst masquerading clinically silent giant cystic pheochromocytoma. *BMJ Case Rep.* 2019;12(9):e230730.

4. Gupta A, Bains L, Agarwal MK, Gupta R. Giant cystic pheochromocytoma: a silent entity. *Urol Ann.* 2016;8(3):384–386.

5. Wang HL, Sun BZ, Xu ZJ, Lei WF, Wang XS. Undiagnosed giant cystic pheochromocytoma: a case report. *Oncol Lett.* 2015;10(3):1444–1446.

Skull Base and Neck Paragangliomas: Considerations for the Endocrinologist

Paragangliomas (PGLs) arise from paraganglia in the parasympathetic and sympathetic chains, which track along large blood vessels. PGLs can be found from the skull base and inner ear to the scrotum. Most skull base and neck PGLs have a parasympathetic origin and are biochemically nonfunctioning. However, 3%–5% of skull base and neck PGLs are of sympathetic origin and can hypersecrete dopamine and/or norepinephrine.[1] The considerations for the endocrinologist when seeing a patient with a skull base and/or neck PGL include addressing the following questions: (1) Is the PGL hypersecreting catecholamines; (2) does the patient have a germline pathogenic variant in a gene that predisposes to PGLs; (3) does the PGL have associated metastatic disease; and (4) are there additional PGLs elsewhere in the body?

Case Report

The patient was a 46-year-old woman seen in endocrine consultation for a large right neck glomus vagale PGL. She had noticed "a knot in my right neck" for about 10 years. It had been attributed by physicians to "swollen glands" over the years. Recently she developed symptoms of episodic heart racing. In addition, although usually normotensive, she had episodic elevated blood pressure (e.g., 188/110 mmHg). To investigate the neck mass, magnetic resonance imaging (MRI) was performed elsewhere and detected a large right glomus vagale PGL. On physical examination her body mass index was 26.8 kg/m^2, blood pressure was 140/86 mmHg, and heart rate was 77 beats per minute. Palpation of the neck revealed a mass high in the neck that extended under the angle of the mandible.

INVESTIGATIONS

The plasma fractionated metanephrines and 24-hour urine for fractionated metanephrines and catecholamines were normal (Table 44.1). Skull base and neck PGLs should always be screened for dopamine hypersecretion.[1-3] A clinical pearl not well known to most endocrinologists is that because of the high sulfation rate of dopamine at the kidney, 24-hour urine for measurement of dopamine may be unreliable. Thus either plasma dopamine or methoxytyramine should be measured. Plasma catecholamines were obtained from in indwelling cannula after the patient was in the supine position and rested condition for 30 minutes. Despite the normal 24-hour urinary excretion of dopamine, the plasma dopamine concentration was more than 19-fold above the upper limit of the reference range (see Table 44.1).

TABLE 44.1 Laboratory Tests		
Biochemical Test	**Result**	**Reference Range**
Sodium, mmol/L	139	135–145
Potassium, mmol/L	4.2	3.6–5.2
Creatinine, mg/dL	0.9	0.6–1.1
Plasma metanephrine, nmol/L	1.1	<0.5
Plasma normetanephrine, nmol/L	14.0	<0.9
Plasma norepinephrine, pg/mL	388	<750
Plasma epinephrine, pg/mL	<25	<111
Plasma dopamine, pg/mL	575	<30
24-Hour urine:		
Metanephrine, mcg	129	<400
Normetanephrine, mcg	263	<900
Norepinephrine, mcg	35	<80
Epinephrine, mcg	5.7	<20
Dopamine, mcg	333	<400

All patients with PGLs should be offered germline genetic testing for pathogenic variants in the succinate dehydrogenase subunits (SDHx).[4] She proved to have a pathogenic variant in SDH subunit B (*SDHB*; p.V140F).

Skull base and neck MRI showed a 2.8 × 5.3 × 2.9–cm right glomus vagale PGL (Fig. 44.1). As the result of her *SDHB* mutation, risk for more than one PGL, and potential for metastases from her known neck PGL, 123-I metaiodobenzylguanidine (MIBG) scintigraphy and MRI of the abdomen and pelvis were obtained. No additional PGLs or sites of metastatic disease were found.

TREATMENT

Treatment with phenoxybenzamine was started at 10 mg per day and titrated for a low-normal systolic blood pressure. Three days later, metoprolol extended release was added for a target heart rate of 80 beats per minute. Preoperative tumor embolization was planned. In addition to α- and β-adrenergic blockade, α-methyl-paratyrosine (metyrosine) was added to her treatment program 4 days before the ablation. Metyrosine blocks tyrosine hydroxylase and inhibits the synthesis of catecholamines and was added in an effort to attenuate a potential massive release of dopamine with the embolization.[3,5,6] Selective catheterization of branches off the right ascending pharyngeal artery and two branches of the right occipital artery was performed with microcatheter technique, and tumor embolization was completed with polyvinyl alcohol foam particles (250–350 μm). Approximately 80% of the tumor was embolized. Fortunately, blood pressure control was acceptable during and after the embolization.

Surgery was performed the day after embolization. The tumor could be seen originating from the vagus nerve (Fig. 44.2). Great care was taken to protect as much as possible the vagus, hypoglossal, cervical sympathetic, and spinal accessory nerves.

OUTCOME AND FOLLOW-UP

After the surgery she had hypoglossal and vagal nerve dysfunction and right vocal cord paralysis. The day after surgery she had injection laryngoplasty into the right vocal cord with Cymetra (a micronized particulate injectable form of acellular human dermis) to achieve medialization and to improve her voice and swallowing.

At her last follow-up (1 year after surgery), her plasma fractionated catecholamines remained normal (including dopamine, <10 pg/mL [normal, <30]). The concept of life-long surveillance to look for PGL recurrence of metastatic disease was reinforced. She was informed that metastatic disease can appear as much as 50 years after surgery.[7] She was also counseled on the need for long-term surveillance for new PGLs associated with her *SDHB* pathogenic variant. We advised the following: (1) annual biochemical testing

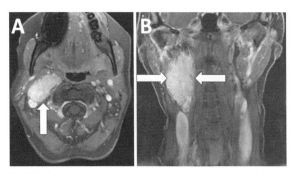

Fig. 44.1 Axial (A) and coronal (B) magnetic resonance images of the neck. Within the right neck there was a large (2.8 × 5.3 × 2.9 cm) hypervascular mass (*arrows*) displacing the internal and external carotid arteries anteriorly and consistent with a glomus vagale paraganglioma.

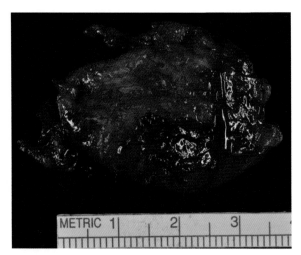

Fig. 44.2 Gross pathology photograph of right neck vagal paraganglioma forming a 3.3 × 2.5 × 1.2–cm tan-red fibrous mass. On immunohistochemistry the tumor cells were positive for synaptophysin and chromogranin. The S-100 immunostain highlighted the sustentacular cells.

with plasma fractionated metanephrines and catechol-amines for life, (2) MRI of her skull base and neck annually for 5 years and then every 2–3 years thereafter, (3) MRI of the abdomen and pelvis every 2–3 years, (4) MRI of the chest every 5 years, and (5) total body imaging with either 18-F fluorodeoxyglucose positron emission tomography (PET) CT or gallium 68 (68-Ga) 1,4,7,10-tetraazacyclododecane-1,4,7,10-tetraacetic acid (DOTA)-octreotate (DOTATATE) PET CT every 5 years to screen for metastatic disease or PGLs not detected with MRI.

Key Points

- All patients with skull base and neck PGLs should be screened for dopamine hypersecretion with measurement of plasma fractionated catecholamines or plasma methoxytyramine. Because of the high sulfation rate of dopamine at the kidney, 24-hour urine for measurement of dopamine may not be reliable in some patients with dopamine-secreting tumors. However, when 24-hour urinary dopamine is >700 mcg, it is diagnostic of a dopamine-secreting tumor (see Case 37) or a patient taking an interfering medication (e.g., levodopa).
- All patients with PGLs should be offered germline genetic testing.
- Patients with dopamine-secreting PGLs should be prepared for surgery exactly the same way patients with norepinephrine or epinephrine tumors are prepared—with α- and β-adrenergic blockade.
- If preoperative embolization of a functioning PGL is planned, the patient should be prepared with α-methyl-para-tyrosine (metyrosine) to deplete the PGL of catecholamine stores.

REFERENCES

1. Erickson D, Kudva YC, Ebersold MJ, et al. Benign paragangliomas: clinical presentation and treatment outcomes in 236 patients. *J Clin Endocrinol Metab.* 2001;86(11):5210–5216.
2. Foo SH, Chan SP, Ananda V, Rajasingam V. Dopamine-secreting phaeochromocytomas and paragangliomas: clinical features and management. *Singapore Med J.* 2010;51(5):e89–e93.
3. Dubois LA, Gray DK. Dopamine-secreting pheochromocytomas: in search of a syndrome. *World J Surg.* 2005;29(7):909–913.
4. Neumann HPH, Young WF Jr., Eng C. Pheochromocytoma and paraganglioma. *N Engl J Med.* 2019;381(6):552–565.
5. Butz JJ, Weingarten TN, Cavalcante AN, et al. Perioperative hemodynamics and outcomes of patients on metyrosine undergoing resection of pheochromocytoma or paraganglioma. *Int J Surg.* 2017;46:1–6.
6. Deljou A, Kohlenberg JD, Weingarten TN, et al. Hemodynamic instability during percutaneous ablation of extra-adrenal metastases of pheochromocytoma and paragangliomas: a case series. *BMC Anesthesiol.* 2018;18(1):158.
7. Hamidi O, Young WF Jr., Iñiguez-Ariza NM, et al. Malignant pheochromocytoma and paraganglioma: 272 patients over 55 years. *J Clin Endocrinol Metab.* 2017;102(9):3296–3305.

Cardiac Paraganglioma

Catecholamine-secreting tumors (pheochromocytoma and paraganglioma [PPGL]) can be found in the midline from the inner ear to the scrotum. However, most (≈85%) are located in the adrenal glands and 95% are between the diaphragm and pubis. Cardiac PGL is an unusual and challenging location. Such a case is reported herein.

Case Report

The patient was a 43-year-old woman who had been diagnosed with multiple PGLs 13 years before the current consultation. However, she previously declined surgical intervention because of the operative risks. She went on to have three pregnancies; two were successful live births, and cesarean deliveries were performed as the result of marked hypertension in the third trimester. Her hypertension was poorly controlled on a calcium channel blocker (amlodipine 5 mg daily) and a combined β- and α-adrenergic blocker (labetalol 400 mg twice daily). She also had insulin-requiring type 2 diabetes mellitus under poor glycemic control. On physical examination her body mass index was 24.5 kg/m², blood pressure 124/81 mmHg, and heart rate 75 beats per minute. The patient was not in respiratory distress, and examination of her heart and lungs was normal. She wanted to reconsider surgical management of her PGLs.

INVESTIGATIONS

The plasma fractionated metanephrines and 24-hour urine for fractionated metanephrines and catecholamines unequivocally confirmed the diagnosis of catecholamine-secreting PPGL (Table 45.1). Chest magnetic resonance imaging (MRI) showed a 6.8 × 4.3–cm hypervascular pericardial PGL in the right atrioventricular groove that encased 50% of the ascending aorta and also encased the origin of the right coronary artery (Fig. 45.1). Abdominal computed tomography (CT) angiography showed a 4.7 × 3.3–cm organ of Zuckerkandl PGL and a 1.9-cm urinary bladder PGL (Fig. 45.2). F-18 fluorodeoxyglucose positron emission tomography CT showed the three known PGLs and no evidence of additional paragangliomas or metastatic disease (Fig. 45.3). The patient proved to have a large gene deletion in succinate dehydrogenase subunit B (deletion of exons 3–8).

TREATMENT

It was decided to address the cardiac paraganglioma first. Doxazosin 1 mg twice daily was added to her medication program and titrated for a low-normal systolic blood pressure. She was started on a high-sodium diet for volume expansion and to prevent orthostasis.

TABLE 45.1 Laboratory Tests		
Biochemical Test	Result	Reference Range
Sodium, mmol/L	140	135–145
Potassium, mmol/L	5.3	3.6–5.2
Creatinine, mg/dL	0.61	0.6–1.04
Glycosylated hemoglobin, %	9.4	4.2–5.6
Plasma metanephrine, nmol/L	0.21	<0.5
Plasma normetanephrine, nmol/L	28.0	<0.9
24-Hour urine:		
Metanephrine, mcg	230	<400
Normetanephrine, mcg	9859	<900
Norepinephrine, mcg	2744	<80
Epinephrine, mcg	8.2	<20
Dopamine, mcg	1036	<400

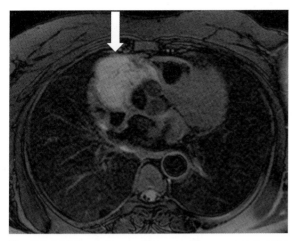

Fig. 45.1 Axial image from cardiac magnetic resonance imaging showed a 6.8 × 4.3–cm hypervascular pericardial mass (*arrow*) in the right atrioventricular groove that extended from the right cardiophrenic angle inferiorly to the periascending aorta space superiorly. The mass caused external compression to the right atrium and ventricle and encased approximately 50% of the ascending aortic diameter and also encased the right coronary artery from its origin.

Blood pressure was monitored daily. To decrease the cardiac PGL catecholamine stores, treatment with α-methylparatyrosine (metyrosine) was started 4 days before surgery at an escalating daily dosage (250 mg every 6 hours on day 1; 500 mg every 6 hours on day 2; 750 mg every 6 hours on day 3; 1000 mg every 6 hours on day 4; and 1000 mg orally on morning of surgery). The patient was placed on cardiopulmonary bypass for 56 minutes while the cardiac PGL was resected. The right atrioventricular groove PGL surrounded the right coronary artery at its origin; however, it did not invade the vessel, and the PGL (Fig. 45.4) was resected without injury to the right coronary artery. A large portion of the right atrium was resected and repaired primarily. Postoperative complications included a right plural effusion and paroxysmal atrial fibrillation.

OUTCOME AND FOLLOW-UP

Six months after surgery her blood pressure was well controlled on α- and β-adrenergic blockade. She no longer required insulin treatment for diabetes mellitus, and her glycosylated hemoglobin improved to 6.4%. At the time of this report, the patient had not returned for resection of the abdominal and urinary bladder PGLs. This patient was operated in 2019 and not included in

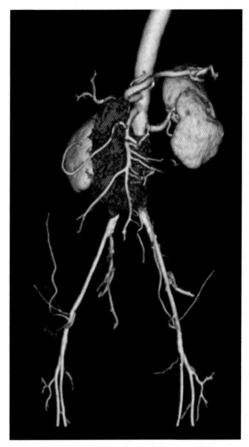

Fig. 45.2 Coronal image from computed tomography angiography showed a 4.7 × 3.3–cm organ of Zuckerkandl paraganglioma (*colored in purple*) closely associated with the infrarenal abdominal aorta and involved approximately 50% of the anterior, posterior, and right-sided aortic wall without invasion into the lumen. There was also partial encasement of the inferior vena cava involving 50% of the anterior and left-sided vessel wall. The mass also encased the proximal inferior mesenteric artery.

our review of 22 patients with intrathoracic PGL operated from 2000 to 2015.[1] Sixteen patients (73%) had functioning tumors (11, noradrenergic; 4, mixed noradrenergic and dopaminergic; 1, dopaminergic). All patients with functioning tumors received preoperative adrenergic blockade, and 13 (59%) were prepared for surgery with metyrosine. Ten patients required cardiopulmonary bypass. Of these, one patient had uncontrollable bleeding and died intraoperatively. Median follow-up was 8.2 years (range, 2.1–17.2). Six patients subsequently had metastatic disease, and of them one died 6 years after the operation.[1]

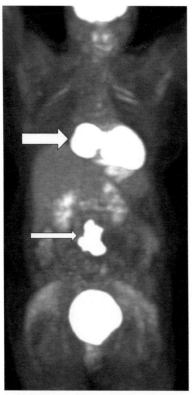

Fig. 45.3 F-18 fluorodeoxyglucose positron emission tomography computed tomography coronal image showed three intensely hypermetabolic paragangliomas: (1) hypermetabolic (maximum standard unit value [SUVmax] 21.3) $7 \times 5.3 \times 6.9$–cm right anterior pericardial mass (*large arrow*); (2) hypermetabolic (SUVmax 25.4) $5.8 \times 5 \times 4.2$–cm lobulated mass (*small arrow*) involving the infrarenal aortocaval region with extension to the aortic bifurcation; and (3) 2×1.7–cm intensely hypermetabolic (SUVmax 15.9) mass along the anterior-inferior wall the urinary bladder (obscured by urinary bladder on this coronal image).

Key Points

- All patients with a PGL should have total body imaging to detect additional PGLs.

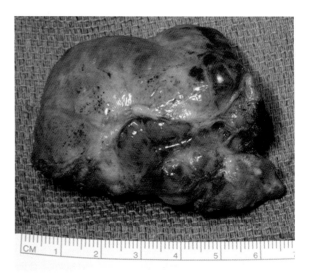

Fig. 45.4 Gross pathology photograph of cardiac paraganglioma. It consisted of a gray-tan, well-circumscribed, rubbery mass measuring $7.0 \times 5.3 \times 3.5$ cm with a focally hemorrhagic and solid cut surface.

- All patients with PGL should be offered germline genetic testing to detect pathogenic variants in genes that predispose to PGL.
- Cardiac PGLs are potentially resectable but represent a high-risk subset of patients and should be referred to centers with experience in managing this rare subtype.
- Preoperative treatment with a tyrosine hydroxylase inhibitor is helpful in the surgical management of cardiac PGLs.

REFERENCE

1. Gurrieri C, Butz JJ, Weingarten TN, et al. Resection of intrathoracic paraganglioma with and without cardiopulmonary bypass. *Ann Thorac Surg*. 2018;105(4):1160–1167.

Pheochromocytoma in Multiple Endocrine Neoplasia Type 2B

Multiple endocrine neoplasia type 2B (MEN2B) is an autosomal dominant disorder with age-related penetrance, and it represents approximately 5% of all MEN2 cases. MEN2B is characterized by medullary thyroid carcinoma (MTC) in all patients, adrenergic (epinephrine and metanephrine predominant) pheochromocytoma in 50%, mucocutaneous neuromas (typically involving the tongue, lips, and eyelids) in most patients, and by skeletal deformities (e.g., kyphoscoliosis, lordosis), joint laxity, myelinated corneal nerves, and intestinal ganglioneuromas.[1,2] MEN2B-associated tumors are caused by mutations in the rearranged during transfection (RET) protein's intracellular domain. A single methionine-to-threonine missense pathogenic variant in exon 16 (p.Met918Thr; c.2753T>C) of the *RET* protooncogene is responsible for more than 95% of MEN2B cases. Another pathogenic variant, alanine to phenylalanine at codon 883 in exon 15 of the *RET* protooncogene, has been found in 4% of MEN2B cases.

Case Report

The patient was a 19-year-old man who had been troubled by episodic tachycardia of 10 minutes duration and occurring every other day for the past 1 year. At age 12 he was diagnosed with MEN2B when an ophthalmologist detected enlarged corneal nerves, which led to germline genetic testing that documented a pathogenic variant in the *RET* protooncogene (p.Met918Thr; c.2753T>C). As with most patients with MEN2B, no one else in the family carried the mutation.[1,2] Other stigmata of MEN2B were clearly evident, including mucocutaneous neuromas of the lips and tongue (Fig. 46.1). At age 12 he underwent thyroidectomy for bilateral multicentric medullary thyroid carcinoma (MTC). Four lymph

nodes contained metastatic MTC. The preoperative serum calcitonin concentration was 970 pg/mL and after surgery it improved to 41 pg/mL (normal, <15.9 pg/mL). At 15 years of age he underwent right adrenalectomy for multifocal pheochromocytoma ($2 \times 1.5 \times 1.2$ cm and 0.5 cm). He took no regular medications. What was of the most concern to the patient was the tongue mucocutaneous neuromas that were a constant irritation because he would inadvertently bite them. His blood pressure was 118/55 mm Hg, heart rate 68 beats per minute, and body mass index 18.6 kg/m^2.

INVESTIGATIONS

Preoperative laboratory studies are shown in Table 46.1. The levels of metanephrine in the blood and urine were diagnostic of an adrenergic pheochromocytoma. Serum calcitonin was elevated at 168 pg/mL (normal, <15.9 pg/mL) and consistent with metastatic MTC. Adrenal computed tomography (CT) scan showed a multinodular left adrenal gland (Fig. 46.2). Neck ultrasound and CT of the chest, abdomen, and pelvis did not localize the sites of persistent MTC.

TREATMENT

The patient was prepared with the α-adrenergic blocker phenoxybenzamine 10 mg daily and the β-adrenergic blocker propranolol extended release 60 mg daily. The patient underwent laparoscopic left adrenalectomy. The adrenal gland weighed 12.75 g and contained multifocal pheochromocytoma (Fig. 46.3). During the same anesthetic event the patient had a partial anterior glossectomy ($6.2 \times 3.1 \times 1.7$ cm), which contained more than 10 submucosal neuromas ranging in size from 0.1 to 0.4 cm in diameter. Postoperatively the adrenergic blockade was discontinued and he was dismissed from the hospital on standard glucocorticoid and mineralocorticoid replacement.

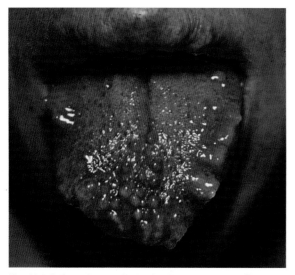

Fig. 46.1 Patient photograph showing innumerable mucocutaneous neuromas of the tongue and upper lip.

TABLE 46.1	Laboratory Tests	
Biochemical Test	**Result**	**Reference Range**
Sodium, mmol/L	141	135–145
Potassium, mmol/L	4.2	3.6–5.2
Creatinine, mg/dL	1.1	0.8–1.3
Plasma metanephrine, nmol/L	1.47	<0.5
Plasma normetanephrine, nmol/L	1.38	<0.9
Serum calcitonin, pg/mL	168	<15.9
24-Hour urine:		
Metanephrine, mcg	490	<400
Normetanephrine, mcg	328	<900
Norepinephrine, mcg	28	<80
Epinephrine, mcg	4.5	<20
Dopamine, mcg	182	<400

OUTCOME AND FOLLOW-UP

The patient recovered well from surgery. When he was last seen 4 years after surgery, plasma fractionated metanephrines were normal. The serum calcitonin remained elevated at 196 pg/mL (normal, <15.9 pg/mL).

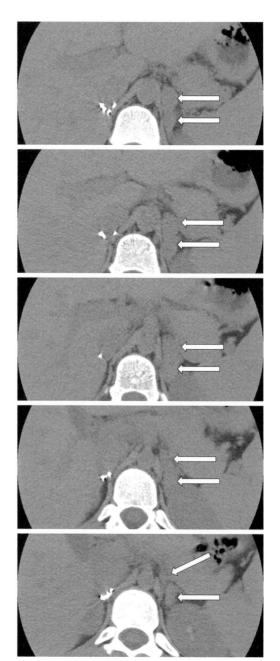

Fig. 46.2 Serial axial (cranial at the top and caudal at the bottom) unenhanced computed tomography scan images showing a 3.0 × 1.3 cm multinodular lipid-poor (42.1 Hounsfield units) left adrenal mass *(arrows)*. Surgical clips from previous right adrenalectomy can be seen in the right adrenal bed.

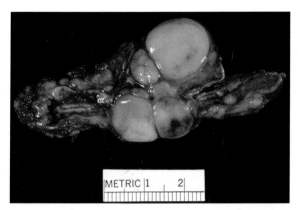

Fig. 46.3 Gross pathology image of the left adrenal gland that weighed 12.75 g (normal, 4–5 g). Eight separate pheochromocytomas can be seen (0.3–1.6 cm in diameter).

Key Points

- Pheochromocytoma in the setting of MEN2B and MEN2A is typically not solitary but rather multifocal and associated with medullary hyperplasia.
- Although there are advocates for cortical-sparing adrenalectomy in patients with MEN2B and MEN2A, a surgeon cannot leave viable cortex without leaving behind adrenal medulla. Thus the risk of recurrent pheochromocytoma in these patients is high, whereas the medullary involvement in von Hippel-Lindau disease is not as diffuse and when technically feasible cortical sparing surgery is indicated.[3] In a study that included both von Hippel-Lindau and MEN2 patients, 13% of those treated with cortical-sparing adrenalectomy developed another pheochromocytoma within the remnant adrenal after a median of 8 years.[4]
- Most patients with MEN2B have de novo mutations and parents and pediatricians are not looking for signs or symptoms of MENB. Thus total thyroidectomy is delayed until a keen clinician suspects MEN2B based on physical examination findings. When total thyroidectomy is not performed in the first year of life, MTC is frequently metastatic and the major cause of morbidity and early mortality.[1,2]

REFERENCES

1. Castinetti F, Waguespack SG, Machens A, et al. Natural history, treatment, and long-term follow up of patients with multiple endocrine neoplasia type 2B: an international, multicentre, retrospective study. *Lancet Diabetes Endocrinol*. 2019;7(3):213–220.
2. Redlich A, Lessel L, Petrou A, Mier P, Vorwerk P. Multiple endocrine neoplasia type 2B: frequency of physical stigmata—results of the GPOH-MET registry. *Pediatr Blood Cancer*. 2020;67(2):e28056.
3. Baghai M, Thompson GB, Young WF Jr, Grant CS, Michels VV, van Heerden JA. Pheochromocytomas and paragangliomas in von Hippel-Lindau disease: a role for laparoscopic and cortical-sparing surgery. *Arch Surg*. 2002;137(6):682–688; discussion 688-9.
4. Neumann HPH, Tsoy U, Bancos I, et al. Comparison of pheochromocytoma-specific morbidity and mortality among adults with bilateral pheochromocytomas undergoing total adrenalectomy vs cortical-sparing adrenalectomy. *JAMA Netw Open*. 2019;2(8):e198898.

Metastatic Paraganglioma: An Approach to Management and the Use of Serial Imaging to Assess the Rate of Tumor Progression

There is no cure for metastatic pheochromocytoma or paraganglioma (PPGL). The first step in the management of metastatic PPGL is to assess the rate of tumor progression and, once determined, provide a proportionate treatment. Herein we demonstrate with a case that although the patient had widely metastatic disease, the rate of progression was slow and minimal therapy was indicated.

Case Report

The patient was a 65-year-old woman seen in endocrine consultation for metastatic paraganglioma (PGL). Twenty years previously (at 45 years of age) she had a 3-cm right carotid body tumor resected. It was clinically nonfunctioning. She had no follow-up neck imaging. Recently she had a pelvic computed tomography (CT) scan performed that incidentally detected multiple boney metastases. Biopsy confirmed metastatic PGL. A F-18 fluorodeoxyglucose (FDG) positron emission tomography (PET)-CT scan showed extensive FDG-avid sclerotic skeletal metastases involving the axial and proximal appendicular skeleton as well as a number of ribs and the right mandible (Fig. 47.1). An I-123 metaiodobenzylguanidine (MIBG) scan showed no uptake in the metastatic PGL. She was asymptomatic and felt well. She went on exercise walks daily and exercised on an elliptical machine for 40 minutes 4 days per week. On physical examination her body mass index

was 21.3 kg/m^2, blood pressure was 127/74 mmHg, and heart rate was 65 beats per minute. There were no areas of tenderness to palpation. She had received multiple opinions and recommendations on treatment options to pursue and seeks another opinion on best management.

INVESTIGATIONS

The laboratory tests confirmed that the metastatic PGL was biochemically nonfunctioning (Table 47.1).

The patient declined germline genetic testing for pathogenic variants in the succinate dehydrogenase subunits.

Magnetic resonance imaging (MRI) of the spine showed multiple metastatic lesions throughout the cervical, thoracic, and lumbar spine (Fig. 47.2). The most extensive involvement was at T2, with replacement of the vertebral body. Prominent lesions were also noted at L2 and L4, without epidural extension (see Fig. 47.2).

TREATMENT

It was clear that this patient had metastatic PGL that predated her carotid body tumor resection 20 years previously. The key question in this asymptomatic 65-year-old woman, despite the extensive metastatic disease, was what was the pace of tumor growth? Treatment with zoledronic acid 4 mg infused intravenously every 3 months was initiated.[1] Follow-up in 1 year was advised. A FDG-PET-CT scan completed 1 year later showed stable metastatic disease (see Fig. 47.1). However, the follow-up spine MRI demonstrated slight

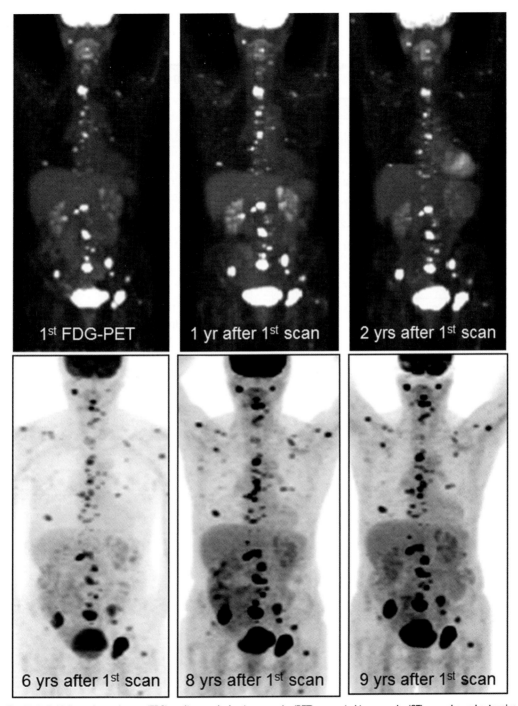

Fig. 47-1 F-18 fluorodeoxyglucose (FDG) positron emission tomography (PET)-computed tomography (CT) scan showed extensive FDG-avid sclerotic skeletal metastases involving the axial and proximal appendicular skeleton as well as a number of ribs and the right mandible. Serial FDG-PET scans show slow progression of disease over 9 years.

anterior epidural tumor extension at T2. Although the patient was asymptomatic, to prevent progression of this tumor in the thoracic spine, which could threaten her quality of life, radiation therapy was advised. A total dose of 4500 cGy in 25 fractions to the T1–T3 vertebral bodies was administered.

OUTCOME AND FOLLOW-UP

Over the subsequent 13 years since her initial visit to Mayo Clinic the spine MRI and FDG-PET-CT scans showed slight progression of disease (see Fig. 47.1). In 2020 and at 78 years of age (33 years after her carotid body tumor surgery), she remained asymptomatic from her metastatic PPGL. Her only tumor-directed treatment had been thoracic spine radiation therapy and zoledronic acid 4 mg infusions every 6 months (decreased frequency as a result of patient intolerance).

Discussion

We have had the most success in extending life with a multimodality, multidisciplinary, and individualized approach to control catecholamine-dependent symptoms, local mass effect symptoms from the tumor, and overall tumor burden.[2] The aggressiveness of the metastatic PPGL should be matched by the escalation in the use of treatment options—a process of "matching the penalty (our treatment) to the crime (the tumor)."[3] Because there is no cure and because

TABLE 47.1 Laboratory Tests

Biochemical Test	Result	Reference Range
Sodium, mmol/L	143	135–145
Potassium, mmol/L	4.2	3.6–5.2
Creatinine, mg/dL	0.7	0.6–1.1
Plasma metanephrine, nmol/L	<0.2	<0.5
Plasma normetanephrine, nmol/L	0.9	<0.9
Plasma norepinephrine, pg/mL	450	<750
Plasma epinephrine, pg/mL	<25	<111
Plasma dopamine, pg/mL	10	<30
24-Hour urine:		
Metanephrine, mcg	107	<400
Normetanephrine, mcg	389	<900
Norepinephrine, mcg	68	<80
Epinephrine, mcg	<2	<20
Dopamine, mcg	156	<400

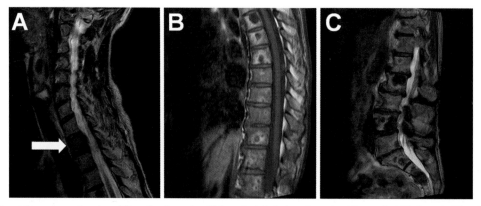

Fig. 47.2 Magnetic resonance imaging of the spine showed multiple metastatic lesions throughout the cervical (A), thoracic (B), and lumbar spine (C). The most extensive involvement was at T2 *(arrow)*, with replacement of the vertebral body. Prominent lesions were also noted at L2 and L4, without epidural extension.

all treatment options carry risk, in patients with indolent disease the best treatment may simply be observation with periodic biochemical testing and imaging. In patients with a limited number of metastases (e.g., <6), targeted treatments are preferred over systemic treatment options. Treatment options include observation, surgery, thermal ablation, external radiotherapy, somatostatin analogs, cytotoxic chemotherapy, tyrosine kinase inhibitors, therapeutic doses of high-specific activity I-131 metaiodobenzylguanidine (I-131 MIBG), and peptide receptor radiotherapy.[3] Using this approach at Mayo Clinic, the median overall and disease-specific survivals for metastatic PPGL are 24.6 and 33.7 years, respectively.[2]

Metastatic lesions should be resected, if possible, to decrease tumor burden.[4] Skeletal metastatic lesions that are painful or threaten structural function can be treated with external radiotherapy, thermal ablation, or approached surgically. If the metastatic PPGL is considered aggressive and tumor burden has exceeded that which can be managed with targeted treatment options, cytotoxic chemotherapy with cyclophosphamide, vincristine, and dacarbazine (CVD) can provide disease stabilization (see Case 50).

Key Points

- There is no cure for metastatic PPGL.
- The first step in managing metastatic PPGL is to determine the pace of progression of the disease and then match it to a proportionate treatment.
- In many patients with slowly progressive metastatic PPGL, observation is the optimal treatment strategy.
- Serial imaging with FDG-PET can be very helpful in assessing total tumor burden and rate of disease progression.

REFERENCES

1. Jeon HL, Oh IS, Baek YH, et al. Zoledronic acid and skeletal-related events in patients with bone metastatic cancer or multiple myeloma. *J Bone Miner Metab.* 2020;38(2):254–263.
2. Hamidi O, WF Young Jr., Iniguez-Ariza NM, et al. Malignant pheochromocytoma and paraganglioma: 272 patients over 55 years. *J Clin Endocrinol Metab.* 2017;102(9):3296–3305.
3. Young WF. Metastatic pheochromocytoma: in search of a cure. *Endocrinology.* 2020;161(3):1–4.
4. Strajina V, Dy BM, Farley DR, et al. Surgical treatment of malignant pheochromocytoma and paraganglioma: retrospective case series. *Ann Surg Oncol.* 2017;24(6): 1546–1550.

Metastatic Pheochromocytoma: Role for Ga-68 DOTATATE PET-CT

There is no cure for metastatic pheochromocytoma or metastatic paraganglioma (PPGL). The first step in the management of metastatic PPGL is to assess the rate of tumor progression and, once determined, provide a proportionate treatment. Herein we demonstrate the role for gallium 68 (Ga-68) 1,4,7,10-tetraazacyclododecane-1,4,7,10-tetraacetic acid (DOTA)-octreotate (DOTATATE) positron emission tomography (PET) computed tomography (CT) in assessing total tumor burden.

Case Report

The patient was a 58-year-old woman seen in endocrine consultation for metastatic pheochromocytoma. She underwent left adrenalectomy 3 years previously for the removal of a 3-cm adrenal pheochromocytoma. Before surgery both metanephrine and normetanephrine were increased above the upper limit of the reference ranges in the blood and urine and they reportedly normalized postoperatively. She had no other follow-up until the current visit, when she presented with paroxysmal symptoms. Her spells, 15 minutes in duration, started with a shaky sensation followed by head pulsations; she said it felt like "my head is going to pop." There was no family history of pheochromocytoma. She had a history of right thyroid lobectomy for a goiter that proved to be Hashimoto thyroiditis. She had chronic hypertension that was treated with a β-adrenergic blocker (carvedilol 6.25 mg daily), angiotensin-converting enzyme inhibitor (enalapril 5 mg daily), and a mineralocorticoid receptor antagonist (spironolactone 50 mg daily). On physical examination her body mass index was 40.9 kg/m^2, blood pressure 126/74 mmHg, and heart rate 76 beats per minute.

INVESTIGATIONS

The laboratory tests confirmed recurrent pheochromocytoma (Table 48.1). She declined germline genetic testing.

CT scan of the abdomen and pelvis revealed no sign of recurrent pheochromocytoma. F-18 fluorodeoxyglucose (FDG) PET-CT scan showed moderate FDG uptake (maximum standard unit value 5.7) in the left acetabular roof, right thyroidectomy and enlarged residual left thyroid lobe with intense FDG uptake, and focal moderate FDG uptake in the gastric antrum near the pylorus (Fig. 48.1). Thyroid ultrasound confirmed Hashimoto thyroiditis and explained the thyroid FDG uptake. Thus the FDG-PET-CT showed minimal disease and did not adequately account for the markedly abnormal laboratory findings. Magnetic resonance

TABLE 48.1 Laboratory Tests		
Biochemical Test	**Result**	**Reference Range**
Sodium, mmol/L	142	135–145
Potassium, mmol/L	4.8	3.6–5.2
Creatinine, mg/dL	1.1	0.6–1.1
Plasma metanephrine, nmol/L	4.1	<0.5
Plasma normetanephrine, nmol/L	8.0	<0.9
24-Hour urine:		
Metanephrine, mcg	2402	<400
Normetanephrine, mcg	2771	<900
Norepinephrine, mcg	107	<80
Epinephrine, mcg	34	<20
Dopamine, mcg	278	<400

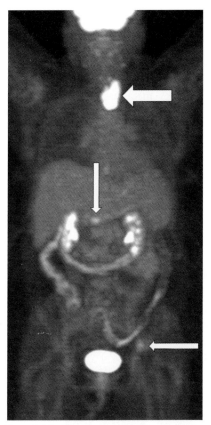

Fig. 48.1 Planar full body image from F-18 fluorodeoxyglucose (FDG) positron emission tomography (PET)-computed tomography (CT) scan. There was moderate FDG uptake (maximum standard unit value [SUVmax] of 5.7) in the left acetabular roof *(small horizontal arrow)*. There was evidence of the prior right thyroidectomy and residual left thyroid lobe was enlarged and had intense FDG uptake *(large arrow)*. There was focal moderate FDG uptake in the gastric antrum near the pylorus *(small vertical arrow)*.

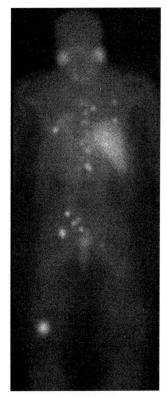

Fig. 48.2 Planar posterior image from I-123 metaiodobenzylguanidine (MIBG) scintigraphy showed innumerable foci of MIBG uptake involving the thorax, abdomen, pelvis, and left thigh.

imaging of the pelvis showed a well-marginated lesion within the left acetabulum that measured 2.3 cm in maximum dimension. In addition, multiple small round areas of T2 hyperintensity were present throughout the pelvis and spine, the largest of which were in the left posterior iliac crest, the left iliac wing, sacrum, and right ilium—all consistent with metastases. The findings on MRI confirmed the suspicion that FDG-PET scan was not detecting the full extent of her disease. I-123 metaiodobenzylguanidine (MIBG) scintigraphy showed innumerable foci of MIBG uptake involving the thorax, abdomen, pelvis, and left thigh (Fig. 48.2). CT of the left femur showed a 2.3 × 2.3 × 2.6–cm marrow replacing lesion in the distal left femoral meta-diaphysis compatible with metastasis.

TREATMENT

The patient was informed that there is no cure for metastatic PPGL.[1] Phenoxybenzamine was added to her antihypertensive program and it prevented further paroxysms. To prevent a pathologic fracture, the large left femur lesion was treated with external beam radiation therapy. Treatment with zoledronic acid 4 mg infused intravenously every 3 months was initiated. However, a key question in the case of this 58-year-old woman was, what was the pace of tumor growth? We suspected that she may have aggressive disease because her 24-hour urine for fractionated metanephrines and catecholamines was reportedly normal after her left adrenalectomy.

OUTCOME AND FOLLOW-UP

She was seen in follow-up 1 year later. There were mild increases in fractionated metanephrines in the blood and urine compared to those at our initial consultation, but the findings on I-123 MIBG scan were stable. It was decided to reassess in another year, at which time the plasma metanephrine and 24-hour urine metanephrine had increased 5.9-fold and 5.1-fold, respectively, from the levels obtained 2 years previously. In addition, the plasma normetanephrine and 24-hour urine normetanephrine increased 2.5-fold and 2.4-fold, respectively. However, I-123 MIBG scintigraphy showed only mild progression of the polyostotic

metastatic disease (Fig. 48.3A). A Ga-68 DOTATATE PET-CT was obtained to see if it would give a better assessment of her overall tumor burden and, compared to I-123 MIBG scintigraphy, Ga-68 DOTATATE PET-CT showed a dramatic increase in the number of visualized boney metastases with marked radiotracer uptake throughout the axial, visualized appendicular skeleton, involving the skull base, sternum, ribs, scapula, and calvarium (Fig. 48.3B). Systemic chemotherapy was initiated with cyclophosphamide, vincristine, and dacarbazine (CVD). CVD chemotherapy for malignant PPGL is associated with complete responses and partial responses based on reductions in tumor volume in 4% and 37% of patients, respectively.[2] CVD

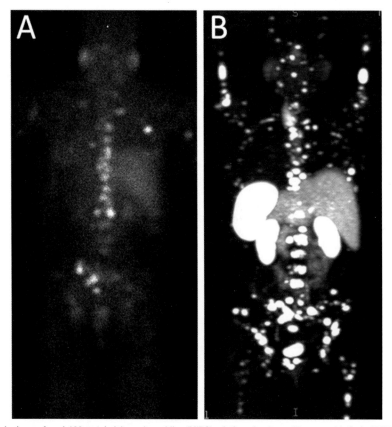

Fig. 48.3 (A) Planar posterior image from I-123 metaiodobenzylguanidine (MIBG) scintigraphy showed innumerable foci of MIBG uptake with moderate progression compared to the scan from 2 years earlier (see Fig. 48.2). (B) Planar posterior image from Ga-68 DOTATATE PET CT scan shows multiple boney metastases with marked radiotracer uptake throughout the axial, visualized appendicular skeleton, involving the skull base, sternum, ribs, scapula, and calvarium. Some of the more DOTATATE-avid sites included: right proximal humerus (standard unit value [SUV] of 36.5); sternum (SUV of 19); left sacrum (SUV of 33.6); L4 (SUV of 29); and T11 (SUV of 34).

chemotherapy is typically administered for 6 months unless new lesions develop or there is a significant (e.g., >25%) increase in size of known tumor sites.

Unfortunately, after a 6-month treatment trial with CVD there was further biochemical progression based on the following: plasma metanephrine 74 nmol/L (normal, <0.5), plasma normetanephrine 56 nmol/L (normal, <0.9), 24-hour urine metanephrine 27,600 mcg (normal, <400 mcg), and 24-hour urine normetanephrine 12,672 mcg (normal, <900 mcg). Subsequent treatment trials that included a somatostatin analog, tyrosine kinase inhibitor, and immunotherapy with pembrolizumab were also ineffective in achieving tumor control. She recently enrolled in a treatment trial with peptide receptor radiotherapy.

Although the median overall and disease-specific survivals for metastatic PPGL at Mayo Clinic are 24.6 and 33.7 years, respectively, approximately 13% of patients have rapidly progressive disease with survivals of <5 years from primary tumor diagnosis.[3]

Key Points

- There is no cure for metastatic PPGL.
- The first step in managing metastatic PPGL is to determine the pace of progression of the disease and then match it to a proportionate treatment.

- Systemic chemotherapy is indicated in those patients with rapidly progressive metastatic PPGL.
- It is important to determine the best total body imaging modality for each patient with metastatic PPGL. Overall, Ga-68 DOTATATE PET-CT has proven to be the most sensitive, followed by FDG-PET and I-123 MIBG. However, there are patients who have DOTATATE nonavid disease and FDG-PET is a superior imaging modality in those cases.

REFERENCES

1. Young WF. Metastatic pheochromocytoma: in search of a cure. *Endocrinology.* 20201;161(3).
2. Niemeijer ND, Alblas G, van Hulsteijn LT, Dekkers OM, Corrsmit EPM. Chemotherapy with cyclophosphamide, vincristine, and dacarbazine for malignant paraganglioma and pheochromocytoma: a systematic review and meta-analysis. *Clin Endocrinol (Oxf).* 2014;81:642–651.
3. Hamidi O, Young WF Jr., Iniguez-Ariza NM, et al. Malignant pheochromocytoma and paraganglioma: 272 patients over 55 years. *J Clin Endocrinol Metab.* 2017;102(9):3296–3305.

Carney Triad (Pentad) and Catecholamine-Secreting Paragangliomas

Carney triad (described in 1977) is a rare, nonfamilial, multitumoral syndrome, with three tumors in the initial description: gastrointestinal stromal tumor (GIST), pulmonary chondroma, and extraadrenal paraganglioma (PGL).[1,2] Subsequently, two other tumors, adrenal cortical adenoma and esophageal leiomyoma, were added as components—thus actually Carney triad is a "pentad."[3] Although it is rare, it is important for endocrinologists to be aware of this disorder because of the links to PGL and adrenocortical tumors.

Case Report

The patient was a 26-year-old woman referred for further management of Carney triad-related neoplasms. The first sign of the triad was at age 17 when she presented with microcytic anemia (hemoglobin 7.0 g/dL) that was treated with iron sulfate. The anemia proved refractory, and esophagogastroduodenoscopy (EGD) performed 1 year before consultation at Mayo Clinic found a large gastrointestinal stromal tumor (GIST), and she underwent an 80% gastrectomy for the removal of a 17-cm GIST. More recently it was noted that she had a mass in her left lingula, which was resected and proved to be a 3.3-cm chondroma. She was also noted to have a 4-cm mass near the aortic arch. She had labile hypertension controlled with a calcium channel blocker (amlodipine 10 mg daily). She had no signs or symptoms of adrenocortical or adrenomedullary hormone excess. On physical examination her body mass index was 28.7 kg/m², blood pressure 138/84 mmHg, and heart rate 96 beats per minute.

INVESTIGATIONS

Chest magnetic resonance imaging (MRI) showed a 4.1 × 3.3–cm precarinal soft tissue mass (Fig. 49.1). The plasma fractionated metanephrines and 24-hour urine for fractionated metanephrines and catecholamines, while not markedly elevated, were consistent with a catecholamine-secreting tumor (Table 49.1). I-123 metaiodobenzylguanidine (MIBG) scintigraphy

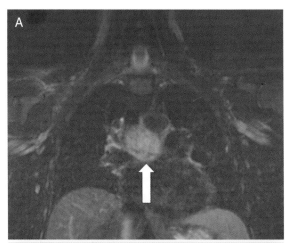

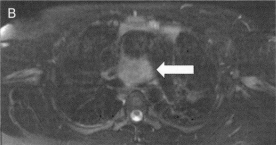

Fig. 49.1 Coronal (A) and axial (B) magnetic resonance imaging of the chest demonstrated a 4.1 × 3.3–cm precarinal soft tissue mass *(arrows)*.

TABLE 49.1 Laboratory Tests

Biochemical Test	Result	Reference Range
Sodium, mmol/L	137	135–145
Potassium, mmol/L	3.9	3.6–5.2
Creatinine, mg/dL	0.8	0.7–1.2
Plasma metanephrine, nmol/L	0.32	<0.5
Plasma normetanephrine, nmol/L	2.23	<0.9
1-mg overnight DST cortisol, mcg/dL	1.5	<1.8
24-hr urine:		
Metanephrine, mcg	104	<400
Normetanephrine, mcg	979	<900
Norepinephrine, mcg	203	<80
Epinephrine, mcg	3.3	<20
Dopamine, mcg	305	<400

DST, Dexamethasone suppression test.

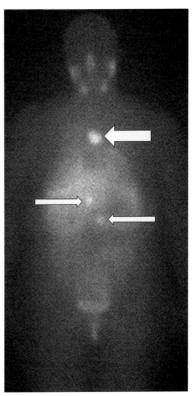

Fig. 49.2 Anterior planar image from I-123 metaiodobenzylguanidine scintigraphy. Intense radiotracer uptake is demonstrated in the precarinal region *(large arrow)* and in two sites *(small arrows)* in the upper abdomen just to the right and left of midline.

colocalized with the precarinal mass and two sites of abnormal uptake were seen in the upper abdomen just to the right and left of midline (Fig. 49.2). MRI of the abdomen demonstrated two retroperitoneal lesions that colocalized with the findings on I-123 MIBG scintigraphy (Fig. 49.3). In addition, the abdominal MRI detected a 2.5-cm right adrenal mass with imaging characteristics consistent with a cortical adenoma (Fig. 49.4). The 1-mg overnight dexamethasone suppression test was normal (see Table 49.1). Finally, EGD showed no sign of residual GIST; however, two asymptomatic 1.5–2.0 cm esophageal leiomyomas were found.

TREATMENT

It was clear that this patient had three PGLs—one in the chest and two in the abdomen. The chest PGL was operated first. She was prepared for surgery by addition of phenoxybenzamine to her calcium channel blocker; phenoxybenzamine was titrated to 10 mg taken three times per day for target low normal systolic blood pressure. Propranolol 60 mg long acting was added for target heart rate of 80 beats per minute. She was encouraged to consume a high-sodium diet. She underwent a left thoracotomy, where a large lobulated mediastinal mass was associated with intense adhesions and resection was associated with profuse bleeding. With considerable difficulty, the mass was separated from the anterior wall of the trachea and the carina, superior vena cava, right pulmonary artery, aorta, and pulmonary trunk. On pathology, the PGL measured 6.5 × 3.0 × 2.7 cm. Five regional lymph nodes were negative for tumor. The postoperative course was complicated by a persistent chylous pericardial effusion that required treatment with a pericardial window.

After resection of the mediastinal PGL, the plasma and 24-hour urine normetanephrine levels remained elevated. Eight months after her thoracotomy she had a laparotomy to remove the two abdominal PGLs. She was prepared with adrenergic blockade as done previously. The right-sided periaortic PGL measured 3.3 × 1.9 × 1.4 cm and the left-sided PGL adjacent to the left renal vein measured 4.5 × 3.0 × 2.3 cm.

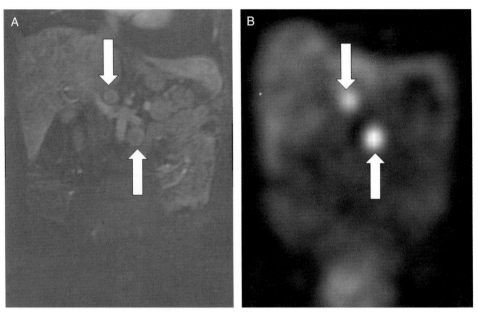

Fig. 49-3 (A) Coronal magnetic resonance imaging (MRI) of the abdomen image demonstrated two retroperitoneal lesions: the largest lesion was located in the left paraaortic retroperitoneum *(arrow)* just inferior to the left renal vasculature and measured 2.5 cm in diameter; the second lesion was located in the right upper retroperitoneum in between the aorta and inferior vena cava approximately at the level of the celiac axis *(arrow)*. (B) The lesions seen on MRI corresponded to findings on I-123 metaiodobenzylguanidine single-photon emission computerized tomography coronal image and confirmed that they were paragangliomas *(arrows)*.

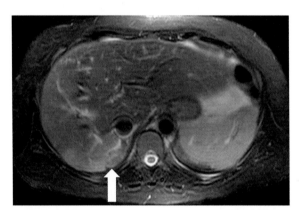

Fig. 49-4 Axial magnetic resonance image shows oblong 2.5 cm right adrenal mass *(arrow)* with imaging characteristics consistent with a cortical adenoma.

OUTCOME AND FOLLOW-UP

Plasma and 24-hour urine normetanephrine levels normalized postoperatively, and antihypertensive medications were no longer required. Follow-up 11 years later showed no imaging or biochemical evidence of recurrent GIST or PGL. She died 18 years after surgery at 44 years of age of an apparent cardiac sudden death.

Discussion

Carney triad is a rare multitumoral syndrome. Approximately 150 cases have been identified.[4] The disorder occurs almost exclusively in young women and is not familial. The patient described herein is the only one known to have five-organ involvement; most patients have two-organ involvement. Thus Carney triad is usually only partially expressed. The gastric GIST is malignant and metastasizes to the liver, peritoneum, and lymph nodes. The lung, adrenal, and esophageal tumors are benign. The PGLs are usually benign. Long-term follow-up shows that the syndrome is a chronic, persistent, and generally indolent condition whose outcome is largely dependent on the behavior of the metastases from the GIST.

The findings from one study suggested that a DNA hypermethylation pattern was correlated with a reduced mRNA expression of *SDHC* and concurrent loss of the SDHC subunit at the protein level.[5] These data suggested epigenetic inactivation of the *SDHC* gene locus with functional impairment of the SDH complex as a plausible mechanism of tumorigenesis in Carney triad.[5]

Key Points

- Although rare, endocrinologists should be aware of the five components of Carney triad, which include PGL, adrenal cortical adenoma, pulmonary chondromas, esophageal leiomyoma, and GIST.
- When adrenalectomy is planned, all patient's adrenal adenomas >1-cm diameter should have case detection testing for subclinical glucocorticoid secretory autonomy preoperatively (see Case 22).

- PGLs in Carney triad can be multiple and located in the chest, abdomen, or pelvis.

REFERENCES

1. Carney JA, Sheps SG, Go VL, et al. The triad of gastric leiomyosarcoma, functioning extra-adrenal paraganglioma and pulmonary chondroma. *N Engl J Med.* 1977;296:1517–1518.

2. Carney JA. The triad of gastric epithelioid leiomyosarcoma, functioning extra-adrenal paraganglioma, and pulmonary chondroma. *Cancer.* 1979;43:374–382.

3. Carney JA, Stratakis CA, Young WF Jr. Adrenal cortical adenoma: the fourth component of the Carney triad and an association with subclinical Cushing syndrome. *Am J Surg Pathol.* 2013 Aug;37(8):1140–1149 .

4. Carney JA. Carney triad. *Front Horm Res.* 2013;41: 92–110.

5. Haller F, Moskalev EA, Faucz FR, et al. Aberrant DNA hypermethylation of SDHC: a novel mechanism of tumor development in Carney triad. *Endocr Relat Cancer.* 2014;21(4):567–577.

Case 50

Metastatic Paraganglioma: Role for Systemic Chemotherapy

There is no cure for metastatic paraganglioma (PGL). The first step in the management of metastatic PGL is to assess the rate of tumor progression and, once determined, provide a proportionate treatment. When the number of metastatic PGL lesions exceeds what can be managed with local/targeted treatments (e.g., ablation and radiation therapies) and the pace of increase in overall tumor bulk becomes excessive, systemic treatment should be considered. The first systemic treatment to consider is cytotoxic chemotherapy with the protocol of cyclophosphamide, vincristine, and dacarbazine (CVD). Although CVD chemotherapy is not curative, it can provide remarkable remissions in disease. Herein we demonstrate the role for chemotherapy with CVD.

Case Report

The patient was a 38-year-old man seen in endocrine consultation for an abdominal paraganglioma (PGL) diagnosed elsewhere on a computed tomography (CT)-guided biopsy. He had been experiencing low back discomfort with jogging, and a lumbar spine magnetic resonance image (MRI) was obtained. Incidentally noted was a retroperitoneal mass. A subsequent CT scan confirmed a 3.7 × 5.5 × 5.5–cm peripherally enhancing solid mass in the retroperitoneum anterior to the inferior vena cava (IVC). He had no paroxysmal symptoms or history of hypertension. He had a niece who was recently diagnosed with metastatic catecholamine-secreting abdominal PGL. On physical examination his body mass index was 29.1 kg/m², blood pressure 142/78 mmHg, and heart rate 54 beats per minute. He was physically fit.

INVESTIGATIONS

The laboratory tests showed that the PGL was nonfunctioning (Table 50.1). Germline genetic testing found a large gene deletion (promotor and exon 1) in succinate dehydrogenase subunit B (*SDHB*). I-123 metaiodobenzylguanidine (MIBG) scintigraphy showed that the PGL was not MIBG-avid.

TREATMENT

Although biochemically nonfunctioning, as a precaution the patient was prepared with adrenergic blockade before open laparotomy. At surgery the PGL was located between the IVC and aorta and was completely resected. Blood pressure and heart rate were stable intraoperatively. Pathology showed the PGL to measure 5.9 × 5.8 × 4.9 cm. He recovered well from surgery and was followed with imaging every 6 months.

TABLE 50.1 Laboratory Tests		
Biochemical Test	**Result**	**Reference Range**
Sodium, mmol/L	143	135–145
Potassium, mmol/L	4.8	3.6–5.2
Creatinine, mg/dL	1.0	0.8–1.3
Plasma metanephrine, nmol/L	<0.2	<0.5
Plasma normetanephrine, nmol/L	0.5	<0.9
24-Hour urine:		
Metanephrine, mcg	132	<400
Normetanephrine, mcg	418	<900
Norepinephrine, mcg	52	<80
Epinephrine, mcg	6.2	<20
Dopamine, mcg	353	<400

OUTCOME AND FOLLOW-UP

Two years postoperatively recurrent disease was found on MRI scan at the original tumor site. F-18 fluorodeoxyglucose (FDG) positron emission tomography (PET)-CT showed a multilobulated 3.6 × 2.7 × 1.6–cm retroperitoneal mass that was intensely FDG avid (maximum standard unit value 22.0). There was FDG-avid metastatic disease in aortocaval lymph nodes just inferior to the mass. No other metastatic disease was evident. The patient underwent his second operation. The recurrent PGL was resected along with a portion of the vena caval wall (patched with a bovine pericardial patch 6 × 2 cm). The pelvis was explored and a 5-mm nodule anterior to sacral promontory was dissected off with electrocautery. Pathologic analysis showed a multinodular PGL (5 × 5 × 2 cm) and a separate PGL nodule (1 × 1 × 0.5 cm). Unfortunately, recurrent disease was found at the original tumor site 1 year later and was treated with radiation therapy (6250 cGy over 25 fractions). The patient then did well on serial follow-up until polyostotic metastatic disease was evident on FDG-PET-CT—7 years after his first surgery. The number of lesions exceeded what could be effectively treated with targeted radiation or ablation therapies, and

CVD chemotherapy was initiated. In a nonrandomized, single-arm trial, the efficacy of chemotherapy with the CVD protocol (cyclophosphamide 750 mg/m² body surface area on day 1, vincristine 1.4 mg/m² on day 1, and dacarbazine 600 mg/m² on days 1 and 2; repeated every 21–28 days) was studied in 14 patients with malignant pheochromocytoma.[1,2] Complete and partial biochemical responses were seen in 79% of patients (median duration, >22 months; range, 6 to >35 months). All responding patients had objective improvement in performance status and blood pressure.[1,2]

A total of 13 cycles of CVD were administered and there was a near complete tumor response (Fig. 50.1). Recurrent disease became evident 2 years after completion of CVD chemotherapy. Over the intervening years there was limited or no tumor response to treatment trials with a somatostatin analog and a tyrosine kinase inhibitor. The FDG-PET-CT scan obtained 13 years after his initial surgery is shown in Fig. 50.2A. CVD chemotherapy was reinitiated and a robust response was documented just 1 month later (Fig. 50.2B). CVD chemotherapy should be continued until there is a plateau in tumor response or tumor progression or near complete tumor response (typically CVD treatment duration is 6–12 months).

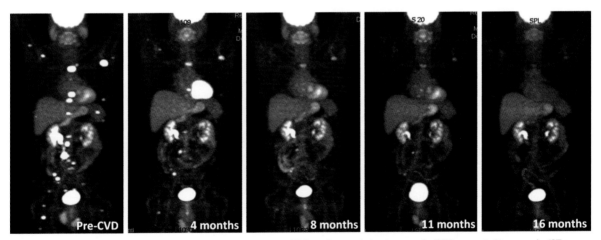

Fig. 50.1 Serial planar full body images from F-18 fluorodeoxyglucose (FDG) positron emission tomography (PET)-computed tomography (CT) scans. The FDG-PET-CT image obtained before CVD chemotherapy is shown on the *left*. Notation on the *bottom right* of each image shows the number of months since starting CVD chemotherapy (left to right). CVD treatment was discontinued at month 14. The FDG-PET-CT at month 16 shows near complete tumor response.

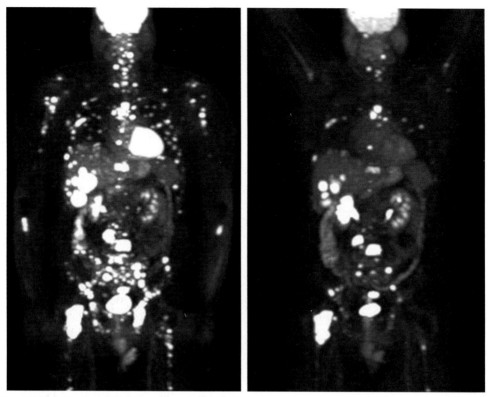

Fig. 50.2 Planar full body images from F-18 fluorodeoxyglucose (FDG) positron emission tomography (PET)-computed tomography (CT) scans. (A) FDG-PET-CT showed innumerable new hypermetabolic lesions throughout the axial and proximal appendicular skeleton. (B) FDG-PET-CT scan after one cycle of CVD chemotherapy showed multiple diffuse hypermetabolic lesions in the axial and proximal appendicular skeleton had decreased in FDG uptake, including resolution of many of the smaller lesions.

Key Points

- There is no cure for metastatic PGL.[3]
- The first step in managing metastatic PPGL is to determine the pace of progression of the disease and then match it to a proportionate treatment.[3]
- Systemic chemotherapy with CVD is indicated in those patients with rapidly progressive metastatic PPGL.
- Although not curative, CVD chemotherapy can provide remarkable remissions of 1–5 years in duration.

REFERENCES

1. Averbuch SD, Steakley CS, Young RC, et al. Malignant pheochromocytoma: effective treatment with a combination of cyclophosphamide, vincristine, and dacarbazine. *Ann Intern Med.* 1988;109(4):267–273.

2. Huang H, Abraham J, Hung E, et al. Treatment of malignant pheochromocytoma/paraganglioma with cyclophosphamide, vincristine, and dacarbazine: recommendation from a 22-year follow-up of 18 patients. *Cancer.* 2008; 113(8):2020–2028.

3. Young WF. Metastatic pheochromocytoma: in search of a cure. *Endocrinology.* 2020;1(3):161.

Cryoablation Therapy for Metastatic Paraganglioma

There is no cure for metastatic pheochromocytoma or metastatic paraganglioma (PPGL). The first step in the management of metastatic PPGL is to assess the rate of tumor progression and, once determined, provide a proportionate treatment. Targeted treatments are preferred over systemic treatment options in patients with a limited number of or slowly progressive metastases. Here we present the use for thermal ablation in treatment of metastatic paraganglioma.

Case Report

The patient was a 47-year-old woman who presented for evaluation of left neck lump. She first noticed the lump approximately 5 years earlier. The lesion had progressively grown since and had become apparent to her friends and family, prompting further evaluation. She was asymptomatic. Her medical history was negative and she was not taking any medications. Family history was positive for a surgery to remove a neck lesion in her father at age 78 and a possible carotid body tumor in her sister.

On physical examination, her body mass index was 27.3 kg/m^2, blood pressure was 141/79 mmHg, and heart rate was 69 beats per minute. She had a 7 × 6–cm left upper neck mass that was mobile and nontender. There was no lymphadenopathy. The rest of the examination was normal.

INVESTIGATIONS

Computed tomography (CT) scan of the neck demonstrated a bilobed enhancing left neck mass measuring 6.2 × 4.2 × 9.5 cm, consistent with carotid body tumor (Fig. 51.1). An F-18 fluorodeoxyglucose (FDG) positron emission tomography (PET)-CT

scan showed intense uptake in the left cervical mass and hypermetabolic lesions in L3 and L5 vertebral bodies, likely representing metastases (Fig. 51.2). The laboratory tests confirmed that the metastatic PGL was biochemically nonfunctioning (Table 51.1).

TREATMENT AND FOLLOW-UP

After a multidisciplinary evaluation by the otorhinolaryngology, neurosurgery, radiation oncology, and interventional radiology specialists, the patient was treated with proton beam radiation therapy of the left cervical mass. Imaging performed 18 months later demonstrated a stable neck mass, and a slight increase in size of the L3 and L5 metastases. At that point she was treated with cryoablation therapy for the L3 and L5 metastases. Another 2 years later, she developed C1, C4, T1, T2, T10, and T12 metastases, all asymptomatic. She was treated with cryoablation of the T3 and T10 metastases—where further progression was considered high risk for symptom development. One year later she demonstrated stable metastatic disease, with no new or progressive metastases across all sites.

The patient declined germline genetic testing for pathogenic variants in the succinate dehydrogenase subunits.

Discussion

Patients with indolent metastatic PPGL may be best served by observation with periodic biochemical testing and imaging. Targeted treatments such as thermal ablation, external radiotherapy, or surgical excision of metastases are preferred over systemic treatment options. Notably, the median overall and disease-specific survivals for metastatic PPGL at Mayo Clinic from 1960 to 2016 were 24.6 and 33.7 years,

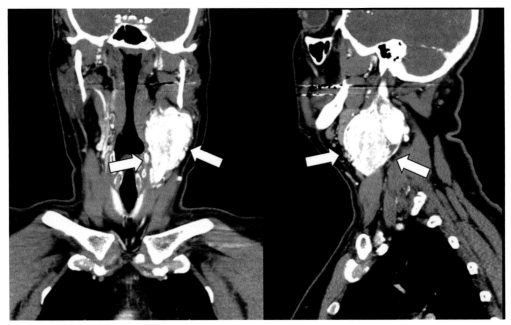

Fig. 51.1 Coronal *(left)* and sagittal *(right)* images from a contrast-enhanced computed tomography (CT) scan of the neck demonstrate a bilobed enhancing left neck mass measuring 6.2 × 4.2 × 9.5 cm.

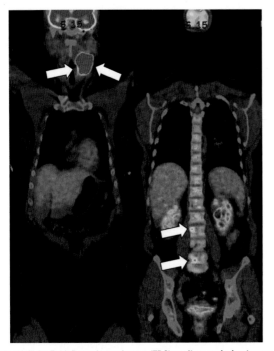

Fig. 51.2 An F-18 fluorodeoxyglucose (FDG) positron emission tomography (PET)-computed tomography (CT) scan showed intense uptake in the left cervical mass *(left)* and hypermetabolic lesions in L3 and L5 vertebral bodies, likely representing metastases *(right)*.

TABLE 51.1 Laboratory Tests

Biochemical Test	Result	Reference Range
Plasma metanephrine, nmol/L	<0.2	<0.5
Plasma normetanephrine, nmol/L	0.36	<0.9
24-Hour urine:		
Metanephrine, mcg	122	<400
Normetanephrine, mcg	297	<900
Norepinephrine, mcg	39	<80
Epinephrine, mcg	4.7	<20
Dopamine, mcg	226	<400

respectively.[1] Thus it is important to consider the long-term potential harm of a specific therapeutic intervention versus potential benefit.

Cryoablation of PPGL metastases can be considered for local symptom control (pain), for treatment of catecholamine excess, or to prevent tumor growth. In a study of 31 patients with 123 PPGL metastases treated with either cryoablation, radiofrequency ablation, or percutaneous ethanol injection, radiographic control was achieved in 86% of lesions.[2] Improvement in pain and catecholamine excess was reported in 92%

of patients who had undergone the procedure. Radiographic progression of the bone metastases treated with cryoablation was observed in 12% of lesions.[2] Appropriate α-adrenergic blockade or therapy with metyrosine needs to be administered before cryoablation in any patient with functioning metastases.[3,4] Cryoablation should be performed by an experienced interventional radiology team. Complications occur in a third of procedures, most mild, such as pain, minor bleeding, and intraprocedural hypertension.[2]

Key Points

- In many patients with slowly progressive metastatic PPGL, observation is the optimal treatment strategy.
- Thermal ablation of bone PPGL metastases is indicated to control tumor-related pain and catecholamine excess or prevent tumor growth.
- α-Adrenergic blockade and/or metyrosine are indicated before thermal ablation of a functioning PPGL metastasis.

REFERENCES

1. Hamidi O, Young Jr WF, Iniguez-Ariza NM, et al. Malignant pheochromocytoma and paraganglioma: 272 patients over 55 years. *J Clin Endocrinol Metab.* 2017;102(9):3296–3305.
2. Kohlenberg J, Welch B, Hamidi O, et al. Efficacy and safety of ablative therapy in the treatment of patients with metastatic pheochromocytoma and paraganglioma. *Cancers (Basel).* 2019;11(2).
3. Gruber LM, Jasim S, Ducharme-Smith A, Weingarten T, Young WF, Bancos I. The role for metyrosine in the treatment of patients with pheochromocytoma and paraganglioma. *J Clin Endocrinol Metab.* 2021;106(6):e2393–e2401.
4. Deljou A, Kohlenberg JD, Weingarten TN, et al. Hemodynamic instability during percutaneous ablation of extra-adrenal metastases of pheochromocytoma and paragangliomas: a case series. *BMC Anesthesiol.* 2018;18(1):158.

Paraganglioma in a Patient With Cyanotic Cardiac Disease

A higher incidence of paraganglioma or pheochromocytoma (PPGL) has been reported in people living at high altitudes, indicating that environmental hypoxia could be a risk factor for development of PPGL. Limited literature suggests that patients with cyanotic congenital heart disease also demonstrate an increased risk for development of PPGL. Herein we share such a case.

Case Report

The patient was a 51-year-old woman with a history of complex cyanotic congenital heart disease who was recently discovered to have a left carotid body tumor after noticing a lump on self-palpation. She was asymptomatic, without signs of catecholamine excess. Family history was negative for PPGL syndromes.

COMPLEX CYANOTIC CONGENITAL HEART DISEASE HISTORY

The patient had been noted to be "blue" on birth. The details of the initial evaluation were not available. At 5 months of age, she underwent a classical Glenn anastomosis. Between age 5 and 6 years, she was treated with the Potts anastomosis (descending aorta to left pulmonary artery anastomosis). Between ages 5 and 34 years, the patient had a gradual reduction in her exercise tolerance and progressive fatigue. At age 35, she had another surgical intervention consisting of atrial septectomy, attempted establishment of pulmonary artery confluence with a homograft right central shunt and patch augmentation of right superior vena cava, and ligation of the left superior vena cava. At age 38, she underwent insertion of a left Blalock-Taussig shunt (left subclavian artery-to-distal left

pulmonary artery graft) with a 7-mm interposition GORE-TEX graft. The shunt resulted in improvement in oxygenation and cardiovascular status.

INVESTIGATIONS

The initial computed tomography (CT) scan of neck demonstrated a 2.0 × 1.8 × 1.9–cm mild to moderately enhancing circumscribed mass within the left carotid bifurcation, consistent with paraganglioma (Fig. 52.1). The laboratory studies were unremarkable, with fractionated catecholamines and metanephrines within the normal range in the 24-hour urine collection (Table 52.1). CT of the abdomen and pelvis did not detect additional PPGLs.

TREATMENT

Surgery was performed without complications; pathologic analysis demonstrated a left 2.1 × 1.8 × 1.5–cm carotid body tumor, which was completely excised (Fig. 52.2), and multiple left jugular lymph nodes were negative for paraganglioma.

FOLLOW-UP

The role for germline mutation testing was discussed, and the patient proceeded with genetic testing for pathogenic variants in succinate dehydrogenase (SDH) B, C, and D subunits, which was negative.

Subsequently, she had imaging follow-up that demonstrated no recurrence at the surgical site but revealed a new right carotid body tumor 2 years later, with mild growth in the following 2 years and stable tumor size for the past 3 years. At the time of the last follow-up, the right carotid paraganglioma measured 10 mm (Fig. 52.3). Biochemical workup was negative for catecholamine excess. After discussion of various management options, conservative follow-up was planned.

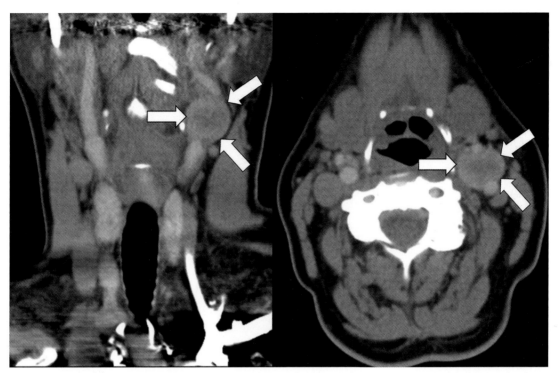

Fig. 52.1 Coronal *(left)* and axial *(right)* images from a contrast-enhanced computed tomography scan of the neck demonstrated a 2 × 1.8 × 1.9–cm mass within the left carotid bifurcation.

TABLE 52.1 Laboratory Tests		
Biochemical Test	**Result**	**Reference Range**
24-Hour urine:		
Metanephrine, mcg	101	<400
Normetanephrine, mcg	288	<900
Norepinephrine, mcg	58	<80
Epinephrine, mcg	6.2	<20
Dopamine, mcg	152	<400

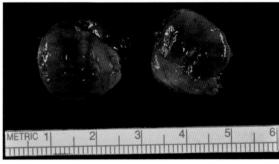

Fig. 52.2 Pathology demonstrated a left 2.1 × 1.8 × 1.5–cm left carotid body paraganglioma.

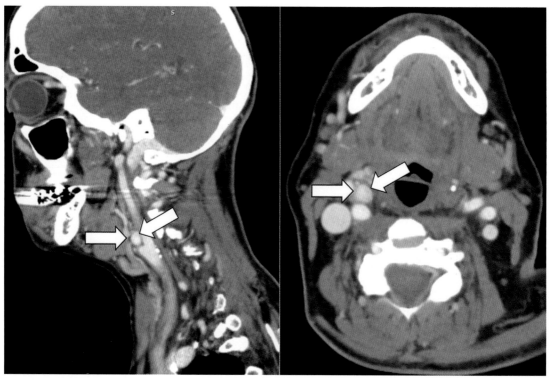

Fig. 52.3 Follow-up imaging 7 years after initial presentation. Sagittal *(left)* and axial *(right)* images from a contrast-enhanced computed tomography scan of the neck demonstrated a 0.8 × 0.8 × 1.0–cm mass within the right carotid bifurcation.

Key Points

- People living at high altitudes are at increased risk for development of PPGL, indicating that environmental hypoxia as a risk factor.[1]
- Patients with cyanotic congenital heart disease (chronic hypoxia) also demonstrate a fivefold increased risk for development of PPGL.[2–4]
- In a small cohort of patients with cyanotic congenital heart disease and PPGL, a high frequency of somatic, gain-of-function *EPAS1* mutations was reported in four out of five patients.[2]

REFERENCES

1. Rodriguez-Cuevas S, Lopez-Garza J, Labastida-Almendaro S. Carotid body tumors in inhabitants of altitudes higher than 2000 meters above sea level. *Head Neck*. 1998;20(5):374–378.
2. Vaidya A, Flores SK, Cheng ZM, et al. EPAS1 mutations and paragangliomas in cyanotic congenital heart disease. *N Engl J Med*. 2018;378(13):1259–1261.
3. Ponz de Antonio I, Ruiz Cantador J, Gonzalez Garcia AE, Oliver Ruiz JM, Sanchez-Recalde A, Lopez-Sendon JL. Prevalence of neuroendocrine tumors in patients with cyanotic congenital heart disease. *Rev Esp Cardiol (Engl Ed)*. 2017;70(8):673–675.
4. Opotowsky AR, Moko LE, Ginns J, et al. Pheochromocytoma and paraganglioma in cyanotic congenital heart disease. *J Clin Endocrinol Metab*. 2015;100(4):1325–1334.

Metastatic Paraganglioma—Role for External Beam Radiation Therapy

There is no cure for metastatic paraganglioma or pheochromocytoma (PPGL). All treatment options are associated with risks and morbidity—many times the side effects of treatment exceed tumor-related morbidity. The first step in the management of metastatic PPGL is to assess the rate of tumor progression and, once determined, provide a proportionate treatment. Herein we demonstrate the role for external beam radiation therapy (EBRT).

Case Report

The patient was a 65-year-old man who had a $4 \times 5 \times 6$–cm periaortic abdominal paraganglioma (PGL) resected elsewhere 12 years previously in 1990. It was found rather incidentally at the time of colonoscopy when the gastroenterologist noted a pulsating mass projecting into the colon. At the time, the patient was asymptomatic except for mild hypertension. After tumor resection (no details of the operative report were available) he was followed with computed tomography (CT) scan once a year for 3 years and annual biochemical testing. His most recent plasma normetanephrine was abnormal and led to the current consultation in 2002. The patient was asymptomatic. On physical examination the body mass index was 28.1 kg/m², blood pressure 130/80 mm Hg, and heart rate 78 beats per minute. He appeared well.

INVESTIGATIONS

The laboratory tests were consistent with a recurrent catecholamine-secreting tumor (Table 53.1). Abdominal CT scan and I-123 metaiodobenzylguanidine (MIBG) scintigraphy detected four sites of recurrent PGL in the upper abdomen with the largest lesion measuring 2.4×2.9 cm (Fig. 53.1).

Germline genetic testing found no pathogenic variants or large gene deletions in succinate dehydrogenase subunits B, C, or D.

TREATMENT

Following α- and β-adrenergic blockade open laparotomy was performed and PGL tissue was found at the crus of the diaphragm ($1.2 \times 0.5 \times 0.5$ cm), adjacent to the portal vein ($2.7 \times 1.8 \times 1.5$ cm), behind the left renal vein ($3.5 \times 2.5 \times 1.8$ cm), and near the right renal artery ($1.8 \times 1.5 \times 1.1$ cm). The pathologist noted that these represented either multiple paragangliomas or seeding from his previous surgery. At follow-up 6 months later, the normetanephrine levels in the blood and urine had normalized.

TABLE 53.1 Laboratory Tests.		
Biochemical Test	**Result**	**Reference Range**
Sodium, mmol/L	143	135–145
Potassium, mmol/L	4.2	3.6–5.2
Creatinine, mg/dL	1.0	0.8–1.3
Plasma metanephrine, nmol/L	<0.2	<0.5
Plasma normetanephrine, nmol/L	1.85	<0.9
24-Hour urine:		
Metanephrine, mcg	139	<400
Normetanephrine, mcg	1434	<900
Norepinephrine, mcg	189	<80
Epinephrine, mcg	5.3	<20
Dopamine, mcg	235	<400

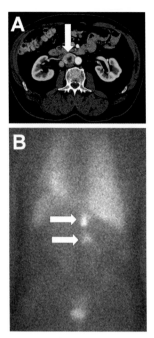

Fig. 53.1 (A) Axial image from abdominal computed tomography (CT) scan shows a 2.4 × 2.9–cm vascular mass *(arrow)* adjacent to the right side of the abdominal aorta and behind the left renal vein. Three addition masses were seen: a 1.5 × 1.8–cm mass just to the right of the larger mass, a 0.8 × 0.7–cm mass adjacent to the crus of the right hemidiaphragm, and a 1.4 × 2.6–cm lesion between the caudate lobe of the liver and the crus of the diaphragm. (B) Planar posterior I-123 metaiodobenzylguanidine image showed intense tracer uptake in the right upper abdomen near the midline just inferior to the liver and a second focus of less intense uptake slightly inferior *(arrows)*. The single-photon emission CT images showed two additional sites of abnormal tracer uptake that colocalized with the findings on CT scan.

OUTCOME AND FOLLOW-UP

The patient was informed that at his first surgery in 1990 he likely had tumor capsule rupture and retroperitoneal seeding. Annual biochemical testing remained normal. Despite normal biochemistry, in 2006 (4 years after the laparotomy to resect recurrent PGL) at screening colonoscopy, his blood pressure rose to 190/110 mm Hg. CT and I-123 MIBG colocalized two sites of disease in right upper quadrant above the right kidney (2.2 cm) and near the diaphragm (2.6 cm). Following adrenergic blockade, the patient underwent his third laparotomy. The surgery was complicated by extensive adhesions, and to remove the recurrent PGL, a right nephrectomy was

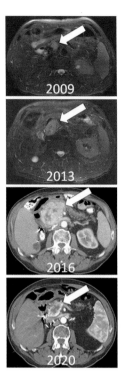

Fig. 53.2 Serial axial computed tomography (CT) images over 10 years of peripancreatic malignant paraganglioma *(arrows)*. The images from 2009 and 2013 were magnetic resonance images and the 2016 and 2020 images were CT scans. External beam radiation therapy was administered following the 2016 scan. The 2020 CT image showed the enhancing centrally necrotic mass has decreased in size from 7.2 × 5.7 × 8.0 cm to 3.0 × 3.0 × 5.1 cm.

necessary. At pathologic analysis recurrent PGL was confirmed, forming three nodules (3.0 × 2.9 × 2.0 cm; 2.5 × 2.0 × 1.5 cm; 0.8 × 0.6 × 0.6 cm). Six months after surgery the levels of fractionated metanephrines in the blood and urine remained normal.

In 2009 (19 years after his initial operation), surveillance imaging detected recurrent PGL (2 cm) adjacent to the pancreatic head (Fig. 53.2). Levels of fractionated metanephrines in the blood and urine remained normal. The patient was asymptomatic. A fourth laparotomy was deemed to carry high risk, and observation was advised. Over the next 4 years the recurrent PGL slowly enlarged and in 2013 it measured 5.8 cm (see Fig. 53.2). I-123 MIBG scintigraphy colocalized with this site of recurrent PGL, and no other areas of abnormal uptake were seen. The patient was asymptomatic and levels of fractionated metanephrines in the blood and urine remained normal.

In 2016 (at 79 years of age and 26 years after his initial operation), the patient presented with right upper quadrant abdominal pain. Biochemical testing was abnormal: plasma normetanephrine 3.9 nmol/L (normal, <0.9), 24-hour urine normetanephrine 2023 mcg (normal, <900), and 24-hr urine norepinephrine 357 mcg (normal, <80). Abdominal CT showed the peripancreatic metastatic PGL had enlarged to 7.2 × 5.7 × 8.0 cm (see Fig. 53.2). A F-18 fluorodeoxyglucose (FDG) positron emission tomography (PET)-CT scan showed that the large mass and two adjacent nodules were FDG avid (Fig. 53.3). The patient was treated with EBRT (3000 cGy over five fractions). Within weeks the abdominal pain resolved.

In 2020, 30 years after his first PGL-related surgery, 4 years after EBRT, and at 83 years of age, the patient remained pain free and was asymptomatic with respect to his malignant PGL. Biochemical testing had improved with a plasma normetanephrine concentration of 2.7 nmol/L (normal, <0.9). An abdominal CT scan showed that the enhancing centrally necrotic mass had decreased in size to 3.0 × 3.0 × 5.1 cm and the adjacent 1.9-cm aortocaval retroperitoneal mass was stable in size (see Fig. 53.2).

Discussion

We recently reported our experience with EBRT in the management of metastatic PPGL.[2] The cohort included 41 patients with 107 sites treated. The primary tumor was PGL in 63% of the patients. Indications for EBRT were local tumor control (66%), pain (22%), or spinal cord compression (12%). Treatment sites included bone (69%), soft tissue (30%), and liver (1%). The median EBRT dose was 40 Gy (range, 6.5–70 Gy). Overall survival at 5 years was 65%. Local tumor control at 5 years was 81% for all lesions. For the symptomatic lesions, symptoms improved in 94% of patients.[1]

Key Points

- There is no cure for metastatic PGL.[2]
- The first step in managing metastatic PPGL is to determine the pace of progression of the disease and then match it to a proportionate treatment.[2]

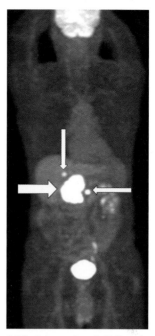

Fig. 53.3 Planar full-body image from F-18 fluorodeoxyglucose (FDG) positron emission tomography computed tomography scan from 2016 showed a large mass *(large arrow)* centered in the region of the pancreatic head (maximum standard unit value of 19.1). In addition, two FDG-avid nodules *(small arrows)* were between the large mass and the adjacent abdominal aorta and along the right hemidiaphragm posteriorly.

- Systemic chemotherapy is indicated in those patients with either rapidly progressive metastatic PPGL or excessive tumor bulk.
- EBRT should be considered for metastatic PPGL where there are focal lesions that are either painful or associated with risk if left untreated (e.g., pathologic bone fracture). EBRT is a very effective treatment option in these settings—a degree of efficacy that is a surprise to many clinicians.

REFERENCES

1. Breen W, Bancos I, Young WF Jr, et al. External beam radiation therapy for advanced/unresectable malignant paraganglioma and pheochromocytoma. *Adv Radiat Oncol.* 2017;3(1):25–29.
2. Young WF. Metastatic pheochromocytoma: in search of a cure. *Endocrinology.* 2020 Mar 1; 161(3):1.

Corticotropin-Dependent Hypercortisolism

Corticotropin (ACTH)-dependent hypercortisolism presents with a wide range of clinical features (Box F.1). Not all patients with symptomatic Cushing syndrome (CS) have the classic physical examination signs. No single feature is 100% sensitive and specific to the diagnosis of CS; however, development of supraclavicular fat pads, wide purple-red striae, and proximal myopathy are rare outside of CS.

Most patients with ACTH-dependent hypercortisolism will have an ACTH-secreting pituitary tumor. However, approximately 10%–15% of patients with ACTH-dependent hypercortisolism have an ectopic source of ACTH secretion (Box F.2). The most common neoplasms associated with ectopic ACTH secretion are bronchial carcinoid (≈25%), pancreatic neuroendocrine tumor (≈16%), occult and unlocalized tumor (≈16%), small cell lung cancer (≈11%), medullary thyroid carcinoma (≈9%), other neuroendocrine tumors (≈7%), thymic carcinoid (≈5%), and pheochromocytoma (≈3%).[1-4] A very rare entity is ectopic corticotropin releasing hormone (CRH) syndrome (<1%) as a result of neuroendocrine tumors secreting purely CRH or CRH and ACTH.[5,6]

Once ACTH-dependent hypercortisolism is diagnosed, the next step is to determine whether hypercortisolism is due to pituitary or ectopic origin (Box F.3). Because most ACTH-dependent hypercortisolism is of pituitary origin, proceeding with magnetic resonance imaging (MRI) of the pituitary gland is reasonable as the next step in management. When a clear-cut pituitary tumor is found on MRI in a woman with slowly progressive and mild-to-moderate ACTH-dependent hypercortisolism, proceeding directly to

transsphenoidal pituitary surgery (TSS) is a reasonable next step. Notably, up to 50% of patients with pituitary ACTH-dependent hypercortisolism do not demonstrate clearly visible pituitary tumors.[7,8]

Inferior petrosal sinus sampling (IPSS) can be used to determine the source of ACTH secretion. The patient must have active hypercortisolism on the day of IPSS, otherwise the test results are invalid and cannot be used. Pituitary-dependent disease is confirmed when the central to peripheral ACTH gradients are >2-to-1 at baseline and >3-to-1 after CRH administration.[9,10] In nearly all patients with pituitary-dependent CS the central-to-peripheral ACTH gradients markedly exceed these cutoffs. The diagnosis of pituitary-dependent hypercortisolism is supported by finding the CRH-stimulated increment in ACTH to

---

BOX F.1 CLINICAL PRESENTATION OF CORTICOTROPIN-DEPENDENT HYPERCORTISOLISM

Obesity, weight gain
Abdominal fat redistribution
Dorsocervical fat pads
Supraclavicular pads
Striae (wide purple-red striae over abdomen, flanks, arms, hips, and breasts)
Proximal myopathy
Thinning of the skin
Easy bruising
Hypertension
Prediabetes, diabetes mellitus type 2
Dyslipidemia
Cardiovascular events
Osteoporosis, fragility fractures
Depression, anxiety

BOX F.2 ETIOLOGY AND PRESENTATION OF SUBTYPES OF CORTICOTROPIN-DEPENDENT HYPERCORTISOLISMJ[2–4]

	Pituitary ACTH-Dependent Hypercortisolism	Ectopic ACTH-Dependent Hypercortisolism
Frequency	85%–90%	10%–15%
Age, years	Usually 20–50	Usually 35–60
Sex, women (%)	70%–80%	50%–60%
Duration of symptoms before diagnosis	Slowly progressing (years)	Rapid onset (months)
Clinical presentation	Mild to moderate cushingoid features (Box F.1)	Muscle loss, myopathy, hypokalemia
Severity of hypercortisolism	Mild-moderate 24-hour urine cortisol: 100–500 mcg/24 h	Severe 24-hour urine cortisol: >1000 mcg/24 h
Magnetic resonance imaging of pituitary gland	50% with visible pituitary lesion	–
Management	Transsphenoidal pituitary surgery	Resection of neuroendocrine tumor or bilateral adrenalectomy if tumor cannot be found

BOX F.3   TESTS USED IN DIAGNOSIS OF CORTICOTROPIN-DEPENDENT HYPERCORTISOLISM

	Pituitary ACTH-Dependent Hypercortisolism	Ectopic ACTH-Dependent Hypercortisolism
Establishing diagnosis of hypercortisolism	Late-night salivary cortisol (elevated) 24-hour UFC excretion (usually <500 mcg/24 h) 1-mg overnight DST (may not be needed)	Late-night salivary cortisol (frequently very high) 24-hour UFC excretion (frequently >500–1000 mcg/24 h) 1-mg overnight DST (usually not needed)
Establishing ACTH-dependence	Mid-normal to elevated plasma ACTH High-normal to elevated DHEA-S	High to very high plasma ACTH Elevated DHEA-S
Localization of hypercortisolism	MRI of pituitary: first step IPSS: not needed in setting of clearly visible pituitary adenoma	In a patient with known neuroendocrine tumor further testing may not be necessary IPSS (selected patients) Localization studies: CT of chest, Ga-68 DOTATATE PET-CT

ACTH, Corticotropin; *CT,* computed tomography; *DHEA-S,* dehydroepiandrosterone sulfate; *DOTATATE,* 1,4,7,10-tetraazacyclodo-decane-1,4,7,10-tetraacetic acid octreotate; *DST,* dexamethasone suppression test; *IPSS,* inferior petrosal sinus sampling; *MRI,* magnetic resonance imaging; *PET,* positron emission tomography; *UFC,* urinary free cortisol.

be >50% from baseline and the increment in cortisol to be >20% from baseline.[11,12] Notably, IPSS is less reliable in diagnosing the location of ACTH secreting tumor within the pituitary gland, as demonstrated in a study where ACTH gradient lateralization ratio of ≥1.4 between the two inferior petrosal sinuses accurately predicted the location only in 68% of cases.[13] IPSS carries small but serious risks, including brain stem injury (0.2%),[14] other serious complications such as venous subarachnoid hemorrhage, lower extremity deep venous thrombosis in 2%,[15] and transient sixth nerve palsies in another 2%.[16]

TSS is the procedure of choice to treat pituitary-dependent hypercortisolism. In a large series of 215 patients who underwent TSS for CS, surgical remission was achieved in 85.6%.[17] Actuarial recurrence rates of CS after initially successful TSS at 1, 2, 3, and 5 years were 0.5%, 6.7%, 10.8%, and 25.5%, respectively. The median time to recurrence was 39 months.[17]

There is no standard imaging protocol in patients with ectopic ACTH secretion. As the majority of neuroendocrine tumors are located in the lung, computed tomography (CT) of the chest is the logical the first step. Ga-68 1,4,7,10-tetraazacyclododecane-1,4,7,10-tetraacetic acid (DOTA)-octreotate (DOTATATE) positron emission tomography (PET)–CT, when available, has the best overall sensitivity and specificity for locating a neuroendocrine tumor.[18] However, the tumor may not be found in up to 9%–27% of patients with ectopic ACTH secretion. Although resecting the culprit neuroendocrine tumor should be attempted when possible, it is important not to delay therapy for severe hypercortisolism when this proves difficult. In these cases, bilateral adrenalectomy can be lifesaving.

Bilateral adrenalectomy is usually used when cure of ACTH-dependent hypercortisolism is not possible through removing the primary tumor. Bilateral adrenalectomy results in immediate cure of the hypercortisolism state, but it does require lifelong glucocorticoid and mineralocorticoid replacement; thus appropriate education of patients in regard to the management of adrenal insufficiency is important.[19] When bilateral adrenalectomy is performed for treatment of pituitary-dependent hypercortisolism, patients need monitoring for Nelson-Salassa syndrome.[20–22]

Curative surgery for ACTH-dependent hypercortisolism results in temporary adrenal insufficiency that needs to be properly treated. Cosyntropin testing is not needed to assess the recovery of the hypothalamic-pituitary-adrenal (HPA) axis.[23] At our institution, we simply check a morning serum cortisol concentration before the morning dose of hydrocortisone and this assesses hypothalamic CRH production, pituitary ACTH secretion, and adrenal cortisol secretion.[23] The periodic postoperative measurement of the morning serum cortisol concentration when the patient is on a single morning dosage of hydrocortisone is a simple and inexpensive way to monitor the recovery of the HPA axis.

Patients uniformly report that the glucocorticoid withdrawal symptoms after the cure of CS are worse than the CS itself. In addition, most patients report symptoms of glucocorticoid withdrawal that may last months and is characterized by fatigue, arthralgias, myalgias, headaches, insomnia, anxiety, and depression.[23] All patients need appropriate counseling in regard to both adrenal insufficiency management and symptoms of glucocorticoid withdrawal syndrome.[19]

REFERENCES

1. Lindholm J, Juul S, Jorgensen JO, et al. Incidence and late prognosis of Cushing's syndrome: a population-based study. *J Clin Endocrinol Metab*. 2001;86(1):117–123.
2. Isidori AM, Kaltsas GA, Pozza C, et al. The ectopic adrenocorticotropin syndrome: clinical features, diagnosis, management, and long-term follow-up. *J Clin Endocrinol Metab*. 2006;91(2):371–377.
3. Aniszewski JP, Young WF Jr., Thompson GB, Grant CS, van Heerden JA. Cushing syndrome due to ectopic adrenocorticotropic hormone secretion. *World J Surg*. 2001;25(7):934–940.
4. Ilias I, Torpy DJ, Pacak K, Mullen N, Wesley RA, Nieman LK. Cushing's syndrome due to ectopic corticotropin secretion: twenty years' experience at the National Institutes of Health. *J Clin Endocrinol Metab*. 2005;90(8):4955–4962.
5. Carey RM, Varma SK, Drake CR Jr., et al. Ectopic secretion of corticotropin-releasing factor as a cause of Cushing's syndrome. A clinical, morphologic, and biochemical study. *N Engl J Med*. 1984;311(1):13–20.
6. O'Brien T, Young WF Jr., Davila DG, et al. Cushing's syndrome associated with ectopic production of corticotrophin-releasing hormone, corticotrophin and vasopressin by a phaeochromocytoma. *Clin Endocrinol (Oxf)*. 1992;37(5):460–467.
7. Invitti C, Pecori Giraldi F, de Martin M, Cavagnini F. Diagnosis and management of Cushing's syndrome: results of an Italian multicentre study. Study Group of the Italian Society of Endocrinology on the Pathophysiology of the Hypothalamic-Pituitary-Adrenal Axis. *J Clin Endocrinol Metab*. 1999;84(2):440–448.
8. Chowdhury IN, Sinai N, Oldfield EH, Patronas N, Nieman LK. A change in pituitary magnetic resonance imaging protocol detects ACTH-secreting tumours in patients with previously negative results. *Clin Endocrinol (Oxf)*. 2010;72(4):502–506.
9. Findling JW, Aron DC, Tyrrell JB, et al. Selective venous sampling for ACTH in Cushing's syndrome: differentiation between Cushing disease and the ectopic ACTH syndrome. *Ann Intern Med*. 1981;94(5):647–652.
10. Oldfield EH, Chrousos GP, Schulte HM, et al. Preoperative lateralization of ACTH-secreting pituitary microadenomas by bilateral and simultaneous inferior petrosal venous sinus sampling. *N Engl J Med*. 1985;312(2):100–103.
11. Nieman LK, Biller BM, Findling JW, et al. The diagnosis of Cushing's syndrome: an Endocrine Society Clinical Practice Guideline. *J Clin Endocrinol Metab*. 2008;93(5):1526–1540.
12. Natt N, Young WF, Jr. The ovine corticotropin-releasing hormone stimulation test in the differential diagnosis of adrenocorticotropic hormone-dependent cushing's syndrome. *Endocr Pract*. 1997;3(3):130–134.
13. Oldfield EH, Doppman JL, Nieman LK, et al. Petrosal sinus sampling with and without corticotropin-releasing

hormone for the differential diagnosis of Cushing's syndrome. *N Engl J Med.* 1991;325(13):897–905.

14. Miller DL, Doppman JL, Peterman SB, Nieman LK, Oldfield EH, Chang R. Neurologic complications of petrosal sinus sampling. *Radiology.* 1992;185(1):143–147.

15. Bonelli FS, Huston 3rd, J, Carpenter PC, Erickson D, Young WF Jr, Meyer FB. Adrenocorticotropic hormone-dependent Cushing's syndrome: sensitivity and specificity of inferior petrosal sinus sampling. *AJNR Am J Neuroradiol.* 2000;21(4):690–696.

16. Lefournier V, Martinie M, Vasdev A, et al. Accuracy of bilateral inferior petrosal or cavernous sinuses sampling in predicting the lateralization of Cushing's disease pituitary microadenoma: influence of catheter position and anatomy of venous drainage. *J Clin Endocrinol Metab.* 2003;88(1):196–203.

17. Patil CG, Prevedello DM, Lad SP, et al. Late recurrences of Cushing's disease after initial successful transsphenoidal surgery. *J Clin Endocrinol Metab.* 2008;93(2):358–362.

18. Isidori AM, Sbardella E, Zatelli MC, et al. Conventional and nuclear medicine imaging in ectopic Cushing's syndrome: a systematic review. *J Clin Endocrinol Metab.* 2015;100(9):3231–3244.

19. Bancos I, Hahner S, Tomlinson J, Arlt W. Diagnosis and management of adrenal insufficiency. *Lancet Diabetes Endocrinol.* 2015;3(3):216–226.

20. Assie G, Bahurel H, Coste J, et al. Corticotroph tumor progression after adrenalectomy in Cushing's Disease: a reappraisal of Nelson's Syndrome. *J Clin Endocrinol Metab.* 2007;92(1):172–179.

21. Osswald A, Plomer E, Dimopoulou C, et al. Favorable long-term outcomes of bilateral adrenalectomy in Cushing's disease. *Eur J Endocrinol.* 2014;171(2):209–215.

22. Graffeo CS, Perry A, Carlstrom LP, et al. Characterizing and predicting the Nelson-Salassa syndrome. *J Neurosurg.* 2017;127(6):1277–1287.

23. Hurtado MD, Cortes T, Natt N, Young WF Jr., Bancos I. Extensive clinical experience: hypothalamic-pituitary-adrenal axis recovery after adrenalectomy for corticotropin-independent cortisol excess. *Clin Endocrinol (Oxf).* 2018;89(6):721–733.

Corticotropin-Dependent Cushing Syndrome Can Be Frequently Misdiagnosed

Corticotropin (ACTH)-dependent hypercortisolism is commonly due to an ACTH-secreting pituitary adenoma (80%–90%).[1] Most patients with ACTH-dependent hypercortisolism are women with slowly progressive mild to moderate Cushing syndrome (CS) who will have an ACTH-secreting pituitary tumor. The mean time from symptom onset to diagnosis in patients with pituitary CS is more than 3 years,[2] and the diagnosis is frequently confused with polycystic ovarian syndrome. When a clear-cut pituitary tumor is found on magnetic resonance imaging (MRI) in a woman with slowly progressive and mild-to-moderate ACTH-dependent CS, proceeding directly to transsphenoidal pituitary surgery (TSS) is a reasonable next step.

Case Report

The patient was a 33-year-old woman who was referred for evaluation and management of a pituitary adenoma. The pituitary lesion was incidentally discovered on a recent MRI of the brain that was performed due to severe headaches several times a week ("15/10" in intensity). Her medical history was positive for polycystic ovarian syndrome diagnosed 5 years ago (based on symptoms of weight gain and hirsutism), newly diagnosed diabetes mellitus type 2, mild hypertension, and anxiety. Since high school, she had gradually gained 140 pounds in weight and noticed progressive development of dorsocervical and supraclavicular pads. Her menstrual cycles were irregular. Her medications included alprazolam, 0.25 mg as needed for anxiety; metformin, 500 mg twice a day; and liraglutide, 1 mg daily for treatment of diabetes mellitus

type 2. On physical examination, her blood pressure was 132/88 mmHg, and her body mass index (BMI) was 46.6 kg/m². She was obese. She had mild supraclavicular pads, a dorsocervical pad, mild facial rounding, and mild facial erythema. She did not have signs of easy bruising, thinning of the skin, striae, or proximal myopathy. Clinical examination suggested a pretest probability of CS to be moderate.

INVESTIGATIONS

The baseline laboratory test results are shown in Table 54.1. The serum cortisol concentrations were increased and lacked diurnal variation. The 24-hour urine free cortisol excretion and the 1-mg

TABLE 54.1 Laboratory Tests

Biochemical Test	Result	Reference Range
8 AM serum cortisol, mcg/dL	15	7–25
4 PM serum cortisol, mcg/dL	12	2–14
1-mg overnight DST cortisol mcg/dL	18	<1.8
24-Hour UFC, mcg	138	<45
Late night salivary cortisol, ng/dL	78	≤100
ACTH, pg/mL	53	10–60
DHEA-S, mcg/dL	246	31–228
Prolactin, ng/mL	15.7	3–27
IGF1, ng/mL	240	59–279
Free thyroxine, ng/dL	1.2	09–1.7

ACTH, Corticotropin; *DHEA-S,* dehydroepiandrosterone sulfate; *DST,* dexamethasone suppression test; *IGF1,* insulinlike growth factor 1; *UFC,* urinary free cortisol.

overnight dexamethasone suppression test (DST) were abnormal, while the late-night salivary cortisol concentration was within normal ranges. The laboratory profile, in conjunction with the clinical presentation, confirmed ACTH-dependent CS. Workup for pituitary dysfunction otherwise was negative. Head MRI showed an $8 \times 10 \times 7$–mm pituitary adenoma in the left aspect of pituitary gland (Fig. 54.1).

TREATMENT

The patient was advised that her slow clinical course and mild-to-moderate degree of CS along with the visible pituitary adenoma on head MRI were most consistent with pituitary-dependent CS. The patient was advised that inferior petrosal sinus sampling (IPSS) was considered unnecessary and she should proceed with TSS. Following the TSS, immunohistochemistry of the pituitary tissue confirmed a corticotroph adenoma; the tumor cells strongly expressed ACTH and chromogranin.

OUTCOME AND FOLLOW-UP

The serum cortisol concentration the morning after surgery was 4.8 mcg/dL, confirming an initial cure. The patient was discharged from the hospital on hydrocortisone 30 mg on waking and 20 mg at noon with a plan for taper. She developed severe glucocorticoid withdrawal syndrome with arthralgias, myalgias, severe fatigue, exacerbation of anxiety, and new-onset

depression. Her hydrocortisone taper was slowed down in response to her marked withdrawal symptoms. She had a slow recovery of the hypothalamic-pituitary-adrenal (HPA) axis, with serum cortisol concentrations as follows: 4.8 mcg/dL 3 months after surgery; 5.2 mcg/dL 1 year after surgery; 8 mcg/dL 16 months after surgery; and 9.8 mcg/dL 19 months after surgery. At last follow-up she was taking 10 mg of hydrocortisone every morning. Cosyntropin testing is not needed to assess the recovery of the hypothalamic-pituitary-adrenal (HPA) axis. At our institution, we simply check a morning serum cortisol concentration before the morning dose of hydrocortisone, and this assesses hypothalamic corticotropin-releasing hormone production, pituitary ACTH secretion, and adrenal cortisol secretion.[3]

Discussion

In this case, the patient presented with unrecognized and long-standing ACTH-dependent hypercortisolism due to a pituitary adenoma. Eventually, she was diagnosed with CS, but only following the incidental discovery of a pituitary adenoma. Until then, her symptoms were attributed to polycystic ovarian syndrome (including weight gain, hirsutism, and diabetes mellitus type 2). In a systematic review of 5367 patients with CS, mean time from symptom onset to diagnosis was 14 months for ectopic ACTH CS, 30 months for adrenal-dependent CS, and 38 months

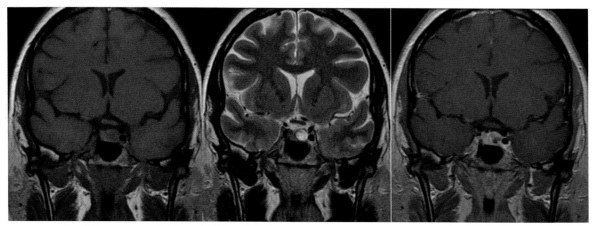

Fig. 54.1 Coronal images from head magnetic resonance imaging showed an $8 \times 10 \times 7$–mm pituitary adenoma.

for pituitary-dependent CS—a time lag that reflects the difficulties with making an accurate diagnosis. The time lag from symptom onset to the diagnosis of CS is likely due to nonspecific and mild symptoms that overlap with other conditions.[2]

The biochemical workup in our patient was consistent with ACTH-dependent hypercortisolism based on high-normal serum ACTH and dehydroepiandrosterone sulfate concentrations abnormal 1-mg overnight DST, and elevated 24-hour urinary free cortisol excretion. Notably, the late-night salivary cortisol concentration was not abnormal. In a systematic review and metaanalysis of diagnostic tests for CS, the sensitivity of late-night salivary cortisol concentration for the diagnosis of CS was 95% and specificity was 90%.[4] As no single test has 100% accuracy for CS diagnosis, it is important to combine clinical suspicion of CS with several biochemical tests to confirm hypercortisolism.

Curative surgery for pituitary-dependent CS leads to adrenal insufficiency. Thus it is important to ensure that patients are initiated and educated on glucocorticoid replacement therapy.[5] Recovery of the HPA axis likely depends on the duration and degree of untreated hypercortisolism before curative surgery.[6–8] Factors such as age, gender, BMI, subtypes of CS, duration of symptoms, clinical and biochemical severity, and postoperative glucocorticoid dose have been reported to affect the HPA axis recovery.[3,6–8] Regular reassessment of the HPA axis should be performed in all patients with adrenal insufficiency following curative surgery for CS. Recovery of the HP axis takes months to years.[3,6,8]

Glucocorticoid withdrawal syndrome (GWS) is a withdrawal reaction that occurs due to a decrease in supraphysiologic glucocorticoid concentrations.[9] The mechanism of GWS is multifactorial and is mediated by the central noradrenergic and dopaminergic system, decrease in proopiomelanocortin-related peptides due to chronic suppression of the HPA axis, and rebound increase in cytokines such as interleukin (IL)-6, tumor necrosis factor alpha, IL-1b, and prostaglandins, which occur with decreased glucocorticoid levels.[9] Patients often feel unwell with flu-like symptoms including anorexia, nausea, emesis, lethargy, somnolence, arthralgia, myalgia, fever, and postural hypotension.[9] The symptoms and signs may be prolonged, and

despite the glucocorticoid replacement, patients fail to immediately restore physical well-being and quality of life.[10] Thus it is important to properly counsel patients about GWS before curative surgery.

Key Points

- The diagnosis of CS is usually delayed, sometimes for years, due to a mild and nonspecific presentation. CS should be considered in any woman with symptoms of weight gain, hirsutism, and irregular menses.
- Both false-positive and false-negative results can occur in any tests for hypercortisolism, and thus the diagnosis of CS should be based on both clinical evaluation as well as a combination of biochemical tests.[4]
- Most women with mild-to-moderate ACTH-dependent CS that is slow in onset will have pituitary-dependent disease. When a definite non–prolactin-secreting pituitary tumor is found on MRI in these patients, it is reasonable to consider proceeding directly to TSS.
- The periodic postoperative measurement of the morning serum cortisol concentration when the patient is on a single morning dosage of hydrocortisone is a simple and inexpensive way to monitor the recovery of the HPA axis.
- Patients uniformly report that the glucocorticoid withdrawal symptoms following the cure of CS are worse than the CS itself.

REFERENCES

1. Nieman LK, Biller BM, Findling JW, et al. The diagnosis of Cushing's syndrome: an Endocrine Society Clinical Practice Guideline. *J Clin Endocrinol Metab.* 2008;93(5):1526–1540.

2. Rubinstein G, Osswald A, Hoster E, et al. Time to diagnosis in Cushing's syndrome: a meta-analysis based on 5367 patients. *J Clin Endocrinol Metab.* 2020;105(3):dgz136.

3. Hurtado MD, Cortes T, Natt N, Young WF Jr, Bancos I. Extensive clinical experience: hypothalamic-pituitary-adrenal axis recovery after adrenalectomy for corticotropin-independent cortisol excess. *Clin Endocrinol (Oxf).* 2018;89(6):721–733.

4. Galm BP, Qiao N, Klibanski A, Biller BMK, Tritos NA. Accuracy of laboratory tests for the diagnosis of Cushing syndrome. *J Clin Endocrinol Metab.* 2020;105(6):2081–2094.

5. Bancos I, Hahner S, Tomlinson J, Arlt W. Diagnosis and management of adrenal insufficiency. *Lancet Diabetes Endocrinol*. 2015;3(3):216–226.

6. Berr CM, Di Dalmazi G, Osswald A, et al. Time to recovery of adrenal function after curative surgery for Cushing's syndrome depends on etiology. *J Clin Endocrinol Metab*. 2015;100(4):1300–1308.

7. Klose M, Jorgensen K, Kristensen LO. Characteristics of recovery of adrenocortical function after treatment for Cushing's syndrome due to pituitary or adrenal adenomas. *Clin Endocrinol (Oxf)*. 2004;61(3):394–399.

8. Prete A, Paragliola RM, Bottiglieri F, et al. Factors predicting the duration of adrenal insufficiency in patients successfully treated for Cushing disease and nonmalignant primary adrenal Cushing syndrome. *Endocrine*. 2017;55(3): 969–980.

9. Hochberg Z, Pacak K, Chrousos GP. Endocrine withdrawal syndromes. *Endocr Rev*. 2003;24(4):523–538.

10. Dorn LD, Burgess ES, Friedman TC, Dubbert B, Gold PW, Chrousos GP. The longitudinal course of psychopathology in Cushing's syndrome after correction of hypercortisolism. *J Clin Endocrinol Metab*. 1997;82(3):912–919.

Corticotropin-Dependent Cushing Syndrome: Role for Inferior Petrosal Sinus Sampling

Most patients with corticotropin (ACTH)-dependent Cushing syndrome (CS) will have an ACTH-secreting pituitary tumor. However, approximately 10%–15% of patients with ACTH-dependent CS have an ectopic source of ACTH secretion (see Cases 58, 59, 60, 61, 62, and 63). When a clear-cut pituitary tumor is found on magnetic resonance imaging (MRI) in a woman with slowly progressive and mild-to-moderate ACTH-dependent CS, proceeding directly to transsphenoidal pituitary surgery (TSS) is a reasonable next step. However, when the pituitary appears normal on MRI, it is important to distinguish between ectopic and eutopic ACTH-dependent CS. The high-dose dexamethasone suppression test has proven to lack accuracy in making this distinction. Use of inferior petrosal sinus sampling (IPSS) to localize the source (pituitary versus ectopic) of ACTH secretion has been the most important technological advance for evaluation of CS over the past four decades.[1-3] Herein we present a case in which IPSS played a key role in directing a cure of CS.

Case Report

The patient was a 51-year-old woman who was referred for evaluation and management of CS. Her signs and symptoms consistent with CS included secondary amenorrhea of 2 years duration, progressive facial plethora over the past 2 years, diabetes mellitus and hypertension diagnosed 9 years previously, osteoporosis diagnosed 5 years previously, scalp hair thinning and marked curling of her hair, easy bruising, and poor wound healing. Although her weight had been fairly stable, she said "I weigh less but feel fatter." She has lost weight from the extremities

but gained abdominal girth. She had been experiencing difficulty walking up stairs. Her medications included glipizide, 10 mg twice daily; metformin, 1000 mg twice daily; sitagliptin, 100 mg daily; alendronate, 70 mg weekly; hydrochlorothiazide, 25 mg daily; and simvastatin 20 mg daily. On physical examination her body mass index was 32.2 kg/m^2, blood pressure was 121/79 mmHg, and heart rate 80 beats per minute. She appeared cushingoid with supraclavicular and dorsocervical fat pads, a round and plethoric face, and noticeable scalp hair loss (Fig. 55.1). Her extremities were relatively thin and she had proximal muscle weakness.

INVESTIGATIONS

The baseline laboratory test results are shown in Table 55.1. The serum cortisol concentrations were increased and lacked diurnal variation. The 24-hour urine free cortisol excretion and salivary cortisol concentration were more than twofold elevated above the respective upper limits of the reference ranges. The goal of laboratory testing is to build a wall of evidence to either refute or confirm the diagnosis of CS.[4] Thus based on the clinical presentation and baseline laboratory findings, CS was confirmed.[4] No additional testing (e.g., 1-mg overnight dexamethasone suppression test or a formal 2-day low-dose dexamethasone suppression testing) was needed. The serum ACTH concentration was high-normal and confirmed that CS was ACTH dependent. A head MRI showed a 3 × 5 × 7–mm region of relative diminished enhancement in left anterior aspect of pituitary (Fig. 55.2); although somewhat heterogeneous and not classic, the findings were consistent with a microadenoma. The serum prolactin concentration was normal (Table 55.1). A preoperative screening chest radiograph showed a small

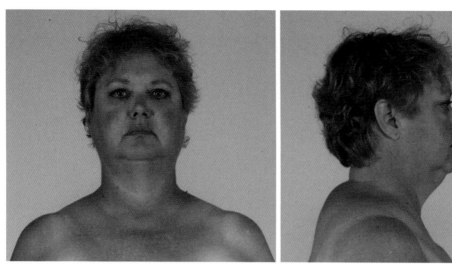

Fig. 55.1 Photographs show full plethoric face, supraclavicular and dorsocervical fat pads, scalp hair thinning, and curly hair that was new for her.

TABLE 55.1 Laboratory Tests

Biochemical Test	Result	Repeat Test Result	Reference Range
Sodium, mEq/L	141		135–145
Potassium, mEq/L	4.1		3.6–5.2
Fasting plasma glucose, mg/dL	96		70–100
Glycosylated hemoglobin, %	7.7		4–6
Creatinine, mg/dL	0.7		0.6–1.1
eGFR, mL/min/BSA	>60		>60
8 AM serum cortisol, mcg/dL	25	15	7–25
4 pm serum cortisol, mcg/dL	25		2–14
24Hour UFC, mcg	284	103	3.5–45
24-Hour urine volume, L	1.7	1.3	Goal <4 L
Late night salivary cortisol, ng/dL	215	198	≤100
ACTH, pg/mL	52	50	10–60
DHEA-S, mcg/dL	138		15–200
Prolactin, ng/mL	11		3–27

ACTH, Corticotropin; *BSA,* body surface area; *DHEA-S,* dehydro-epiandrosterone sulfate; *eGFR,* estimated glomerular filtration rate; *UFC,* urinary free cortisol.

nodule in the left upper lung laterally. A subsequent chest computed tomography (CT) scan showed a 7-mm noncalcified nodule in the left upper lobe laterally that corresponded to the finding described on the chest radiograph (Fig. 55.3). The patient was advised that her slow clinical course and mild-to-moderate degree of CS along with the apparent pituitary adenoma on head MRI were most consistent with pituitary-dependent CS. However, the nodule found on chest CT raised the possibility of an ACTH-secreting bronchial carcinoid tumor—the clinical and biochemical presentation of which can mimic pituitary-dependent CS. IPPS was advised, and the results are shown in Box 55.1. Baseline serum cortisol concentrations on the day of IPSS confirmed active CS. The patient must have active CS on the day of IPSS—otherwise the test results are invalid and cannot be used to direct patient care.[5] The central-to-peripheral ACTH gradient from the right IPS was 13.3-to-1 before corticotropin-releasing hormone (CRH) administration and 36.6-to-1 after CRH administration. Pituitary dependent-disease is confirmed when these gradients are >2-to-1 at baseline and >3-to-1 after CRH administration.[1–3] In nearly all patients with pituitary-dependent CS the central-to-peripheral ACTH gradients markedly exceed these cutoffs (as was the case for this patient); when the gradients are just above the cut-offs, we worry that the patient may actually have ectopic CS. In addition, the peripheral CRH stimulation test

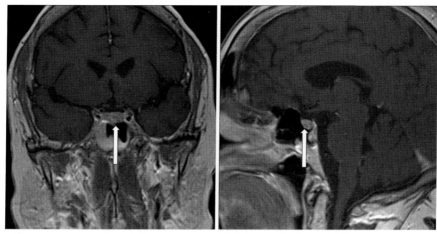

Fig. 55.2 Coronal *(left)* and sagittal *(right)* images from head magnetic resonance imaging showed a 3 × 5 × 7–mm region of relative diminished enhancement in anterior aspect of pituitary *(arrows)*. The apparent lesion had a more h eterogeneous in appearance on the coronal images. These findings could be consistent with a pituitary microadenoma.

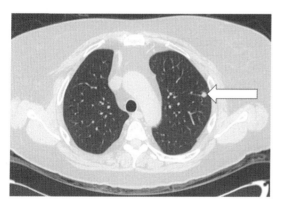

Fig. 55.3 Axial image from chest computed tomography scan showed a 7-mm noncalcified nodule *(arrow)* in the left upper lobe laterally.

BOX 55.1 INFERIOR PETROSAL SINUS SAMPLING[a]

	ACTH, pg/mL		Cortisol, mcg/dL	
	Right IPS	PV	Left IPS	PV
–5 minutes	423	32	57	14
–1 minute	403	30	54	14
+2 minutes	987	28	70	13
+5 minutes	1370	32	52	13
+10 minutes	1155	37	59	13
+30 minutes		54		22
+45 minutes		59		26
+60 minutes		55		28

[a]Simultaneous IPSS completed before (–5 and –1 minutes) and after (+2, +5, and +10 minutes) administration of corticotropin-releasing hormone (CRH) (1 mcg per kg body weight; maximum dose of 100 mcg). Peripheral vein sampling was continued through 60 minutes after CRH administration. *ACTH,* Corticotropin; *IPS,* inferior petrosal sinus; *IPSS,* inferior petrosal sinus sampling; *PV,* peripheral vein.

showed a 90% increase in ACTH concentration from baseline and a 100% increase in cortisol concentration from baseline. The diagnosis of pituitary-dependent CS is supported by finding the CRH-stimulated increment in ACTH to be >50% from baseline and the increment in cortisol to be >20% from baseline.[6] Thus pituitary-dependent CS was confirmed.

TREATMENT

The patient underwent transsphenoidal surgery, and on entering the sella the tumor was immediately visible and removed. Immunohistochemistry of the pituitary tissue confirmed a corticotroph adenoma; the tumor cells strongly expressed ACTH and chromogranin. The serum cortisol concentration the morning after surgery was 1.6 mcg/dL, confirming an initial cure. The patient was dismissed from the hospital on prednisone 10 mg twice daily with a plan for taper. We tell all patients before surgery that although CS is associated with marked debilitating signs and symptoms, recovering from CS is worse!

OUTCOME AND FOLLOW-UP

Follow-up 3 months later showed some of the signs and symptoms of CS had resolved, and the patient was struggling markedly with glucocorticoid withdrawal symptoms on her tapered dosage of prednisone 5 mg daily. She had lost 20 pounds of weight. Her glycosylated hemoglobin had improved to 5.4%, and two of her diabetes medications had been discontinued. Her morning serum cortisol was 5.4 mcg/dL. Because of the marked steroid withdrawal symptoms, the dosage of prednisone was increased for several weeks and a slower taper schedule was provided until prednisone was replaced with hydrocortisone 15 mg every morning and an 8 AM serum cortisol concentration (obtained before the morning dose of hydrocortisone) was measured every 6 weeks. Nine months after surgery the serum cortisol concentration was >10 mcg/dL, and treatment with hydrocortisone was discontinued. Cosyntropin testing is not needed to assess the recovery of the hypothalamic-pituitary-adrenal (HPA) axis.[7] Simply check a morning serum cortisol concentration before the morning dose of hydrocortisone and this assesses hypothalamic CRH production, pituitary ACTH secretion, and adrenal cortisol secretion.[7]

Last follow-up was 10 years after surgery. Her annual 24-hour urine cortisol measurements remained normal. Her weight decreased from 198 pounds preoperatively to a nadir of 164 pounds postoperatively. Diabetes mellitus and hypertension resolved. Follow-up chest imaging showed long-term stability of the lung nodule. She specifically highlighted the observation that the curliness of her hair resolved after surgery. Her friend had a horse with CS and one of the main symptoms was new onset of curly hair . . .

Key Points

- Most women with mild-to-moderate ACTH-dependent CS that is slow in onset will have pituitary-dependent disease. When a definite non–prolactin-secreting pituitary tumor is found on MRI in these patients, it is reasonable to consider proceeding directly to TSS.
- There is a subset of patients with ectopic ACTH syndrome caused by bronchial carcinoid tumors that has mild-to-moderate CS that can mimic pituitary-dependent disease. Thus there should be a low threshold to pursue IPSS—especially if there are imaging findings that are suspicious for an ectopic source of ACTH secretion (e.g., a lung nodule).
- For IPSS to be valid, the patient must have active CS on the day of IPSS.
- Pituitary-dependent CS is confirmed when the IPSS central-to-peripheral gradients are >2-to-1 at baseline and >3-to-1 after CRH administration. In nearly all patients with pituitary-dependent CS the central-to-peripheral ACTH gradients markedly exceed these cutoffs; when the gradients are just above the cutoffs, we worry that the patient may actually have ectopic CS.
- The periodic postoperative measurement of the morning serum cortisol concentration when the patient is on a single morning dosage of hydrocortisone is a simple and inexpensive way to monitor the recovery of the HPA axis.
- Patients uniformly report that the glucocorticoid withdrawal symptoms after the cure of CS are worse than CS itself.

REFERENCES

1. Findling JW, Aron DC, Tyrrell JB, et al. Selective venous sampling for ACTH in Cushing's syndrome: differentiation between Cushing disease and the ectopic ACTH syndrome. *Ann Intern Med.* 1981;94(5):647–652.

2. Manni A, Latshaw RF, Page R, Santen RJ. Simultaneous bilateral venous sampling for adrenocorticotropin in pituitary-dependent Cushing's disease: evidence for lateralization of pituitary venous drainage. *J Clin Endocrinol Metab.* 1983;57(5):1070–1073.

3. Oldfield EH, Chrousos GP, Schulte HM, et al. Preoperative lateralization of ACTH-secreting pituitary microadenomas by bilateral and simultaneous inferior petrosal venous sinus sampling. *N Engl J Med.* 1985;312(2):100–103.

4. Nieman LK, Biller BM, Findling JW, et al. The diagnosis of Cushing's syndrome: an Endocrine Society Clinical Practice Guideline. *J Clin Endocrinol Metab.* 2008;93(5):1526–1540.

5. Yamamoto Y, Davis DH, Nippoldt TB, Young WF Jr, Huston J 3rd, Parisi JE. False-positive inferior petrosal sinus sampling in the diagnosis of Cushing's disease. Report of two cases. *J Neurosurg.* 1995;83(6):1087–1091.

6. Natt N, Young WF Jr. The ovine corticotropin-releasing hormone stimulation test in the differential diagnosis of adrenocorticotropic hormone-dependent Cushing's syndrome. *Endocr Pract.* 1997;3(3):130–134.

7. Hurtado MD, Cortes T, Natt N, Young WF Jr, Bancos I. Extensive clinical experience: hypothalamic-pituitary-adrenal axis recovery after adrenalectomy for corticotropin-independent cortisol excess. *Clin Endocrinol (Oxf).* 2018;89(6):721–733.

Corticotropin-Dependent Cushing Syndrome: When Inferior Petrosal Sinus Sampling Is Not Needed

Most patients with corticotropin (ACTH)-dependent Cushing syndrome (CS) will have an ACTH-secreting pituitary tumor. When a clear-cut pituitary tumor is found on magnetic resonance imaging (MRI) in a woman with slowly progressive and mild-to-moderate ACTH-dependent CS, proceeding directly to transsphenoidal pituitary surgery (TSS) is a reasonable next step. Herein we present such a case in which inferior petrosal sinus sampling (IPSS) was not needed.

Case Report

The patient was a 26-year-old woman who was referred for a second opinion on whether she might have CS. She developed very subtle signs and symptoms of glucocorticoid excess over the past 2 1/2 years. With plans for fertility, she stopped her oral contraceptive pill 3 years ago and has not had a menstrual period since. She sought consultation with a reproductive endocrinologist, and the serum prolactin concentration was normal, but the serum dehydroepiandrosterone sulfate (DHEA-S) concentration was elevated (Table 56.1). Her symptoms included insomnia (routinely woke between 11:30 PM and 1:30 AM and she felt "wired"), new-onset acne, mild hirsutism, and a 10-pound weight gain with distribution above her clavicles, in her face, and on her abdomen. She was diagnosed with new-onset hypertension 1 year ago. She had been working hard to prevent further weight gain with a high-intensity exercise program 5 days a week for 45 minutes. Her only medication was α-methyldopa, 500 mg daily. On physical examination her body mass index was 21.8 kg/m^2, blood pressure was 138/97 mmHg,

and heart rate 96 beats per minute. She did not appear overtly cushingoid. Her skin was normal and there were no purple-red striae. Her abdomen was flat. Compared to her old photographs, she did have supraclavicular fullness (Fig. 56.1). She had good muscle tone and no proximal muscle weakness.

INVESTIGATIONS

The laboratory test results are shown in Table 56.1. The serum cortisol concentrations were high-normal, but diurnal variation was intact. On repeated measurements the 24-hour urine free cortisol excretion and salivary cortisol concentration were more than twofold elevated above the respective upper limits of the reference ranges. An 8-mg overnight dexamethasone suppression test (DST) was performed before referral to Mayo Clinic and was remarkably abnormal (see Table 56.1). Thus based on her symptoms, the finding of supraclavicular fat pads, and the laboratory findings, CS was confirmed.[1] The serum ACTH concentration was high-normal and confirmed that CS was ACTH dependent. Head MRI showed a 2-mm apparent pituitary adenoma (Fig. 56.2). The patient was advised that her slow clinical course and very mild degree of signs and symptoms of CS along with the apparent pituitary adenoma on head MRI were diagnostic of pituitary-dependent CS. We advised her that IPSS does carry some risk and was not needed in her case. Brain stem injury has been reported to occur in 1 out of 508 (0.2%) patients undergoing IPSS at the National Institutes of Health.[1] In our early Mayo Clinic series of IPSS (1990–97) in 92 patients we had 2 (2%) serious complications (venous subarachnoid hemorrhage, lower extremity deep venous thrombosis).[2] In a series of 86 patients who had IPSS in Grenoble, France, 2 (2%) patients had transient sixth nerve palsies.[3]

TABLE 56.1 Laboratory Tests

Biochemical Test	Result	Repeat Test Result	Repeat Test Result	Reference Range
Sodium, mEq/L	142			135–145
Potassium, mEq/L	4.0			3.6–5.2
Fasting plasma glucose, mg/dL	85			70–100
Glycosylated hemoglobin, %	5.2			4–6
Creatinine, mg/dL	0.7			0.6–1.1
eGFR, mL/min per BSA	>60			>60
8 AM serum cortisol, mcg/dL	23	15	22.9	7–25
4 PM serum cortisol, mcg/dL	14			2–14
24-Hour UFC, mcg	111	296	103	3.5–45
24-Hour urine volume, L	3.7	2.4	3.1	Goal <4 L
Late night salivary cortisol, ng/dL	190	210		≤100
ACTH, pg/mL	80	50	88	10–60
DHEA-S, mcg/dL	687	502	561	44–332
Prolactin, ng/mL	10			3–27
8-mg overnight DST, mcg/dL	2.1			Undetectable

ACTH, Corticotropin; *BSA,* body surface area; *DHEA-S,* dehydroepiandrosterone sulfate; *DST,* dexamethasone suppression test; *eGFR,* estimated glomerular filtration rate; *UFC,* urinary free cortisol.

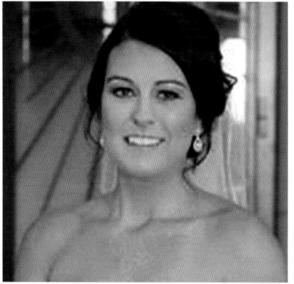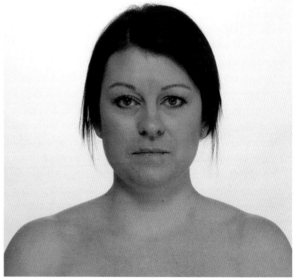

Fig. 56.1 Photographs from 3 years previously *(left)* and at time of consultation *(right)* show the development of supraclavicular fat pads—a subtle but important clinical clue.

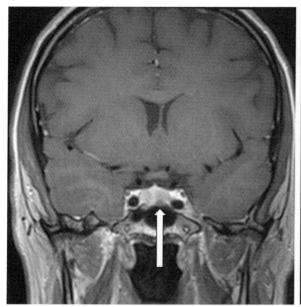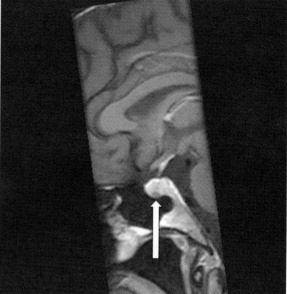

Fig. 56.2 Coronal *(left)* and sagittal *(right)* images from gadolinium-enhanced head magnetic resonance imaging showed at the base of the pituitary gland on the left there was a 2-mm hypointense and hypoenhancing region *(arrows)* consistent with a pituitary microadenoma.

TREATMENT

The patient underwent TSS. On entering the sella, there was a small tumor on the left side of the pituitary gland, as predicted by the MRI. The specimens provided to pathology did not show a definitive adenoma on hematoxylin and eosin and reticulin staining. Immunohistochemistry of the pituitary tissue showed a mixture of cell types within the anterior hypophysis when stained with growth hormone, prolactin, thyroid-stimulating hormone, α-subunit, follicle-stimulating hormone, luteinizing hormone, and ACTH. The serum cortisol concentration the morning after surgery was 7.0 mcg/dL, and the patient was symptomatic with diffuse myalgias. Because the serum cortisol was not <2.0 mcg/dL,[4] we were concerned that she might not be in remission. The patient was discharged from the hospital on prednisone 10 mg in the morning and 5 mg in the afternoon with a plan to taper the total dosage by 2.5 mg every week until a maintenance dose of 5 mg every morning.

OUTCOME AND FOLLOW-UP

Two weeks after surgery her morning serum cortisol concentration was 2.6 mcg/dL. Once the prednisone dosage reached 5 mg every morning, she was switched to hydrocortisone 20 mg every morning for 2 weeks and then 15 mg every morning thereafter. At her 4-month postoperative follow-up visit and before her morning dose of hydrocortisone, her serum cortisol concentration was 2.9 mcg/dL. She had lost 10 pounds "without even trying." Her face was thinner and the supraclavicular fat pads resolved. Her blood pressure normalized, and treatment with α-methyldopa was discontinued. Her menstrual cycles restarted. Six months after surgery before her morning dose of hydrocortisone, the serum cortisol concentration was 9.3 mcg/dL. Nine months after surgery, the morning serum cortisol concentration was >10 mcg/dL, and hydrocortisone was discontinued. One year after surgery, the 24-hour urinary free cortisol was normal. Eighteen months after surgery she delivered a healthy baby boy. Four years after surgery she remained well with normal blood pressure and had recently delivered her second child. Annual 24-hour urinary free cortisol excretion remained normal.

As demonstrated in this case, cosyntropin testing is not needed to assess the recovery of the hypothalamic-pituitary-adrenal (HPA) axis.[5] Simply check a morning serum cortisol concentration before the morning dose of hydrocortisone, and this assesses hypothalamic CRH production, pituitary ACTH secretion, and adrenal cortisol secretion.[5]

Key Points

- Distinguishing between mild CS and pseudo-CS is one of the most difficult challenges for the endocrinologist. There should never be a rush to make this distinction. The endocrinologist needs to build a wall of evidence to support the diagnosis of CS.

- Not all patients with symptomatic CS have the classic physical examination signs, and old photographs can be invaluable, as they were in the case described here.

- Although dorsocervical fat pads may develop with weight gain in people without CS, the development of supraclavicular fat pads is quite specific for CS.

- In some patients with cured pituitary-dependent CS, the corticotroph adenoma is not seen on pathology specimens, as was the situation with our case. In a report of 29 patients with pituitary-dependent CS and no confirmation of tumor on pathology, 19 (66%) had a long-term cure.[6] The authors speculated that this phenomenon is to the result of one or more of the following: (1) the tumor was removed but not provided for histologic evaluation; (2) the tumor was not sampled in the specimen provided to the pathologist; (3) the adenomas may have been lost in the suction apparatus or in the surgical field; and/or (4) the adenoma was too small to be detected on routine histology.[6]

REFERENCES

1. Miller DL, Doppman JL, Peterman SB, Nieman LK, Oldfield EH, Chang R. Neurologic complications of petrosal sinus sampling. *Radiology*. 1992;185(1): 143–147.

2. Bonelli FS, Huston 3rd J, Carpenter PC, Erickson D, Young Jr WF, Meyer FB. Adrenocorticotropic hormone-dependent Cushing's syndrome: sensitivity and specificity of inferior petrosal sinus sampling. *AJNR Am J Neuroradiol*. 2000;21(4):690–696.

3. Lefournier V, Martinie M, Vasdev A, et al. Accuracy of bilateral inferior petrosal or cavernous sinuses sampling in predicting the lateralization of Cushing's disease pituitary microadenoma: influence of catheter position and anatomy of venous drainage. *J Clin Endocrinol Metab*. 2003;88(1):196–203.

4. Biller BM, Grossman AB, Stewart PM, et al. Treatment of adrenocorticotropin-dependent Cushing's syndrome: a consensus statement. *J Clin Endocrinol Metab*. 2008;93(7):2454–2462.

5. Hurtado MD, Cortes T, Natt N, Young WF Jr, Bancos I. Extensive clinical experience: hypothalamic-pituitary-adrenal axis recovery after adrenalectomy for corticotropin-independent cortisol excess. *Clin Endocrinol (Oxf)*. 2018;89(6):721–733.

6. Sheehan JM, Lopes MB, Sheehan JP, Ellegala D, Webb KM, Laws ER Jr. Results of transsphenoidal surgery for Cushing's disease in patients with no histologically confirmed tumor. *Neurosurgery*. 2000;47(1):33–36; discussion 37-9.

Severe Corticotropin-Dependent Cushing Syndrome From a Pituitary Adenoma

Most patients with corticotropin (ACTH)-dependent Cushing syndrome (CS) will have an ACTH-secreting pituitary microadenoma—50% of which are so small that they cannot be seen on magnetic resonance imaging (MRI). Pituitary-dependent CS is typically associated with mild-to-moderate CS, and 24-hour urinary free cortisol (UFC) excretion is typically 100–500 mcg and very rarely >1000 mcg. When patients with ACTH-dependent CS present with spontaneous hypokalemia and 24-hour UFC >1000 mcg, the clinician should suspect an ectopic ACTH-secreting tumor. However, there is a subset of patients with pituitary-dependent CS who have large pituitary adenomas and the clinical presentation can overlap with that of ectopic ACTH secretion. Herein we present such a case.

Case Report

The patient was a 28-year-old woman who was self-referred for possible CS. She experienced a 62-pound centrally distributed weight gain over 3 years. She had noticed a rounding and redness of her face, hirsutism on her cheeks and upper lip, and acne on her arms. She had marked weakness in her legs when going up stairs. Recently, she was diagnosed with mild hyperglycemia and placed on metformin. Elevated blood pressure readings were noted on her last few blood pressure checks. She had also developed secondary amenorrhea. As a registered nurse, she raised the possibility of CS to explain her signs and symptoms. Her medications included metformin 500 mg twice daily and ranitidine 150 mg daily. Amlodipine and metoprolol were added to treat her hypertension. On physical examination her body mass index was 38.9 kg/m^2, blood pressure was 138/98 mmHg, and heart rate 76 beats per minute. She appeared markedly cushingoid compared to photographs taken 3 years previously (Fig. 57.1). She had a full round and plethoric face. She had marked supraclavicular and dorsocervical fat pads. Her lower extremities were thinner than the rest of her body. There were thin red striae on her flanks.

INVESTIGATIONS

The laboratory test results are shown in Table 57.1. She had spontaneous hypokalemia. The cortisol concentrations in the blood and urine were diagnostic of severe hypercortisolism. The serum concentration of ACTH was markedly elevated. Computed tomography of the chest and abdomen did not reveal a neoplasm in the lung, pancreas, or small bowel. However, head MRI did identify an 8-mm right-sided pituitary tumor (Fig. 57.2). The patient was informed that her marked CS was most likely because of a relatively large corticotroph pituitary tumor. We advised that IPSS does carry some risk and was not needed in her case. Brain stem injury has been reported to occur in 1 out of 508 (0.2%) patients undergoing IPSS at the National Institutes of Health.[1] In our early Mayo Clinic series of IPSS (1990–97) in 92 patients we had 2 (2%) serious complications (venous subarachnoid hemorrhage, lower extremity deep venous thrombosis).[2] In a series of 86 patients who had IPSS in Grenoble, France, 2 (2%) patients had transient sixth nerve palsies.[3]

TREATMENT

The patient underwent transsphenoidal surgery, and the tumor on the right side of the sella was immediately encountered. Pathology demonstrated loss of the

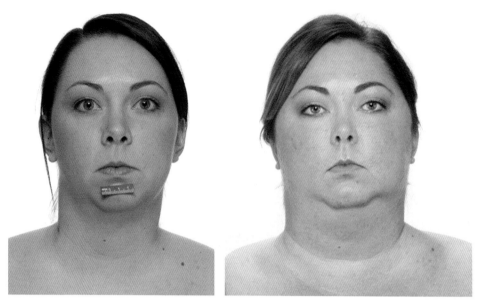

Fig. 57.1 Photographs from 3 years previously (on *left* at the time of nevus-related dermatology photographs) and at time of consultation *(right)* show the development of a full plethoric face, fine lanugo hair on the checks, and supraclavicular fat pads.

TABLE 57.1	Laboratory Tests		
Biochemical Test	Result	Repeat Test Result	Reference Range
Sodium, mEq/L	146		135–145
Potassium, mEq/L	3.5		3.6–5.2
Fasting plasma glucose, mg/dL	102		70–100
Glycosylated hemoglobin, %	5.4		4–6
Creatinine, mg/dL	0.8		0.6–1.04
eGFR, mL/min per BSA	>60		>60
8 AM serum cortisol, mcg/dL	33	42	7–25
4 PM serum cortisol, mcg/dL	33		2–14
24-Hour UFC, mcg	1057		3.5–45
24-Hour urine volume, L	2.1		Goal <4 L
ACTH, pg/mL	192		10–60
DHEA-S, mcg/dL	181		44–332
Prolactin, ng/mL	17.3		4.8–23.3

ACTH, Corticotropin; *BSA,* body surface area; *DHEA-S,* dehydroepiandrosterone sulfate; *eGFR,* estimated glomerular filtration rate; *UFC,* urinary free cortisol.

normal nested pattern on reticulin staining, supporting the diagnosis of pituitary adenoma. On immunohistochemical staining, the adenoma cells were positive for chromogranin and ACTH and negative for growth hormone, prolactin, thyroid-stimulating hormone, α-subunit, follicle-stimulating hormone, and luteinizing hormone. The serum cortisol concentration the morning after surgery was 3.1 mcg/dL, and the patient was symptomatic with diffuse myalgias and nausea. She was discharged from the hospital on prednisone 10 mg in the morning and 10 mg in the afternoon with a plan to taper the total dosage by 2.5 mg every week until reaching a maintenance dose of 5 mg every morning.

OUTCOME AND FOLLOW-UP

Four weeks after surgery the morning serum cortisol concentration was <1.0 mcg/dL. Once the prednisone taper reached 5 mg every morning, she was switched to hydrocortisone 20 mg every morning for 2 weeks and then 15 mg every morning thereafter. At her 4-month postoperative visit and before her morning dose of hydrocortisone, the serum cortisol concentration was <1.0 mcg/dL. She had lost 15 pounds of body weight. Her menses restarted and were regular. Her

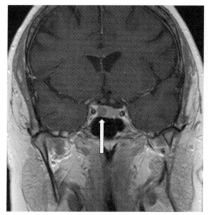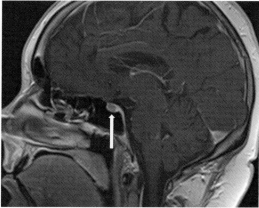

Fig. 57.2 Coronal *(left)* and sagittal *(right)* images from gadolinium-enhanced head magnetic resonance imaging showed an 8-mm hypointense and hypoenhancing right-sided pituitary adenoma *(arrows)*.

blood pressure was low-normal, and treatment with the calcium channel blocker and β-adrenergic blocker was discontinued. Serial serum cortisol levels before her morning dose of hydrocortisone were <1.0 mcg/dL at 6 months, 2.6 mcg/dL at 7 months, 3.9 mcg/dL at 9 months, 4.9 mcg/dL at 10 months, 9.7 mcg/dL at 12 months, and 12 mcg/dL at 15 months after surgery—at which point treatment with hydrocortisone was discontinued. The glucocorticoid taper to 15 mg of hydrocortisone every morning and monitoring the hypothalamic-pituitary-adrenal axis recovery with the periodic measurement of morning serum cortisol is the standard approach at Mayo Clinic.[4] The cosyntropin stimulation test is an unnecessary expense in this setting; it only informs the clinician about adrenal function and not what is needed, which is assessment of hypothalamic and pituitary recovery.[4]

At 1 year after surgery she had lost 49 pounds of body weight, and 24-hour UFC was normal. She was informed of the approximately 25% risk of recurrent CS over time. Subsequent 24-hour UFC measurements were 14, 21, and 18 mcg (normal, <45 mcg) at 2, 3, and 4 years after surgery. In a large series of 215 patients who underwent transsphenoidal surgery for CS, surgical remission was achieved in 85.6%.[5] Actuarial recurrence rates of CS after initially successful transsphenoidal surgery at 1, 2, 3, and 5 years were 0.5%, 6.7%, 10.8%, and 25.5%, respectively. The median time to recurrence was 39 months.[5] Thus we advised annual 24-hour UFC for at least 10 years after surgery.

Key Points

- Most patients with ACTH-dependent CS will have an ACTH-secreting pituitary microadenoma —50% of which are so small that they cannot be seen on MRI.
- Pituitary-dependent CS is typically associated with mild-to-moderate CS, and 24-hour UFC excretion is typically 100–500 mcg and very rarely >1000 mcg. When patients with ACTH-dependent CS present with spontaneous hypokalemia and 24-hour UFC >1000 mcg, the clinician should suspect an ectopic ACTH-secreting tumor.
- Clinicians need to be aware of the subset of patients with pituitary-dependent CS who have large pituitary adenomas, and the clinical presentation can overlap with the severe hypercortisolism associated with ectopic ACTH secretion.
- The risk for recurrent pituitary-dependent CS after an initial surgical cure is approximately 25%, and these patients require annual follow-up for at least 10 years.

REFERENCES

1. Miller DL, Doppman JL, Peterman SB, Nieman LK, Oldfield EH, Chang R. Neurologic complications of petrosal sinus sampling. *Radiology*. 1992;185(1): 143–147.
2. Bonelli FS, Huston J 3rd, Carpenter PC, Erickson D, Young WF Jr, Meyer FB. Adrenocorticotropic hormone-dependent Cushing's syndrome: sensitivity and specificity of inferior petrosal sinus sampling. *AJNR Am J Neuroradiol*. 2000;21(4):690–696.

3. Lefournier V, Martinie M, Vasdev A, et al. Accuracy of bilateral inferior petrosal or cavernous sinuses sampling in predicting the lateralization of Cushing's disease pituitary microadenoma: influence of catheter position and anatomy of venous drainage. *J Clin Endocrinol Metab*. 2003;88(1):196–203.

4. Hurtado MD, Cortes T, Natt N, Young WF Jr, Bancos I. Extensive clinical experience: hypothalamic-pituitary-adrenal axis recovery after adrenalectomy for corticotropin-independent cortisol excess. *Clin Endocrinol (Oxf)*. 2018;89(6):721–733.

5. Patil CG, Prevedello DM, Lad SP, et al. Late recurrences of Cushing's disease after initial successful transsphenoidal surgery. *J Clin Endocrinol Metab*. 2008;93(2):358–362.

Ectopic Cushing Syndrome Associated With Multiple Endocrine Neoplasia Type 2B

Approximately 15% of patients with corticotropin (ACTH)-dependent Cushing syndrome (CS) have an ectopic source of ACTH secretion, with the most common source being a bronchial carcinoid (≈25%).[1–4] Ectopic CS resulting from medullary carcinoma of the thyroid is rarer (2%–7.5% of ectopic CS cases).[2] In patients with ACTH-dependent CS, rapid onset of CS and a known diagnosis of a metastatic medullary thyroid carcinoma suggest an ectopic origin of CS.

Case Report

The patient was a 31-year-old young man who was referred for management of CS. He was initially diagnosed with medullary thyroid carcinoma 17 years prior and was treated with a total thyroidectomy elsewhere. Subsequently (11 years before Mayo Clinic evaluation), he was diagnosed with a right pheochromocytoma and was treated with right adrenalectomy. At that time, genetic evaluation was pursued, and he was diagnosed with the multiple endocrine neoplasia (MEN) type 2B. The patient developed metastatic medullary thyroid carcinoma and received multiple treatments over the past 10 years, including repeat neck exploration and resection of lymphadenopathy; chemotherapy with vandetanib, cabozantinib, and lenvatinib; as well local radiation therapy for liver metastases.

Five months before evaluation, he started developing symptoms consistent with CS. On physical examination, moon facies, supraclavicular and dorsocervical fat pads, facial erythema, and proximal myopathy were documented. No striae or acne were observed. Multiple mucosal neuromas were visible.

INVESTIGATIONS

The laboratory test results are shown in Table 58.1. ACTH-dependent hypercortisolism was documented based on elevated levels of ACTH, midnight salivary cortisol, and 24-hour urine cortisol. A pituitary origin of ACTH was considered less likely because of the rapid onset of hypercortisolism, suspected link to the metastatic medullary carcinoma, and negative pituitary imaging on review of brain magnetic resonance imaging performed for cancer staging purposes. In addition, on review of abdominal imaging (Fig. 58.1), left adrenal nodularity was demonstrated and suspected to represent pheochromocytoma associated with MEN2B. Workup for catecholamine excess was obtained but was negative (Table 58.1).

TREATMENT

After discussion of options, the patient chose to pursue completion adrenalectomy for treatment of both ectopic CS as well as for possible pheochromocytoma.

TABLE 58.1 Laboratory Tests		
Biochemical Test	Result	Reference Range
4 PM serum cortisol, mcg/dL	18	2–14
ACTH, pg/mL	100	7.2–63
DHEA-S, mcg/dL	144	57–552
24-Hour urine free cortisol, mcg	303	<45
Midnight salivary cortisol, ng/dL	193	<100
Plasma metanephrines, nmol/L	0.45	<0.5
Plasma normetanephrines, nmol/L	0.28	<0.9

ACTH, Corticotropin; *DHEA-S,* dehydroepiandrosterone sulfate.

213

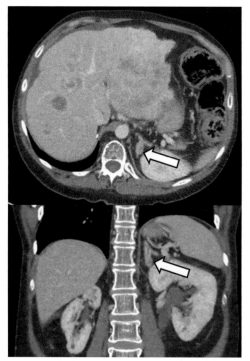

Fig. 58.1 Contrast-enhanced axial *(above)* and coronal *(below)* abdominal computed tomography images showed a nodular left adrenal gland *(arrows)* and absence of the right adrenal gland.

The patient was treated with left laparoscopic adrenalectomy (Fig. 58.2). On histopathology, three pheochromocytomas were diagnosed, measuring 1.0, 1.1, and 1.5 cm in diameter. The patient was initiated on glucocorticoid and mineralocorticoid replacement therapy with resolution of cushingoid features several months after adrenalectomy.

Discussion

Prompt surgical resection of the culprit ACTH source should be pursued when possible. In cases when this is not feasible as the result of an unknown tumor origin (~12%–19%), an anticipated difficult surgery, or, as in this case, metastatic disease, bilateral adrenalectomy is a good therapeutic option.[2,5,6] In this case, biochemically silent multiple small pheochromocytomas were found in the resected left adrenal gland. Biochemically silent pheochromocytomas are more common in patients with smaller tumors and when discovered through genetic-based case detection.[7]

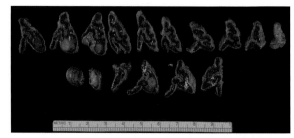

Fig. 58.2 Gross pathology photograph of the left adrenal gland sections. The adrenal gland weighed 10.7 g and demonstrated three white, soft masses located in the medulla, 1.5 cm, 1.1 cm, and 1.0 cm in the largest diameter, which proved to be pheochromocytomas.

Key Points

- Medullary thyroid carcinoma is a rare cause of ectopic CS and should be suspected in a patient with a known diagnosis or predisposition, such as MEN2.
- Bilateral adrenalectomy is an effective treatment of ectopic CS, especially when complete resection of the culprit lesion is not possible.

REFERENCES

1. Lindholm J, Juul S, Jorgensen JO, et al. Incidence and late prognosis of Cushing's syndrome: a population-based study. *J Clin Endocrinol Metab.* 2001;86(1):117–123.
2. Isidori AM, Kaltsas GA, Pozza C, et al. The ectopic adrenocorticotropin syndrome: clinical features, diagnosis, management, and long-term follow-up. *J Clin Endocrinol Metab.* 2006;91(2):371–377.
3. Aniszewski JP, Young WF Jr. Thompson GB, Grant CS, van Heerden JA. Cushing syndrome due to ectopic adrenocorticotropic hormone secretion. *World Journal of Surgery.* 2001;25(7):934–940.
4. Ilias I, Torpy DJ, Pacak K, Mullen N, Wesley RA, Nieman LK. Cushing's syndrome due to ectopic corticotropin secretion: twenty years' experience at the National Institutes of Health. *J Clin Endocrinol Metab.* 2005;90(8):4955–4962.
5. Chow JT, Thompson GB, Grant CS, Farley DR, Richards ML, Young WF Jr. Bilateral laparoscopic adrenalectomy for corticotrophin-dependent Cushing's syndrome: a review of the Mayo Clinic experience. *Clin Endocrinol (Oxf).* 2008;68(4):513–519.
6. Szabo Yamashita T, Sada A, Bancos I, et al. Differences in outcomes of bilateral adrenalectomy in patients with ectopic ACTH producing tumor of known and unknown origin. *Am J Surg.* 2021;221(2):460–464.
7. Gruber LM, Hartman RP, Thompson GB, et al. Pheochromocytoma Characteristics and Behavior Differ Depending on Method of Discovery. *J Clin Endocrinol Metab.* 2019;104(5):1386–1393.

Ectopic Cushing Syndrome Treated With Cryoablation

Most patients with corticotropin (ACTH)-dependent Cushing syndrome (CS) will have an ACTH-secreting pituitary microadenoma. Approximately 15% of patients with ACTH-dependent CS have an ectopic source of ACTH secretion, with the most common source being a bronchial carcinoid tumor (≈25%).[1–4] The tumor may not be found in up to 9%–27% of patients with ectopic ACTH secretion.[1–4] Although resecting the culprit neuroendocrine tumor should be attempted when possible, it is important not to delay therapy for severe hypercortisolism when this proves difficult. In these cases, bilateral adrenalectomy can be lifesaving. Here we present a case in which an alternative therapy for a suspected neuroendocrine tumor avoided bilateral adrenalectomy.

Case Report

The patient was a 69-year-old woman who was referred for management of ACTH-dependent CS. Evaluation was prompted by progressive symptoms of generalized weakness, inability to stand up from a sitting position, lower extremity edema, and easy bruisability. The patient and her family have also noticed some weight loss (mainly as a result of muscle loss) and rounding of the face. At one point, hypokalemia was diagnosed and potassium supplements were initiated. Several months before evaluation at the Mayo Clinic, she was also diagnosed with type 2 diabetes mellitus and required additional medications for hypertension control. CS was suspected, and initial workup suggested ACTH-dependent hypercortisolism (Table 59.1). Localizing studies that included magnetic resonance imaging (MRI) of the pituitary gland, computed tomography (CT) of the chest and abdomen, In-111 pentetreotide scintigraphy, as well as F-18 fluorodeoxyglucose (FDG) positron emission tomography (PET) scan were obtained but failed to localize the culprit lesion. The patient was referred to Mayo Clinic for further management. On physical examination, the patient was sitting in a wheelchair. Skin was found to be thin, with multiple bruises. Her fingernails revealed onychomycosis. She had moon facies without plethora. She had no striae. She had proximal myopathy on examination in both upper and lower extremities. Mild edema was noted.

Medications included glipizide, metformin, hydrochlorothiazide, spironolactone, lisinopril, metoprolol, and potassium chloride.

INVESTIGATIONS

ACTH-dependent hypercortisolism was confirmed (see Table 59.1). Inferior petrosal sinus sampling was performed to determine the subtype of ACTH-dependent hypercortisolism (Box 59.1) and pointed toward an ectopic source.[5,6] Given that a CT of the patient's chest was performed locally, the images were obtained and reexamined. On CT, a 7 × 5–mm right lower lobe nodule was demonstrated (Fig. 59-1).

TREATMENT

In a multidisciplinary team discussion, therapeutic options were considered given the uncertain etiology of ectopic CS, a visible lung nodule that could potentially represent a bronchial carcinoid tumor despite the lack of pentetreotide or FDG avidity, patient's functional status, and the severity of CS. Given that the location of the lung nodule was not amenable to an open wedge or a thoracoscopic wedge resection, other

TABLE 59.1   Laboratory Tests

Biochemical Test	Biochemical Testing at a Local Institution	Biochemical Testing at Our Institution	
	Result (6 months Prior)	Result (At the Time of Evaluation)	Reference Range
8 AM serum cortisol, mcg/dL	56	18	7–25
8-mg overnight DST, mcg/dL	34		<1
ACTH, pg/mL	155	108	10–60
DHEA-S, mcg/dL	115	110	15–157
24-Hour urine free cortisol, mcg (low volume of 800 mL)		47	<45

ACTH, Corticotropin; *DHEA-S,* dehydroepiandrosterone sulfate; *DST,* dexamethasone suppression test.

BOX 59.1   INFERIOR PETROSAL SINUS SAMPLING[a]

	ACTH, pg/mL		Cortisol, mcg/dL	
	Right IPS	PV	Left IPS	PV
−5 minutes	122	94	111	19
−1 minute	120	103	117	18
+2 minutes	195	100	106	19
+5 minutes	233	108	111	18
+10 minutes	183	113	125	19
+30 minutes		108		19
+45 minutes		109		20
+60 minutes		109		19

[a]Simultaneous IPSS completed before (−5 and −1 minutes) and after (+2, +5, and +10 minutes) administration of corticotropin-releasing hormone (CRH) (1 mcg per kg body weight; maximum dose of 100 mcg). Peripheral vein sampling was continued through 60 minutes after CRH administration. *ACTH,* Corticotropin; *IPS,* inferior petrosal sinus; *IPSS,* inferior petrosal sinus sampling; *PV,* peripheral vein.

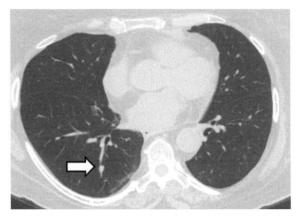

Fig. 59.1 Contrast-enhanced axial chest computed tomography images demonstrated a 7 × 5–mm right lower lobe nodule *(arrow)*.

OUTCOME AND FOLLOW-UP

The hypothalamic-pituitary-adrenal axis recovered 3 months after surgery, and prednisone was discontinued. All signs and symptoms of CS resolved after surgery. At the 3-month follow-up, the patient had lost 12 pounds of weight and noticed improvement in muscle function. She no longer needed to use the wheelchair. Her blood pressure improved and she was able to stop her antihypertensive medications. Four years after treatment, the patient had no recurrence of ACTH-dependent hypercortisolism.

therapeutic options were considered. Bilateral adrenalectomy was scheduled, but the option of cryoablation of the lung nodule was discussed with the patient. The lung nodule was successfully ablated; ACTH concentrations decreased to 13 pg/mL and cortisol concentrations decreased to 6 mcg/dL at 20 hours after the treatment, and glucocorticoid supplementation with prednisone was initiated (Table 59.2).

TABLE 59.2 Serum Cortisol and ACTH Concentrations Before and After Cyroablation of Lung Nodule

	Baseline	2 Hours After Procedure	24 Hours After Procedure	10 Weeks After Procedure, Off Glucocorticoid Therapy	Reference Range
ACTH, pg/mL	108	54	13	32	10–60
Serum cortisol, mcg/dL	18	16	6	14	7–25

ACTH, Corticotropin.

Key Points

- When ectopic ACTH secretion is suspected as the cause of biochemically confirmed CS, the first localization step is CT of the chest, followed by CT of the abdomen and pelvis if chest imaging is negative.
- Most women with mild-to-moderate ACTH-dependent CS that is slow in onset will have pituitary-dependent disease. However, a subset of patients with ectopic ACTH syndrome resulting from bronchial carcinoid tumors present with mild ACTH hypercortisolism.
- In patients with ectopic CS with an unknown source, bilateral adrenalectomy can be lifesaving.
- Cryoablation therapy of the culprit lesion is a potential therapeutic option when surgical resection is deemed difficult or the etiology of the ectopic CS is unclear.

REFERENCES

1. Lindholm J, Juul S, Jorgensen JO, et al. Incidence and late prognosis of Cushing's syndrome: a population-based study. *J Clin Endocrinol Metab.* 2001;86(1):117–123.
2. Isidori AM, Kaltsas GA, Pozza C, et al. The ectopic adrenocorticotropin syndrome: clinical features, diagnosis, management, and long-term follow-up. *J Clin Endocrinol Metab.* 2006;91(2):371–377.
3. Aniszewski JP, Young WF Jr, Thompson GB, Grant CS, van Heerden JA. Cushing syndrome due to ectopic adrenocorticotropic hormone secretion. *World Journal of Surgery.* 2001;25(7):934–940.
4. Ilias I, Torpy DJ, Pacak K, Mullen N, Wesley RA, Nieman LK. Cushing's syndrome due to ectopic corticotropin secretion: twenty years' experience at the National Institutes of Health. *J Clin Endocrinol Metab.* 2005;90(8):4955–4962.
5. Findling JW, Aron DC, Tyrrell JB, et al. Selective venous sampling for ACTH in Cushing's syndrome: differentiation between Cushing disease and the ectopic ACTH syndrome. *Ann Intern Med.* 1981;94(5):647–652.
6. Oldfield EH, Chrousos GP, Schulte HM, et al. Preoperative lateralization of ACTH-secreting pituitary microadenomas by bilateral and simultaneous inferior petrosal venous sinus sampling. *N Engl J Med.* 1985;312(2):100–103.

Cyclical Ectopic Cushing Syndrome

Most patients with corticotropin (ACTH)-dependent Cushing syndrome (CS) will have an ACTH-secreting pituitary microadenoma. Approximately 15% of patients with ACTH-dependent CS have an ectopic source of ACTH secretion.[1–4] The most common neoplasms associated with ectopic ACTH secretion are bronchial carcinoid (≈25%), pancreatic neuroendocrine tumor (≈16%), occult and unlocalized tumor (≈16%), small cell lung cancer (≈11%), medullary thyroid carcinoma (≈9%), other neuroendocrine tumors (≈7%), thymic carcinoid (≈5%), and pheochromocytoma (≈3%).[1] The main clues that a patient may have ectopic ACTH-dependent CS include severe CS as evidenced by spontaneous hypokalemia and 24-hour urinary free cortisol (UFC) >1000 mcg, rapid onset of CS (sometimes so rapid that there is not time to develop the typical physical stigmata of CS), previous diagnosis of a neuroendocrine tumor, and male sex. Herein we present a case of cyclical ectopic secretion of ACTH.

Case Report

The patient was a 71-year-old woman who was referred for management of ACTH-dependent CS.

Evaluation was prompted by the new-onset symptoms of several months duration that included resistant hypertension, bilateral lower extremity edema, uncontrolled diabetes mellitus, and proximal myopathy. She also noticed hirsutism, facial puffiness, thinning of the skin, and easy bruising. Because of muscle weakness, she sustained several falls and was no longer able to live independently. CS was suspected, and she was referred to our institution for further evaluation and management.

The patient's history was remarkable for resolved ACTH-dependent hypercortisolism 2 years prior. At that time, she presented with similar symptoms of difficult to control hypertension, uncontrolled diabetes mellitus, and hypokalemia. Workup at that time confirmed ACTH-dependent hypercortisolism (Table 60.1). Magnetic resonance imaging (MRI) of the pituitary gland was performed at that time and did not reveal a pituitary adenoma. Computed tomography (CT) of the chest and abdomen, as well as In-111 pentetreotide scintigraphy at that time did not reveal a neuroendocrine tumor. Inferior petrosal sinus sampling (IPSS) was scheduled but was cancelled, as repeated workup no longer revealed hypercortisolism (see Table 60.1). Her symptoms resolved several months later and she had no concerns until 2 years later.

TABLE 60.1 Laboratory Tests					
Biochemical Test	30 Months Prior	27 Months Prior	25 Months Prior	Current Evaluation	Reference Range
8 AM serum cortisol, mcg/dL	27	11	14	93	7–25
8-mg overnight DST, mcg/dL	27.4				<1
ACTH, pg/mL	254	35		366	10–60
DHEA-S, mcg/dL				211	15–157
24-Hour urine free cortisol, mcg	86	3.9	9	683	<45

ACTH, Corticotropin; *DHEA-S,* dehydroepiandrosterone sulfate; *DST,* dexamethasone suppression test.

On physical examination, the patient was sitting in a wheelchair. Her skin was found to be thin, with multiple bruises. She had moon facies, facial plethora, supraclavicular pads, and a mild dorsocervical pad. She had no striae. Facial hirsutism and mild androgenic alopecia were observed. She had proximal myopathy on examination in both upper and lower extremities. Bilateral 1+ lower extremity edema was noted.

INVESTIGATIONS

ACTH-dependent hypercortisolism was confirmed (see Table 60.1). IPSS was performed to determine the subtype of ACTH-dependent hypercortisolism (Box 60.1) and pointed toward an ectopic source. CT of abdomen was performed and revealed a 1.8-cm pancreatic lesion (Fig. 60.1). When compared to the CT scan from 2 years prior, the pancreatic lesion had grown by 1 cm. It was In-111 pentetreotide negative on the initial scan.

Treatment

In a multidisciplinary team discussion, therapeutic options were considered. The pancreatic lesion was considered most likely to represent the culprit neuroendocrine tumor secreting ACTH, despite the negative In-111 pentetreotide uptake. However, the patient was considered a poor surgical candidate for the major surgery that would be required to remove the pancreatic lesion. Bilateral adrenalectomy was considered the best option to treat severe ectopic CS and defer pancreatic surgery. The patient was treated with bilateral laparoscopic adrenalectomy and discharged to a skilled nursing facility for intensive physical therapy. She was initiated on hydrocortisone and fludrocortisone therapy immediately postoperatively.

OUTCOME AND FOLLOW-UP

The patient unexpectedly died 1 month later when she was still at the nursing facility. The family declined to pursue an autopsy.

Discussion

Cyclical ACTH secretion from a neuroendocrine tumor is very rare, with only several case reports in the literature.[5–8] In this case, the initial duration of ACTH-dependent hypercortisolism was only several months long and was followed by a 2-year-long remission period. In a recent study of 1564 patients with CS followed for a median of 2.7 years, mortality was 3%.[9] Of 42 patients who died and the cause of death was known, one-third died as a result of the progression of the underlying disease; one-third died of infections; and one-fifth died of cardiovascular, cerebrovascular, or thromboembolic disease.[9] Ectopic CS, proximal

BOX 60.1 INFERIOR PETROSAL SINUS SAMPLING[a]

	ACTH, pg/mL		Cortisol, mcg/dL	
	Right IPS	**PV**	**Left IPS**	**PV**
–5 minutes	298	279	274	76
–1 minute	301	297	284	79
+2 minutes	294	270	312	75
+5 minutes	283	269	308	72
+10 minutes	290	265	297	77
+30 minutes		352		73
+45 minutes		377		76
+60 minutes		377		71

[a]Simultaneous IPSS completed before (–5 and –1 minutes) and after (+2, +5, and +10 minutes) administration of corticotropin-releasing hormone (CRH) (1 mcg per kg body weight; maximum dose of 100 mcg). Peripheral vein sampling was continued through 60 minutes after CRH administration. *ACTH,* Corticotropin; *IPS,* inferior petrosal sinus; *IPSS,* inferior petrosal sinus sampling; *PV,* peripheral vein.

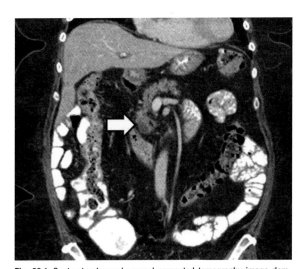

Fig. 60.1 Contrast-enhanced coronal computed tomography image demonstrated a 1.8 × 1.0–cm cystic pancreatic lesion *(arrow)* in the uncinate process.

myopathy, and diabetes mellitus were the key risk factors that were associated with mortality within 90 days from therapy.[9] Patients with severe CS need intense management after curative surgery that includes appropriate management of adrenal insufficiency, control of existent comorbidities such as diabetes mellitus with reevaluation of insulin requirements, and prevention of thromboembolic events.

Key Points

- When ectopic ACTH secretion is suspected as the cause of biochemically confirmed CS, the first localization step is CT of the chest, followed by CT of the abdomen and pelvis if chest imaging is negative.
- Any patient with severe CS should be promptly evaluated and treated.
- Patients with severe CS are at high risk for perioperative morbidity and mortality even after a curative surgery.

REFERENCES

1. Lindholm J, Juul S, Jorgensen JO, et al. Incidence and late prognosis of Cushing's syndrome: a population-based study. *J Clin Endocrinol Metab*. 2001;86(1):117–123.
2. Isidori AM, Kaltsas GA, Pozza C, et al. The ectopic adrenocorticotropin syndrome: clinical features, diagnosis, management, and long-term follow-up. *J Clin Endocrinol Metab*. 2006;91(2):371–377.
3. Aniszewski JP, Young WF Jr, Thompson GB, Grant CS, van Heerden JA. Cushing syndrome due to ectopic adrenocorticotropic hormone secretion. *World journal of surgery*. 2001;25(7):934–940.
4. Ilias I, Torpy DJ, Pacak K, Mullen N, Wesley RA, Nieman LK. Cushing's syndrome due to ectopic corticotropin secretion: twenty years' experience at the National Institutes of Health. *J Clin Endocrinol Metab*. 2005;90(8):4955–4962.
5. Arnaldi G, Mancini T, Kola B, et al. Cyclical Cushing's syndrome in a patient with a bronchial neuroendocrine tumor (typical carcinoid) expressing ghrelin and growth hormone secretagogue receptors. *J Clin Endocrinol Metab*. 2003;88(12):5834–5840.
6. Francia G, Davi MV, Montresor E, Colato C, Ferdeghini M, Lo Cascio V. Long-term quiescence of ectopic Cushing's syndrome caused by ectopic Cushing's syndrome (typical carcinoid) and tumorlets: spontaneous remission or therapeutic effect of bromocriptine? *J Endocrinol Invest*. 2006;29(4):358–362.
7. Meinardi JR, van den Berg G, Wolffenbuttel BH, Kema IP, Dullaart RP. Cyclical Cushing's syndrome due to an atypical thymic carcinoid. *Neth J Med*. 2006;64(1):23–27.
8. Cameron CM, Roberts F, Connell J, Sproule MW. Diffuse idiopathic pulmonary neuroendocrine cell hyperplasia: an unusual cause of cyclical ectopic adrenocorticotrophic syndrome. *Br J Radiol*. 2011;84(997):e14–e17.
9. Valassi E, Tabarin A, Brue T, et al. High mortality within 90 days of diagnosis in patients with Cushing's syndrome: results from the ERCUSYN registry. *Eur J Endocrinol*. 2019;181(5):461–472.

Mild Cushing Syndrome Associated With Ectopic Corticotropin Secretion

Most patients with corticotropin (ACTH)-dependent Cushing syndrome (CS) will have an ACTH-secreting pituitary microadenoma. Approximately 15% of patients with ACTH-dependent CS have an ectopic source of ACTH secretion, with the most common source being a bronchial carcinoid (≈25%).[1–4] The main clues that a patient may have ectopic ACTH-dependent CS include severe CS as evidenced by spontaneous hypokalemia and 24-hour urinary free cortisol (UFC) >1000 mcg, rapid onset of CS, previous diagnosis of a neuroendocrine tumor, and male sex. Rarely, ectopic ACTH-dependent CS presents with symptoms of mild, long-standing hypercortisolism. Herein we present one such case.

Case Report

The patient was a young 18-year-old woman, a high school student, who presented for evaluation of possible CS. Over the 3 years before the current evaluation, she developed slowly progressive symptoms of weight gain, acne, hirsutism, facial fullness, thinning of hair, and some menstrual irregularity. Diagnosis of polycystic ovarian syndrome was made; however, the patient's mother was unconvinced and, after performing additional research, requested an evaluation for CS. Eventually, workup for hypercortisolism was pursued and indeed confirmed ACTH-dependent CS (Table 61.1). Magnetic resonance imaging (MRI) of the pituitary gland was then obtained and did not reveal a pituitary adenoma. At that time, the patient presented to our institution.

On physical examination, she demonstrated rounding of the face; acne on face and torso; hirsutism over face, back, and extremities; and violaceous striae on inner thighs.

She was taking no medications. Notably, the patient was under chronic care by a local pulmonologist for chronic bronchitis, and a recent computed tomography (CT) scan of chest demonstrated evidence of mucous plugging.

INVESTIGATIONS

The laboratory test results are shown in Table 61.1. ACTH-dependent hypercortisolism was documented. A pituitary origin of ACTH was suspected despite a negative MRI of pituitary gland given the mild, long-standing presentation of hypercortisolism. Inferior petrosal sinus sampling was performed to determine the subtype of ACTH-dependent hypercortisolism (Box 61.1) and pointed toward an ectopic source. Given that a CT of the chest was performed locally, the images were obtained and reexamined (Fig. 61.1). On CT, collapse of the right middle lobe was observed, which was interpreted as nonperfused lung related to chronic known infection; also noted were bronchial

TABLE 61.1 Laboratory Tests		
Biochemical Test	Result	Reference Range
4 PM serum cortisol, mcg/dL	16	2–14
1-mg overnight DST, mcg/dL	20.8	<1.8
8-mg overnight DST, mcg/dL	11.8	<1
ACTH, pg/mL	109	7.2–63
DHEA-S, mcg/dL	263	44–332
24-Hour urine free cortisol, mcg	158	<45
Midnight salivary cortisol, ng/dL	458	<100

ACTH, Corticotropin; *DHEA-S,* dehydroepiandrosterone sulfate; *DST,* dexamethasone suppression test.

BOX 61.1 INFERIOR PETROSAL SINUS SAMPLING[a]

	ACTH, pg/mL		Cortisol, mcg/dL	
	Right IPS	PV	**Left IPS**	PV
–5 minutes	98	63	92	16
–1 minute	85	63	74	16
+2 minutes	101	70	102	16
+5 minutes	109	84	95	17
+10 minutes	110	96	98	18
+30 minutes		96		16
+45 minutes		94		16
+60 minutes		89		16

[a]Simultaneous IPSS completed before (–5 and –1 minutes) and after (+2, +5, and +10 minutes) administration of corticotropin-releasing hormone (CRH) (1 mcg per kg body weight; maximum dose of 100 mcg). Peripheral vein sampling was continued through 60 minutes after CRH administration. *ACTH,* Corticotropin; *IPS,* inferior petrosal sinus; *IPSS,* inferior petrosal sinus sampling; *PV,* peripheral vein.

wall thickening, endobronchial plugging, and clustered micronodularity in the lower lobes. Ga-68 1,4,7,10-tetraazacyclododecane-1,4,7,10-tetraacetic acid (DOTA)-octreotate (DOTATATE) positron emission tomography (PET)-CT imaging was obtained and demonstrated a 1.8-cm neuroendocrine tumor in the right middle lobe (see Fig. 61.1).

TREATMENT

The patient was treated with a right middle lobectomy and thoracic lymphadenectomy (Fig. 61.2). On histopathology an atypical carcinoid tumor 1.9 cm in greatest dimension was confirmed, without visceral pleural invasion and negative margins. Subcarinal and right lower paratracheal lymph nodes were negative for tumor. Immunoperoxidase stain for ACTH was performed on paraffin sections of the right middle lobe tumor with tumor cells showing focal cytoplasmic positivity.

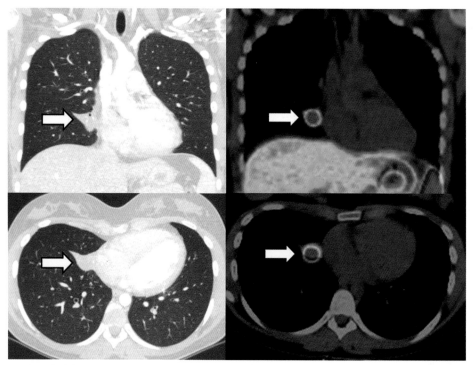

Fig. 61.1 Contrast-enhanced axial and coronal chest computed tomography (CT) images *(left)* showed collapse of the right middle lobe, which could represent nonperfused lung related to chronic infection, or mask an underlying lesion *(arrows)*. Ga-68 1,4,7,10-tetraazacyclododecane-1,4,7,10-tetraacetic acid-octreotate positron emission tomography-CT *(right)* axial and coronal images demonstrated a right middle lobe pulmonary neuroendocrine tumor. The tumor, 1.8 cm with increased tracer activity (11.7 standard unit value), was located in the area of collapsed right middle pulmonary lobe.

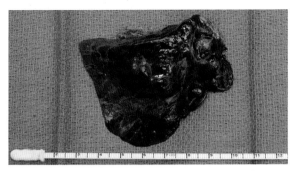

Fig. 61.2 Gross pathology photograph of the 1.9-cm neuroendocrine tumor.

OUTCOME AND FOLLOW-UP

Postoperative blood levels of ACTH and cortisol were low (Table 61.2), confirming resolution of ACTH-dependent hypercortisolism. The hypothalamic-pituitary-adrenal (HPA) axis recovered 1 year after surgery and exogenous glucocorticoids were discontinued. All signs and symptoms of CS resolved after surgery. Two years after treatment, the patient had no recurrence of neuroendocrine tumor or ACTH-dependent hypercortisolism.

TABLE 61.2   Laboratory Tests After Surgery

	Before Surgery	1 Day After Surgery	6 Weeks After Surgery	5 Months After Surgery	1 Year After Surgery	2 Years After Surgery	Reference Range
ACTH, pg/mL	109	5.7	<5	22	27	19	7.2–63
8 AM serum cortisol, mcg/dL	16	5	1	9.6	11	12	7–25

ACTH, Corticotropin.

Key Points

- When ectopic ACTH secretion is suspected as the cause of biochemically confirmed CS, the first localization step is CT of the chest, followed by CT of abdomen and pelvis if chest imaging is negative.
- For inferior petrosal sinus sampling (IPSS) to be valid, patients must have active CS on the day of IPSS.
- Ectopic CS is confirmed when the IPSS central-to-peripheral gradients are <2-to-1 at baseline and <3-to-1 after CRH administration.[5,6]
- Most women with mild-to-moderate ACTH-dependent CS that is slow in onset will have pituitary-dependent disease. However, a subset of patients with ectopic ACTH syndrome resulting from bronchial carcinoid tumors present with mild ACTH hypercortisolism.

REFERENCES

1. Lindholm J, Juul S, Jorgensen JO, et al. Incidence and late prognosis of Cushing's syndrome: a population-based study. *J Clin Endocrinol Metab.* 2001;86(1):117–123.
2. Isidori AM, Kaltsas GA, Pozza C, et al. The ectopic adrenocorticotropin syndrome: clinical features, diagnosis, management, and long-term follow-up. *J Clin Endocrinol Metab.* 2006;91(2):371–377.
3. Aniszewski JP, Young WF Jr, Thompson GB, Grant CS, van Heerden JA. Cushing syndrome due to ectopic adrenocorticotropic hormone secretion. *World Journal of Surgery.* 2001;25(7):934–940.
4. Ilias I, Torpy DJ, Pacak K, Mullen N, Wesley RA, Nieman LK. Cushing's syndrome due to ectopic corticotropin secretion: twenty years' experience at the National Institutes of Health. *J Clin Endocrinol Metab.* 2005;90(8):4955–4962.
5. Findling JW, Aron DC, Tyrrell JB, et al. Selective venous sampling for ACTH in Cushing's syndrome: differentiation between Cushing disease and the ectopic ACTH syndrome. *Ann Intern Med.* 1981;94(5):647–652.
6. Oldfield EH, Chrousos GP, Schulte HM, et al. Preoperative lateralization of ACTH-secreting pituitary microadenomas by bilateral and simultaneous inferior petrosal venous sinus sampling. *N Engl J Med.* 1985;312(2):100–103.

Bilateral Adrenal Cryoablation in Corticotropin-Dependent Cushing Syndrome

Most patients with corticotropin (ACTH)-dependent Cushing syndrome (CS) will have an ACTH-secreting pituitary microadenoma. When the pituitary appears normal on magnetic resonance imaging (MRI), it is important to distinguish between ectopic and pituitary ACTH-dependent CS. Use of inferior petrosal sinus sampling (IPSS) can help localize the source (pituitary versus ectopic) of ACTH secretion. Pituitary-dependent CS is typically associated with mild to moderate CS, and 24-hour urinary free cortisol (UFC) excretion is typically 100–500 mcg and very rarely >1000 mcg. When patients with ACTH-dependent CS present with spontaneous hypokalemia and 24-hour UFC >1000 mcg, the clinician should suspect an ectopic ACTH-secreting tumor. A subset of patients with pituitary-dependent CS who have large pituitary adenomas demonstrate the clinical presentation that overlaps with ectopic ACTH secretion. Here we present a case of severe ACTH-dependent CS in a patient with negative MRI and IPSS suggesting a pituitary source, who was treated with bilateral adrenal cryoablation.

Case Report

The patient was a 69-year-old woman who was referred for management of ACTH-dependent CS. Evaluation was prompted by the new onset of symptoms of 3 months, duration that included progressive weakness with proximal myopathy, severe bilateral edema, uncontrolled hypertension, new-onset hypokalemia, cognitive decline, and several falls resulting in a fracture. She also noticed rounding of the face, thinning of the skin, and easy bruising. CS was suspected, and she was referred to our institution for further evaluation and management.

On physical examination, the patient was sitting in a wheelchair. Blood pressure was 150/82 mmHg, heart rate was 63 beats per minute, and weight was 108 kg. Her skin was found to be thin, with multiple bruises. She had moon facies, supraclavicular pads, and a mild dorsocervical pad. She had no striae. She had proximal myopathy on examination in both upper and lower extremities. Bilateral 3+ edema was noted.

At the time of evaluation, hypertension was treated with five drugs (spironolactone, metoprolol succinate, losartan, hydrochlorothiazide, and hydralazine), and hypokalemia was treated with 80 mEq of potassium chloride per day.

INVESTIGATIONS

ACTH-dependent hypercortisolism was diagnosed (Table 62.1). MRI of the pituitary gland was performed at that time and did not reveal a pituitary adenoma. Ectopic CS was suspected due to the rapid onset of symptoms and severity of hypercortisolism, especially in light of negative pituitary imaging. Computed tomography (CT) of the chest was obtained and demonstrated an indeterminate 9-mm lung nodule in the posterior lateral left lung base. This nodule was previously noted on a CT of the chest 3 years prior, but was smaller, measuring 6 mm. A gallium-68 (Ga-68) 1,4,7,10-tetraazacyclododecane-1,4,7,10-tetraacetic acid (DOTA)-octreotate (DOTATATE) positron emission tomography (PET)-CT scan was obtained and

TABLE 62.1 Laboratory Tests

Biochemical Test	Result	Reference Range
8 AM serum cortisol, mcg/dL	48	7–25
ACTH, pg/mL	128	7.2–63
DHEA-S, mcg/dL	86	9.7–159
24-Hour urine free cortisol, mcg	803	<45
Late night salivary cortisol, ng/dL	2820, 1560	<100

ACTH, Corticotropin; DHEA-S, dehydroepiandrosterone sulfate.

BOX 62.1 INFERIOR PETROSAL SINUS SAMPLING[a]

	ACTH, pg/mL		Cortisol, mcg/dL	
	Right IPS	PV	Left IPS	PV
–5 minutes	68	66	60	43
–1 minute	74	83	88	46
+2 minutes	177	27	160	43
+5 minutes	544	44	242	43
+10 minutes	580	64	393	42
+30 minutes		113		43
+45 minutes		111		39
+60 minutes		107		43

[a]Simultaneous IPSS completed before (–5 and –1 minutes) and after (+2, +5, and +10 minutes) administration of corticotropin-releasing hormone (CRH) (1 mcg per kg body weight; maximum dose of 100 mcg). Peripheral vein sampling was continued through 60 minutes after CRH administration. *ACTH,* Corticotropin; *IPS,* inferior petrosal sinus; *IPSS,* inferior petrosal sinus sampling; *PV,* peripheral vein.

demonstrated no uptake in the 9-mm lung nodule. Given the negative localization workup, it was decided to proceed with IPSS that demonstrated a pituitary origin of ACTH secretion (Box 62.1). Ultrasound of lower extremities was obtained and was negative for deep venous thrombosis.

TREATMENT

While pursuing the imaging workup, the patient was initiated on anticoagulation and antibiotic therapy for prophylaxis against opportunistic infections and thrombotic events. In a multidisciplinary team discussion, therapeutic options were considered. Pituitary exploration was discussed. The likelihood of a curative surgery was estimated to be around 50%, and the risk of pituitary insufficiency of around 25%. Bilateral adrenalectomy was considered; however, this was deemed to be a procedure with a high risk of morbidity and mortality because of the patient's functional status and previous history of traumatic splenectomy and the two revisional surgeries for bleeding that followed.

After considering the potential lack of success and/or high risk of complications with either pituitary exploration or bilateral adrenalectomy, a nonstandard approach was considered: bilateral cryoablation of adrenal glands. After appropriate α-adrenergic and β-adrenergic blockade, the patient was treated with bilateral cryoablation 13 days after initial evaluation. Serum cortisol was measured 4 hours after the procedure and was significantly decreased from the baseline (baseline, 41 mcg/dL; 4 hours after procedure, 9.1 mcg/dL). Hydrocortisone therapy was immediately initiated, and later fludrocortisone was added.

OUTCOME AND FOLLOW-UP

Two months after bilateral adrenal cryoablation, the patient demonstrated an improvement in her symptoms. She was able to walk, though still occasionally using the wheelchair for long distances. Edema improved (from previous 3+ edema to now mild edema). She was able to stop four of the five antihypertensive medications.

Discussion

Ablation therapy is most commonly used for treatment of adrenal metastases.[1] It is infrequently used for management of ACTH-dependent hypercortisolism and is usually reserved for patients considered poor surgical candidates.[2–4] As catecholamine release occurs with ablation of adrenal medullary tissue, patients should be appropriately treated with preprocedural α-adrenergic blockade.[2]

Key Points

- Any patient with severe CS should be promptly evaluated and treated.
- Patients with severe CS are at high risk for perioperative morbidity and mortality even after a curative surgery.

- Pituitary-dependent CS is typically associated with mild to moderate CS, and 24-hour UFC excretion is typically 100–500 mcg. When patients with ACTH-dependent CS present with spontaneous hypokalemia and 24-hour UFC >500–1000 mcg, the clinician should suspect an ectopic ACTH-secreting tumor, especially in the setting of a negative MRI of the pituitary.
- Bilateral adrenalectomy is the treatment of choice in patients with severe ACTH-dependent CS when resection of the culprit lesion is not possible.
- Bilateral adrenal cryoablation is an effective treatment option and should be performed only after optimal α-adrenergic blockade.

REFERENCES

1. Espinosa De Ycaza AE, Welch TL, Ospina NS, et al. Image-guided thermal ablation of adrenal metastases: hemodynamic and endocrine outcomes. *Endocr Pract*. 2017;23(2):132–140.
2. Rosiak G, Milczarek K, Konecki D, Otto M, Rowinski O, Zgliczynski W. Percutaneous bilateral adrenal radiofrequency ablation in severe adrenocorticotropic hormone-dependent Cushing syndrome. *J Clin Imaging Sci*. 2020;10:60.
3. Zener R, Zaleski A, Van Uum SH, Gray DK, Mujoomdar A. Successful percutaneous CT-guided microwave ablation of adrenal gland for ectopic Cushing syndrome. *Clin Imaging*. 2017;42:93–95.
4. Chan C, Roberts JM. Ectopic ACTH syndrome complicated by multiple opportunistic infections treated with percutaneous ablation of the adrenal glands. *BMJ Case Rep*. 2017;2017:221580.

Cushing Syndrome Associated With Ectopic Corticotropin and Corticotropin-Releasing Hormone–Secreting Pheochromocytoma

Most patients with corticotropin (ACTH)-dependent Cushing syndrome (CS) will have an ACTH-secreting pituitary microadenoma. Approximately 15% of patients with ACTH-dependent CS have an ectopic source of ACTH secretion. The most common neoplasms associated with ectopic ACTH secretion are bronchial carcinoid (≈25%), pancreatic neuroendocrine tumor (≈16%), occult and unlocalized tumor (≈16%), small cell lung cancer (≈11%), medullary thyroid carcinoma (≈9%), other neuroendocrine tumors (≈7%), thymic carcinoid (≈5%), and pheochromocytoma (≈3%).[1] The main clues that a patient may have ectopic ACTH-dependent CS include severe CS as evidenced by spontaneous hypokalemia and 24-hour urinary free cortisol (UFC) >1000 mcg, rapid onset of CS (sometimes so rapid that there is not time to develop the typical physical stigmata of CS), previous diagnosis of a neuroendocrine tumor, and male sex. Herein we present a case of ectopic secretion of ACTH and corticotropin-releasing hormone (CRH) from a pheochromocytoma causing severe CS.

Case Report

The patient was a 49-year-old woman who presented with a 1-month history of lower extremity edema, polydipsia, and polyuria. She had a 6-year history of untreated hypertension. She had no recent weight gain. On physical examination her blood pressure was 210/115 mmHg. She appeared cushingoid with a plethoric face, lanugo-type facial hair, central obesity, red abdominal striae, and edema (Fig. 63.1).

INVESTIGATIONS

The laboratory test results are shown in Table 63.1. Severe hypercortisolism was documented with a 24-hour urinary free cortisol excretion that was more than 100-fold elevated above the upper limit of normal. Although the patient was clearly cushingoid on physical examination, there was a mismatch between the severity of hypercortisolism and the physical stigmata of CS, which was consistent with a short duration of disease. Computed tomography (CT) of the chest and abdomen showed a 4-cm left adrenal mass (Fig. 63.2). The 24-hour urine for total metanephrines and fractionated catecholamines confirmed that the patient had an adrenergic pheochromocytoma (see Table 63.1). Adrenal venous sampling confirmed a gradient of both ACTH and CRH from the left adrenal gland (Box 63.1).

TREATMENT

The hyperglycemia required 80 units of insulin per day. Hypertension was treated with α-adrenergic blockade (phenoxybenzamine) titrated for low-normal systolic blood pressure for age and subsequently β-adrenergic blockade (propranolol) was added and titrated to an average heart rate of 80 beats per minute. The patient received perioperative glucocorticoid coverage. An open laparotomy was performed to resect the left

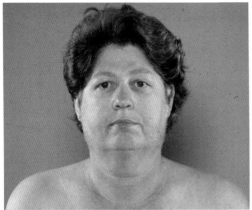 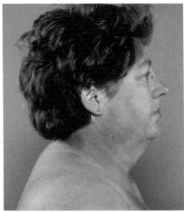

Fig. 63.1 Photographs show neck and facial plethora, fine lanugo hair on the checks, and supraclavicular and dorsocervical fat pads.

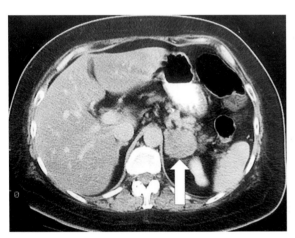

Fig. 63.2 Contrast-enhanced axial computed tomography image shows a vascular 4 × 3–cm left adrenal mass *(arrow).*

adrenal gland. The left adrenal gland showed cortical hyperplasia and contained a typical pheochromocytoma (3.4 × 3.3 × 3.0 cm) (Fig. 63.3). Histologic features showed typical Zellballen formation and monomorphism of tumor cells. Immunohistochemistry was strongly positive for chromogranin, CRH, ACTH, vasopressin, and β-endorphin.

OUTCOME AND FOLLOW-UP

As the signs and symptoms of CS resolved after surgery, treatments for diabetes mellitus and hypertension were discontinued. The hypothalamic-pituitary-adrenal

TABLE 63.1 Laboratory Tests

Biochemical Test	Result	Repeat Test Result	Reference Range
Sodium, mEq/L	139		135–145
Potassium, mEq/L	3.6		3.6–5.2
Fasting plasma glucose, mg/dL	312		70–100
8 AM serum cortisol, mcg/dL	74		7–25
ACTH, pg/mL	550		10–60
CRH, pg/mL	2	11	<34
24-Hour urine:			
Free cortisol, mcg	12,454		<108
Total metanephrines, mcg	5.4		<1.3
Norepinephrine, mcg	476		<80
Epinephrine, mcg	1124		<20
Dopamine, mcg	279		<400

ACTH, Corticotropin; *CRH,* corticotropin-releasing hormone.

BOX 63.1 ADRENAL VENOUS SAMPLING

	Left AV	IVC	Right Renal	Left Renal
ACTH, pg/mL	1400	159	140	140
CRH, pg/mL	83	11	4	4

ACTH, Corticotropin; *AV,* adrenal vein; *CRH,* corticotropin-releasing hormone; *IVC,* inferior vena cava.

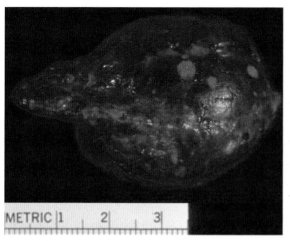 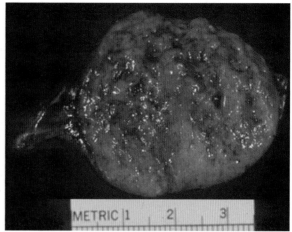

Fig. 63.3 Gross pathology photographs of the left adrenal mass show a dark brown-red tumor capsule *(left)* and a pink-red cut surface *(right)*. The left adrenal gland showed cortical hyperplasia and contained a typical pheochromocytoma (3.4 × 3.3 × 3.0 cm). Histologic features showed typical Zellballen formation and monomorphism of tumor cells. Immunohistochemistry was strongly positive for chromogranin, corticotropin-releasing hormone (CRH), corticotropin (ACTH), vasopressin, and β-endorphin.

(HPA) axis recovered 1 month after surgery, and exogenous glucocorticoids were discontinued. We assumed the rapid recovery of the HPA axis reflected chronic priming of the pituitary gland from pheochromocytoma secretion of CRH. One month after surgery the 24-hour urine for total metanephrines and fractionated catecholamines was normal. Her surgery was in 1990, and we reported her case in the medical literature in 1992.[2] She has been followed annually for 30 years and there has been no recurrence of pheochromocytoma or CS.

Discussion

This patient is one of three at Mayo Clinic who had CS as a result of ectopic ACTH secretion from a pheochromocytoma.[1] A recent publication documented a total of 99 cases of CS resulting from ectopic ACTH- and/or CRH-secreting pheochromocytomas in the world literature (only 4 were documented to hypersecrete CRH).[3] The median age at diagnosis was 49 years with a 2:1 female to male ratio. Most patients presented with clinical CS (n = 79; 81%), hypertension (n = 87; 93%), and/or diabetes (n = 50; 54%). Blood pressure, glucose control, and biochemical parameters improved in nearly all patients postoperatively. Infections were the most common complication. Most patients (n = 70, 88%)

survived to publication (median follow-up 6 months).[3] The 30 years of follow-up documented in the case reported herein is the longest documented recurrence-free follow-up.

Key Points

- Because of the rapidity of onset of hypercortisolism in some patients with CS resulting from ectopic ACTH secretion, there may be a mismatch between the severity of hypercortisolism and the physical stigmata of CS.
- When ectopic ACTH secretion is suspected as the cause of biochemically confirmed CS, the first localization step is CT of the chest, abdomen, and pelvis.
- When a lipid-poor and vascular adrenal mass is found in a patient with ACTH-dependent CS, the clinician should obtain biochemical testing for pheochromocytoma.
- Inferior petrosal sinus sampling may not be needed in patients with ectopic ACTH syndrome where the tumor is found with cross-sectional imaging and is either classic for a certain tumor type (e.g., pheochromocytoma) or is colocalized with octreotide scintigraphy or Ga-68 1,4,7,10-tetraazacyclododecane-1,4,7,10-tetraacetic acid-octreotate-positron emission tomography-CT.

REFERENCES

1. Aniszewski JP, Young WF Jr, Thompson GB, Grant CS, van Heerden JA. Cushing syndrome due to ectopic adrenocorticotropic hormone secretion. *World J Surg.* 2001;25(7):934–940.

2. O'Brien T, Young WF Jr, Davila DG, et al. Cushing's syndrome associated with ectopic production of corticotrophin-releasing hormone, corticotrophin and vasopressin by a phaeochromocytoma. *Clin Endocrinol (Oxf).* 1992;37(5):460–467.

3. Elliott PF, Berhane T, Ragnarsson O, Falhammar H. Ectopic ACTH- and/or CRH-producing pheochromocytomas. *J Clin Endocrinol Metab.* 2021;106(2):598–608.

Cushing Syndrome in the Setting of Multiple Endocrine Neoplasia Type 1

When a patient with multiple endocrine neoplasia type 1 (MEN-1) presents with Cushing syndrome (CS), it may be corticotropin (ACTH) independent (e.g., adenoma, carcinoma, or bilateral macronodular adrenal hyperplasia) or ACTH dependent (e.g., pituitary adenoma, ectopic ACTH secretion from bronchial carcinoid, thymic carcinoid, or pancreatic neuroendocrine tumor).[1,2] Herein we present a patient with MEN-1 who presented with ACTH-dependent CS.

Case Report

The patient was a 20-year-old woman referred for evaluation and management of CS in the setting of MEN-1 (pathogenic variant in menin gene: c.35C>T [p.Pro12Leu]). MEN-1 was diagnosed 6 months before she came to Mayo Clinic when she presented with multiple gland primary hyperparathyroidism requiring two operations and resection of three and a half parathyroid glands. Over 6–12 months before her Mayo Clinic endocrine consultation she experienced the following: 80-pound weight gain, red striae on her medial thighs and abdomen, scalp hair loss, oligomenorrhea, and hirsutism on the jawline and low midline abdomen. She had been diagnosed with polycystic ovarian syndrome and insulin resistance and was treated with metformin 500 mg twice daily. Owing to progression of the aforementioned symptoms listed and weakness going up stairs, 24-hour urinary free cortisol (UFC) excretion was obtained and was elevated at 96 mcg (normal, <45 mcg)—a finding that triggered referral to Mayo Clinic.

On physical examination, body mass index was 37.2 kg/m^2, blood pressure was 118/75 mm Hg, and heart rate 93 beats per minute. She appeared cushingoid based on the following: facial rounding; increased fat deposition in the supraclavicular and dorsocervical areas; excess terminal hair on the cheeks, chin, and low midline abdomen; and pink to darker red striae in vertical orientation across the abdomen and some striae on the upper medial thigh and axillary areas as well. Her appearance was markedly different from that in a photograph taken 2 years earlier (Fig. 64.1).

INVESTIGATIONS

The laboratory test results are shown in Table 64.1. The serum cortisol concentrations showed lack of normal diurnal variation. The 24-hour urine free cortisol (UFC) excretion and salivary cortisol concentrations were more than threefold elevated above the respective upper limits of the reference ranges. The 2-day formal low-dose dexamethasone suppression test (DST) (0.5 mg of dexamethasone every 6 hours × 48 hours) showed marked cortisol suppression in the blood and urine—to levels seen in normal individuals. A recent metaanalysis of 139 studies with 14,140 participants showed that the sensitivity and specificity (95% confidence interval) for the 2-day low-dose DST were 95.3% (91.3%–97.5%) and 92.8% (85.7%–96.5%), respectively.[3] Thus like in all CS-related testing, there are no absolutes and there is no single best test for all patients. Approximately 5% of patients with pituitary-dependent CS will have normal suppression of cortisol with the formal 2-day low-dose DST—the patient presented here is a good example. It is up the clinician to build a wall of evidence to confirm CS before proceeding to subtype evaluation and treatment. In this patient the diagnosis of CS was firm based on clinical signs and symptoms, marked change in physical appearance, and marked elevations in baseline

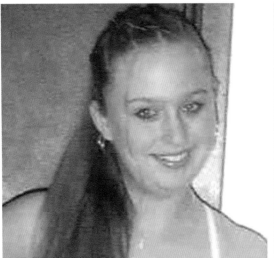 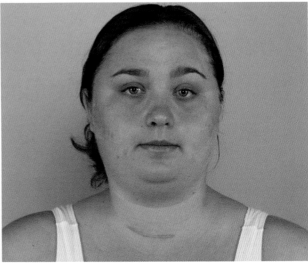

Fig. 64.1 Photographs from 2 years previously *(left)* and at time of consultation *(right)* show the development of facial features consistent with Cushing syndrome (note neck surgical scar from two recent parathyroid operations).

24-hour UFC and late-night salivary cortisols (see Table 64.1).

The serum ACTH concentration was mid-normal and confirmed that CS was ACTH dependent. Head magnetic resonance imaging (MRI) showed there was a 3-mm area of decreased enhancement within the superior left ventral portion of the pituitary gland consistent with a pituitary microadenoma (Fig. 64.2). The blood levels of prolactin and insulin-like growth factor 1 were normal (see Table 64.1). Computed tomography (CT) of the chest did not show any findings that would be consistent with bronchial or thymic carcinoid tumor. The abdominal CT showed at least three tiny calyceal tip stones in the right kidney and innumerable tiny calyceal tip stones in the left kidney, no evidence for a pancreatic neuroendocrine tumor, and normal-appearing adrenal glands. In addition, the pancreatic neuroendocrine tumor markers were all normal. Although in the setting of MEN-1, ACTH-dependent CS might be caused by ectopic ACTH secretion,[1,2] her mild degree of CS, near total dexamethasone suppressibility, and apparent pituitary adenoma on MRI all strongly favored pituitary-dependent disease. In a patient with CS, when 24-hour UFC suppresses more than 90% from baseline with formal 2-day high-dose

DST (2 mg every 6 hours × 48 hours), it is 100% specific for pituitary-dependent CS.[4] Our patient suppressed the 24-hour UFC more than 90% with the formal 2-day low dose DST! We advised that inferior petrosal sinus sampling (IPSS) does carry some risk and was not needed in her case. Brain stem injury has been reported to occur in 0.2% of patients undergoing IPSS.[5] The patient was advised to proceed with transsphenoidal surgery.

TREATMENT

At transsphenoidal surgery, tissue consistent with a pituitary adenoma was quite gelatinous and completely removed. The vast majority of the pituitary gland was preserved. The specimens provided for pathologic analysis showed anterior pituitary tissue with changes suggestive of corticotroph cell hyperplasia. Crooke's hyaline changes consistent with hypercortisolism were present focally. There was no evidence of adenoma. The serum cortisol concentration the morning after surgery was 1.6 mcg/dL, and the patient was symptomatic with nausea and diffuse myalgias. The patient was discharged from the hospital on prednisone 10 mg in the morning and 5 mg in the afternoon with a plan to taper the total dosage by 2.5 mg every week until a maintenance dose of 5 mg every morning.

TABLE 64.1 Laboratory Tests

Biochemical Test	Result	Repeat Test Result	Reference Range
Sodium, mEq/L	138		135–145
Potassium, mEq/L	4.1		3.6–5.2
Fasting plasma glucose, mg/dL	75		70100
Creatinine, mg/dL	0.8		0.6–1.1
eGFR, mL/min per BSA	>60		>60
Calcium, mg/dL	9.6		8.9–10.1
Phosphorus, mg/dL	3.5		2.5–4.5
8 AM serum cortisol, mcg/dL	14		7–25
4 PM serum cortisol, mcg/dL	22		2–14
24-Hour UFC, mcg	206	96	3.5–45
24-Hour urine volume, L	2.2	2.4	Goal <4 L
Late night salivary cortisol, ng/dL	320	286	≤100
ACTH, pg/mL	26	42	10–60
DHEA-S, mcg/dL	320		44–332
Prolactin, ng/mL	13		327
IGF-1, ng/mL	147		122–384
Chromogranin A, ng/mL	84		<225
HPP, pg/mL	<40		<228
Glucagon, pg/mL	48		<80
Gastrin, pg/mL	13		<100
2-Day low-dose DST:			
8 AM serum cortisol, mcg/dL	1.4		<1.8
24-Hour UFC, mcg	6.8		<10

ACTH, Corticotropin; *BSA,* body surface area; *DHEA-S,* dehydroepiandrosterone sulfate; *DST,* dexamethasone suppression test; *eGFR,* estimated glomerular filtration rate; *HPP,* human pancreatic polypeptide; *IGF-1,* insulinlike growth factor 1; *UFC,* urinary free cortisol.

OUTCOME AND FOLLOW-UP

Two months after surgery her morning serum cortisol concentration was 4.1 mcg/dL; she had lost 11 pounds of weight, had more energy, and could walk around the mall without getting exhausted. Once the prednisone dosage reached 5 mg every morning, she was switched to hydrocortisone 20 mg every morning for 2 weeks and then 15 mg every morning thereafter. At her 9-month postoperative follow-up, before her morning dose of hydrocortisone, her serum cortisol concentration was 9.6 mcg/dL. She had lost 25 pounds of body weight and most of her signs and symptoms of CS had resolved. Her menstrual cycles were regular. One year after surgery, the morning serum cortisol concentration was >10 mcg/dL, and hydrocortisone was discontinued. Two years after surgery, the 24-hour urinary free cortisol was normal. Four years after surgery she delivered a healthy baby boy. In addition to annual surveillance testing for MEN-1–related neoplasms, the patient was advised to complete an annual 24-hour urine collection for UFC.

As demonstrated in this case, cosyntropin testing is not needed to assess the recovery of the hypothalamic-pituitary-adrenal axis.[6] Simply check a morning serum cortisol concentration before the morning dose of hydrocortisone, and this assesses hypothalamic CRH production, pituitary ACTH secretion, and adrenal cortisol secretion.[6] Once the morning serum cortisol concentration is >10 mcg/dL, hydrocortisone replacement can be discontinued (assuming the patient is not taking a medication that increases cortisol binding globulin such as oral estrogen).

Primary corticotroph hyperplasia (not related to ectopic corticotropin-releasing hormone secretion) is a rare cause of ACTH-dependent CS and has not been previously described in a patient with MEN-1.[7,8] As noted earlier, annual follow-up will be important to detect recurrent CS if it should occur.

Key Points

- CS in the setting of MEN-1 is particularly challenging. CS may be ACTH independent (e.g., adrenal adenoma, carcinoma, or bilateral macronodular adrenal hyperplasia) or ACTH dependent (e.g., pituitary adenoma, ectopic ACTH secretion from bronchial carcinoid, thymic carcinoid, or pancreatic neuroendocrine tumor).

- No one case detection test for CS is infallible. The patient described herein had suppression in 24-hour UFC and serum cortisol with the 2-day formal low-dose DST to a degree that most

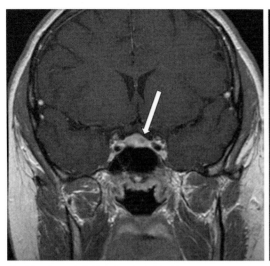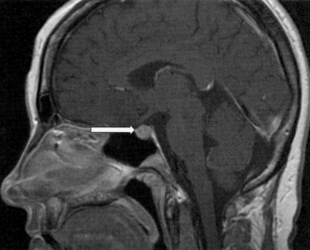

Fig. 64.2 Coronal *(left)* and sagittal *(right)* images from gadolinium-enhanced head magnetic resonance imaging showed within the superior left ventral portion of the pituitary gland there was a 3-mm area of decreased enhancement *(arrows)* consistent with a pituitary microadenoma.

clinicians would accept as excluding the diagnosis of CS.

- In the setting of ACTH-dependent CS, if the 24-hour UFC excretion suppresses more than 90% with the 2-day formal low- or high-dose DST, the patient has pituitary-dependent disease.

REFERENCES

1. Simonds WF, Varghese S, Marx SJ, Nieman LK. Cushing's syndrome in multiple endocrine neoplasia type 1. *Clin Endocrinol (Oxf)*. 2012 Mar;76(3):379–386 .

2. Hasani-Ranjbar S, Rahmanian M, Ebrahim-Habibi A. Ectopic Cushing syndrome associated with thymic carcinoid tumor as the first presentation of MEN1 syndrome-report of a family with MEN1 gene mutation. *Fam Cancer*. 2014 Jun;13(2):267-272.

3. Galm BP, Qiao N, Klibanski A, Biller BMK, Tritos NA. Accuracy of laboratory tests for the diagnosis of Cushing syndrome. *J Clin Endocrinol Metab*. 2020;105(6).

4. Flack MR, Oldfield EH, Cutler GB Jr, et al. Urine free cortisol in the high-dose dexamethasone suppression test for the differential diagnosis of the Cushing syndrome. *Ann Intern Med*. 1992;116(3):211–217.

5. Miller DL, Doppman JL, Peterman SB, Nieman LK, Oldfield EH, Chang R. Neurologic complications of petrosal sinus sampling. *Radiology*. 1992;185(1): 143–147.

6. Hurtado MD, Cortes T, Natt N, Young WF Jr, Bancos I. Extensive clinical experience: hypothalamic-pituitary-adrenal axis recovery after adrenalectomy for corticotropin-independent cortisol excess. *Clin Endocrinol (Oxf)*. 2018;89(6):721–733.

7. Schnall AM, Kovacs K, Brodkey JS, Pearson OH. Pituitary Cushing's disease without adenoma. *Acta Endocrinol (Copenh)*. 1980;94(3):297–303.

8. Young WF Jr, Scheithauer BW, Gharib H, Laws ER Jr, Carpenter PC. Cushing's syndrome due to primary multinodular corticotrope hyperplasia. *Mayo Clin Proc*. 1988;63(3):256–262.

Other Adrenal Masses

As highlighted in the pages of this book, the evaluation and management of patients with adrenal masses can be both challenging and humbling. In this section we highlight case examples of other common and uncommon benign and malignant adrenal masses that have not been included in the sections on the incidentally discovered adrenal mass, primary aldosteronism, Cushing syndrome, adrenal cortical carcinoma, pheochromocytoma, androgen excess, and adrenal disorders in pregnancy. In Olmsted County, the standardized incidence rates for image-detected adrenal mass increased from 4.4 per 100,000 person-years in 1995 to 47.8 in 2017.[1] This more than 10-fold rise in incidence was due to the more widespread use of cross-sectional computed imaging. All clinicians should be aware of the differential diagnosis for incidentally discovered apparent adrenal masses—many of which are highlighted in this section.

Image-Specific Diagnoses

In some cases, the image characteristics on cross-sectional imaging are diagnostic. For example, the presence of macroscopic fat mixed with myeloid elements is diagnostic of adrenal myelolipoma (see Cases 65, 82, and 86). Adrenal hemorrhage is another example where the clinical presentation combined with the cross-sectional image phenotype is diagnostic (see Cases 67 and 68). In addition, adrenal stones (see Case 70) and simple adrenal cysts (see Case 71) have classic image-based findings.

Image Phenotypes Highly Suspicious for Underlying Diagnoses

In other cases, the cross-sectional computed images, although not diagnostic, can be highly suspicious for the underlying etiology. Some examples of this situation include pure ganglioneuroma (see Case 74), adrenal lymphoma (see Case 77), metastatic disease to the adrenals (see Cases 79 and 80), and congenital adrenal hyperplasia (see Cases 82 and 86).

Pseudo-Adrenal Masses

We also highlight several examples where the findings on cross-sectional imaging can fool the radiologist and the endocrinologist—where the mass is actually not adrenal in origin (see examples under Case 85).

REFERENCE

1. Ebbehoj A, Li D, Kaur RJ, et al. Epidemiology of adrenal tumours in Olmsted County, Minnesota, USA: a population-based cohort study. *Lancet Diabetes Endocrinol.* 2020;8(11):894–902.

Adrenal Myelolipoma: A Computed Tomography Diagnosis

Adrenal myelolipoma is a benign adrenocortical tumor composed of adipose tissue and bone marrow elements; it is reported in one out of 500–1250 autopsy cases.[1] Adrenal myelolipoma is typically diagnosed in the fifth and sixth decades of life with no sex predilection. Although large myelolipomas can lead to mass effect symptoms, most are asymptomatic and detected incidentally on cross-sectional imaging performed for other reasons. There are a few types of adrenal masses in which the imaging phenotype is diagnostic. Herein we share such a case.

Case Report

The patient was a 52-year-old man referred for evaluation of an incidentally discovered right adrenal mass. This patient was well until 1 month previously when he had signs and symptoms of pulmonary embolism that was confirmed on a chest computed tomography (CT) study. The chest CT scan incidentally discovered a large right adrenal mass (14 × 9 × 13 cm) that was predominately fat density (Fig. 65.1). He had a history of hypertension controlled on a calcium channel blocker (amlodipine 5 mg daily) and a diuretic (hydrochlorothiazide 12.5 mg daily). The question was whether compression of the inferior vena cava by the right adrenal mass predisposed the patient to pulmonary embolism. Doppler ultrasound of the lower extremities was normal. His only other medication at the time of our consultation was warfarin. On physical examination his body mass index was 31.9 kg/m^2, blood pressure was 133/85 mmHg, and heart rate 56 beats per minute. There was no right upper quadrant abdominal discomfort.

INVESTIGATIONS

The laboratory studies were normal, including the 24-hour urine excretion of fractionated metanephrines and serum 17-hydroxyprogesterone (Table 65.1).

TREATMENT

Because of his relatively young age, general good health, and the possibility that the large right adrenal mass predisposed him to pulmonary emboli, we advised resection. We suggested that he complete a full 6 months of anticoagulation before the elective operation. We repeated the CT scan before surgery, and the right adrenal mass was unchanged in size and configuration. The patient underwent an uneventful laparoscopic right adrenalectomy. The adrenal mass weighed 211 g (normal adrenal gland weight, 4–5 g) and was a typical myelolipoma that measured 13.5 × 12 × 9 cm.

OUTCOME AND FOLLOW-UP

The patient recovered well from surgery and was advised to have a follow-up abdominal CT scan in 1 year.

Discussion

We recently published a retrospective study of 305 consecutive patients with 321 myelolipomas (median largest lesional diameter, 2.3 cm).[2] The median age at diagnosis was 63 years (range, 25–87). Most myelolipomas (86%) were incidentally detected. Only 12% were resected, and all but two of those were >6 cm in diameter. Tumor growth of ≥1 cm on follow-up imaging was associated with larger myelolipomas and hemorrhagic changes. We concluded that adrenalectomy should be considered in symptomatic patients with large tumors and when there is evidence of hemorrhage or tumor growth.[2]

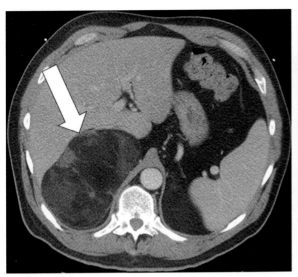 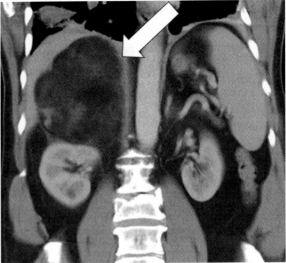

Fig. 65.1 Contrast-enhanced abdominal computed tomography axial (CT) *(left)* and coronal *(right)* scan images show a 14 × 9 × 13–cm predominately fat density right adrenal mass *(arrows)* consistent with an adrenal myelolipoma. The unenhanced CT attenuation was −84 Hounsfield units.

TABLE 65.1 **Laboratory Tests**		
Biochemical Test	**Result**	**Reference Range**
Sodium, mmol/L	139	135–145
Potassium, mmol/L	4.3	3.6–5.2
Creatinine, mg/dL	0.8	0.8–1.3
17-Hydroxyprogesterone, ng/dL	80	<220
24-Hour urine:		
Metanephrine, mcg	112	<400
Normetanephrine, mcg	793	<900

Key Points

- The CT scan finding of macroscopic fat in an adrenal mass is diagnostic of an adrenal myelolipoma.

- Most adrenal myelolipomas do not require surgical intervention. However, when observation is chosen, at least one follow-up image should be obtained to document stability.
- All patients with adrenal myelolipomas should be screened for congenital adrenal hyperplasia—especially in the setting of bilateral adrenal myelolipomas (see Case 82).

REFERENCES

1. Olsson CA, Krane RJ, Klugo RC, Selikowitz SMJS. Adrenal myelolipoma. *Surgery*. 1973;73(5):665–670.
2. Hamidi O, Raman R, Lazik N, et al. Clinical course of adrenal myelolipoma: a long-term longitudinal follow-up study. *Clin Endocrinol (Oxf)*. 2020;93(1):11–18.

Adrenal Schwannoma

Adrenal schwannoma is a rare benign tumor with microscopic features of nerve sheath differentiation.[1] Fewer than 100 cases have been reported in the literature. Herein we share a case of a patient with an adrenal schwannoma who presented with acute tumor infarction.

Case Report

The patient was a 77-year-old man who was well until 10 days before our evaluation when he had abrupt onset of nausea, vomiting, and back pain (7/10 in severity). He went to the emergency department, and a computed tomography (CT) scan of the abdomen disclosed a 9.7 cm × 10 cm × 10.6–cm right adrenal mass (Fig. 66.1). He was informed that he had "cancer" and was given intramuscular pain medicine and oral pain medications and sent home. The back pain slowly resolved over 5 days. He had no paroxysmal symptoms, and there was no history of hypertension. His weight had been stable. He had no signs or symptoms of Cushing

syndrome. There was no history of hypokalemia. He had no prior abdominal cross-sectional computed imaging studies. His regular medications included aspirin 81 mg daily and calcium carbonate 600 mg daily. On physical examination his body mass index was 28.2 kg/m², blood pressure 126/60 mmHg, and heart rate 68 beats per minute. He had no stigmata of an adrenal disorder. Heart and lung examinations were normal.

INVESTIGATIONS

The laboratory studies were normal (Table 66.1). There was no biochemical evidence for functioning pheochromocytoma or adrenocortical carcinoma.

TREATMENT

Based on the imaging phenotype on the CT scan we were highly suspect of either a nonfunctioning pheochromocytoma or adrenocortical carcinoma with the presentation of acute tumor infarction. We stopped his aspirin and prepared him for surgery with doxazosin—titrating the dosage to 2 mg twice daily for target

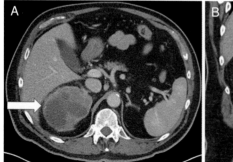 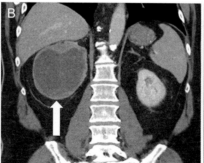 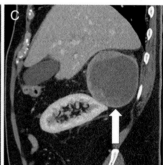

Fig. 66-1 Axial (A), coronal (B), and sagittal (C) images from contrast-enhanced abdominal computed tomography scan showed a 9.7 cm × 10 cm × 10.6–cm right adrenal mass *(arrows)*. The central lucency was consistent with necrosis. The adrenal mass abutted but did not invade the upper pole of the right kidney. The left kidney and left adrenal gland appeared normal.

TABLE 66.1 Laboratory Tests

Biochemical Test	Result	Reference Range
Sodium, mmol/L	139	135–145
Potassium, mmol/L	4.2	3.6–5.2
Fasting plasma glucose, mg/dL	84	70–100
Creatinine, mg/dL	0.8	0.6–1.1
8 AM serum cortisol, mcg/dL	18	7–25
8 AM serum ACTH, pg/mL	41	10–60
DHEA-S, mcg/dL	81.4	25–131
Plasma metanephrine, nmol/L	<0.2	<0.5
Plasma normetanephrine, nmol/L	0.47	<0.9
Plasma aldosterone, ng/dL	<4.0	≤21
Plasma renin activity, ng/mL per hour	2.2	≤0.6–3.0
24-Hour urine:		
Metanephrine, mcg	148	<400
Normetanephrine, mcg	523	<900
Norepinephrine, mcg	47	<80
Epinephrine, mcg	5.5	<20
Dopamine, mcg	301	<400
Cortisol, mcg	51	3.5–45

ACTH, Corticotropin; *DHEA-S,* dehydroepiandrosterone sulfate.

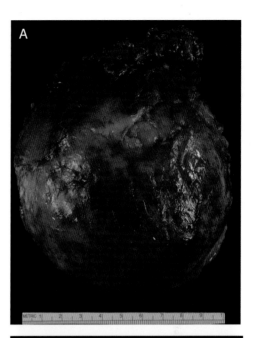

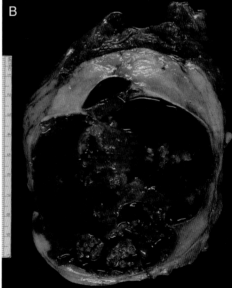

low-normal blood pressure for age. An open laparotomy was performed, and a palpable firm and inflamed mass in the right retroperitoneum was found. Resection was quite difficult because of the inflammation. The tumor was freed off the anterior wall of the kidney and removed intact (Fig. 66.2). At pathology it proved to be a large (11.5 × 9.5 × 6.0 cm) schwannoma that was well circumscribed but centrally infarcted. Most reported adrenal schwannomas are smaller (median tumor size, 6.1 cm), pale yellow to grayish white, and some are cystic.[1,2]

OUTCOME AND FOLLOW-UP

The patient recovered well from surgery and had a follow-up abdominal CT scan 6 months postoperatively that showed no evidence of persistent tumor.

Fig. 66-2 Gross pathology images with intact (A) and bisected (B) adrenal tumor. A schwannoma was identified forming a well-circumscribed but centrally infarcted and cystic necrotic mass measuring 11.5 × 9.5 × 6.0 cm. The tumor was composed of spindle cells. Immunoperoxidase studies showed strong and diffuse expression of S-100 and strong patchy expression of collagen IV. The Ki-67 proliferative index was low (visually <2%). Tumor cells were negative for HMB45, Melan-A, smooth muscle actin, desmin, CD34, keratin AE1/ AE3, ALK, CD3, CD20, and myeloperoxidase.

Key Points

- Adrenal schwannomas need to be considered in the differential diagnosis when a patient presents with a nonfunctioning adrenal mass with a suspicious imaging phenotype on computed imaging.
- Although adrenal schwannomas are benign, when large (e.g., >6 cm), resection should be considered to avoid a future acute presentation as occurred in the case reported here.
- In a series of 17 cases of adrenal schwannoma, all were unilateral, round, or oval solitary tumors, with diameters ranging from 2.5 to 8.8 cm. On CT, adrenal schwannomas were well circumscribed round and lipid poor (mean unenhanced CT attenuation = 30.1 Hounsfield units). Of the 17 cases, 10 showed heterogeneous cystic or hemorrhagic changes.[3]
- Because adrenal schwannomas are benign, following resection they do not require long-term imaging follow-up.

REFERENCES

1. Lam AKY, Just P-A, Lack E, Tissier F, Weiss LM. Schwannoma. In: Lloyd RV, Osamura RY, Kloppel G, Rosai J, eds. *WHO classification of tumours of endocrine organs*. Lyon: International Agency for Research on Cancer (IARC) Press; 2017:176.

2. Mohiuddin Y, Gilliland MG. Adrenal schwannoma: a rare type of adrenal incidentaloma. *Arch Pathol Lab Med*. 2013;137(7):1009–1014.

3. Tang W, Yu XR, Zhou LP, Gao HB, Wang QF, Peng WJ. Adrenal schwannoma: CT, MR manifestations and pathological correlation. *Clin Hemorheol Microcirc*. 2018;68(4):401–412.

Trauma-Related Unilateral Adrenal Hemorrhage

Unilateral adrenal hemorrhage is unusual and usually is related to a unilateral adrenal mass or trauma. In one series, adrenal hematoma was detected in 1.9% of 2692 trauma patients who underwent computed tomography (CT).[1] Compared with the other trauma patients, the patients with adrenal hematomas had more severe injuries associated with higher mortality.[1] Herein we present a case of a patient with unilateral adrenal hemorrhage caused by blunt force trauma.

Case Report

Four weeks before coming to Mayo Clinic, this 61-year-old man was using a four-wheel all-terrain vehicle on a hunting trip. He had a rollover accident and landed on his chest and sustained four right-sided rib fractures. Most of his pain was localized to his right posterior flank. In the emergency department a CT with contrast was performed of his head, chest, and abdomen. Nondisplaced fractures of the right fifth, sixth, seventh, and eighth ribs were noted. In addition, a 4.5 × 2.7 cm right adrenal mass was found (Fig. 67.1). It took about 4 weeks for the right flank pain to resolve. He had no paroxysmal symptoms and there was no history of hypertension. His weight had been stable. The patient had no signs or symptoms of Cushing syndrome. There was no history of hypokalemia. He had no prior abdominal cross-sectional computed imaging studies. The patient took no regular medications. On physical examination his body mass index was 28.2 kg/m^2, blood pressure 110/72 mmHg, and heart rate 65 beats per minute. He had no stigmata of an adrenal disorder. Heart and lung examinations were normal.

INVESTIGATIONS

The laboratory studies were normal (Table 67.1). There was no clinical or biochemical evidence of adrenal gland dysfunction.

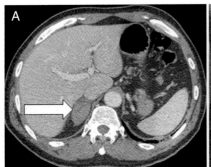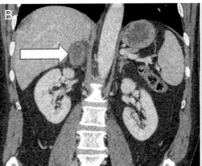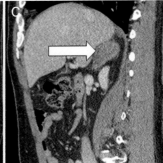

Fig. 67.1 Axial (A), coronal (B), a sagittal (C) images from a contrast-enhanced abdominal computed tomography (CT) scan showed a 4.1 × 2.7–cm right adrenal mass *(arrows)*. With contrast administration the CT attenuation was 60 Hounsfield units. The entire right adrenal was involved. There was some fat stranding above and lateral to the adrenal mass. The left adrenal gland appeared normal.

TABLE 67.1 Laboratory Tests		
Biochemical Test	**Result**	**Reference Range**
Sodium, mmol/L	142	135–145
Potassium, mmol/L	4.4	3.6–5.2
8 AM serum cortisol, mcg/dL	10.5	7–25
8 AM serum ACTH, pg/mL	20	10–60

ACTH, Corticotropin.

TREATMENT

Based on the history of trauma, right-sided rib fractures, and the imaging phenotype on the CT scan, we were highly suspicious of blunt force trauma–induced right adrenal gland hemorrhage.[2] We could not exclude a preceding right adrenal mass. A follow-up computed image 4 months posttrauma was advised.

OUTCOME AND FOLLOW-UP

The follow-up magnetic resonance imaging completed 4 months after his accident documented near complete resolution of the right adrenal gland mass and confirmed our suspicion of a right adrenal gland hemorrhage (Fig. 67.2).

Key Points

- Traumatic adrenal injury may be seen in up to 2% of people with blunt abdominal trauma.[1]
- Usually adrenal hemorrhage that is associated with blunt force trauma is unilateral, self-limiting, and requires no intervention. However, if the hemorrhage is not localized and massive, transarterial embolization may be indicated.[2]
- Blunt force trauma–induced adrenal injury typically appears as a discrete round to oval hematoma expanding the adrenal gland with a typical maximum lesional diameter of 2.5–4.0 cm.[1-3] Associated CT findings included "stranding" of the periadrenal fat caused by blood.
- Unilateral adrenal hemorrhage is usually not associated with significant medical sequelae. Adrenal insufficiency should not occur unless the hemorrhage is bilateral. On long-term follow-up, the adrenal gland with the hemorrhage may develop eggshell calcification (see Case 70).
- In patients with unilateral adrenal hemorrhage, it is important to exclude an underlying neoplasm—thus follow-up imaging to document hemorrhage resolution is important.

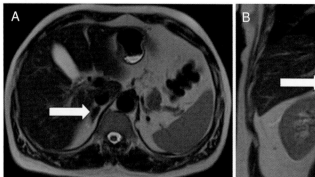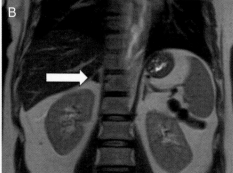

Fig. 67-2 Axial (A) and coronal (B) images from abdominal magnetic resonance imaging (MRI) scan obtained 4 months after the CT scan shown in Fig. 67.1. The MRI shows near complete resolution of the right adrenal gland hemorrhage. The remaining adrenal gland is slightly thickened.

REFERENCES

1. Rana AI, Kenney PJ, Lockhart ME, et al. Adrenal gland hematomas in trauma patients. *Radiology*. 2004;230(3):669–675.

2. Ikeda O, Urata J, Araki Y, et al. Acute adrenal hemorrhage after blunt trauma. *Abdom Imaging*. 2007;32(2):248–252.

3. Burks DW, Mirvis SE, Shanmuganathan K. Acute adrenal injury after blunt abdominal trauma: CT findings. *AJR Am J Roentgenol*. 1992;158(3):503–507.

Bilateral Adrenal Hemorrhage

Fortunately, bilateral adrenal hemorrhage is a rare event. In situations of physiologic stress (e.g., postoperative state or sepsis), blood flow to the adrenal glands and cortisol production are markedly increased—the adrenal glands become edematous and susceptible to hemorrhage, hypotension, and venous infarction. Thus the typical clinical settings for bilateral adrenal hemorrhage include the postoperative period, trauma, neoplastic infiltration of the adrenal glands, anticoagulation therapy, and coagulopathies such as antiphospholipid-antibody syndrome. Typically, primary adrenal insufficiency, if present, is a permanent deficit. The case presented herein highlights the evolution of adrenal hemorrhage on computed tomography (CT) and the potential to recover adrenocortical function.

Case Report

This 68-year-old woman presented to the emergency department with severe left flank pain. Eleven days previously she had undergone left total knee arthroplasty. Following the orthopedic procedure she was placed on a 7-day course of low-molecular-weight heparin for deep venous thrombosis (DVT) prophylaxis. She had no history of DVT or blood clotting disorder. An abdominal CT scan was obtained in the emergency department and showed bilateral adrenal masses with imaging characteristics consistent with bilateral adrenal hemorrhage (Fig. 68.1).

INVESTIGATIONS

Laboratory testing showed hyponatremia, high-normal serum potassium concentration, and low serum cortisol concentration (Table 68.1). The next study

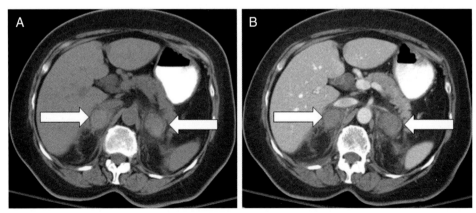

Fig. 68.1 Axial images from unenhanced (A) and contrast-enhanced (B) abdominal computed tomography (CT) scan showed bilateral heterogeneous adrenal masses *(arrows)* that did not have the imaging characteristics of benign adrenal adenomas. The left adrenal mass measured 3.3 × 2.6 cm and the right mass 3.0 × 2.7 cm. The unenhanced CT attenuations were 59.7 Hounsfield units (HU) on the right and 49.3 HU on the left. There was soft tissue thickening or edema of the adjacent mesenteric fat bilaterally. After contrast administration, there was minimal enhancement. Given the imaging characteristics, the clinical presentation, and the recent history of anticoagulation, this likely represented bilateral adrenal hemorrhage.

TABLE 68.1 Laboratory Tests

Biochemical Test	Result	Reference Range
Sodium, mEq/L	121	135–145
Potassium, mEq/L	4.9	3.6–5.2
Creatinine, mg/dL	0.9	0.6–1.1
eGFR, mL/min per BSA	>60	>60
7:50 AM serum cortisol, mcg/dL	3.1	7–25
Aldosterone, ng/dL	<1	≤21 ng/dL
Plasma metanephrine, nmol/L	0.31	<0.5
Plasma normetanephrine, nmol/L	1.09	<0.9

BSA, Body surface area; *eGFR,* estimated glomerular filtration rate.

obtained in the hospital was a 250-mcg cosyntropin stimulation test that showed serum cortisol concentrations of 5.3, 6.1, and 6.4 mcg/dL obtained at baseline and 30 and 60 minutes post-cosyntropin, respectively. Serum corticotropin, although indicated in this setting, was not measured.

TREATMENT

Her blood pressure was normal. She was treated with stress dose glucocorticoids and discharged from the hospital on hydrocortisone 20 mg twice daily. Endocrine consultation was obtained as an outpatient, and her hydrocortisone dosage was decreased to 20 mg in the morning and 10 mg in the afternoon. In addition, treatment with 0.05 mg of fludrocortisone daily was initiated.

OUTCOME AND FOLLOW-UP

Serial abdominal CT scans were obtained and showed near total resolution of the hemorrhagic adrenal masses 3 months later and total resolution 2.5 years later (Fig. 68.2). Although primary adrenal insufficiency is frequently permanent in this setting, it should be reassessed over time. The dosage of hydrocortisone was tapered to a single morning dose of 15 mg in an effort to determine if adrenocortical function would recover. The serial 8 AM serum cortisol concentrations (obtained 24 hours after last dose of hydrocortisone) were 4.9 mcg/dL, 6.3 mcg/dL, 11 mcg/dL, 15 mcg/dL, 17 mcg/dL, and 14 mcg/dL at 1, 3, 6, 8, 10, and 19 months, respectively, following the bilateral adrenal hemorrhage.

Hydrocortisone and fludrocortisone replacement was discontinued 6 months after the adrenal hemorrhage. The 250-mcg cosyntropin stimulation test was obtained at the 19-month time point and was normal with a baseline cortisol concentration of 12 mcg/dL and rose to 17 mcg/dL and 20 mcg/dL at 30 and 60 minutes, respectively. After fludrocortisone was discontinued, the serum sodium and potassium concentrations remained normal; in addition, the serum aldosterone concentration was normal at 8.4 ng/dL and plasma renin activity was normal at 1.6 ng/mL per hour. She continued to do well until progressive dementia was diagnosed 10 years later and she passed away with dementia-related complications at 80 years of age and 12 years after her bilateral adrenal gland hemorrhage.

Discussion

In 2001, our center reported on a 25-year experience with adrenal hemorrhage.[1] Of the 141 cases of adrenal gland hemorrhage, 55% were bilateral. Historically, bilateral adrenal hemorrhage was most frequently associated with the Waterhouse-Friderichsen syndrome of meningococcal septicemia. However, bilateral adrenal hemorrhage in the current era is more commonly associated with the following: postoperative period, trauma, neoplastic infiltration of the adrenal glands, anticoagulation therapy, and coagulopathies such as antiphospholipid-antibody syndrome.[1–+3] The vascular supply to and venous drainage from the adrenal glands predisposes to hemorrhagic necrosis. In situations of physiologic stress such as the postoperative state or sepsis, blood flow to the adrenal glands and cortisol production are markedly increased—the adrenal glands become edematous and susceptible to hemorrhage, hypotension, and venous infarction.[4]

Key Points

- Fortunately, bilateral adrenal hemorrhage is a rare event. However, when it does occur, it can cause life-threatening primary adrenal failure if not recognized and treated.
- Bilateral adrenal hemorrhage is associated with meningococcal and other forms of septicemia, the postoperative period, trauma, neoplastic infiltration of

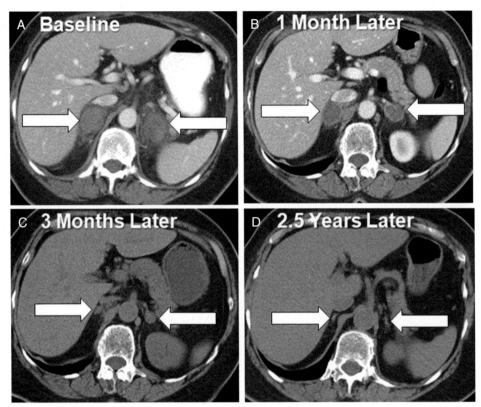

Fig. 68.2 Serial axial computed tomography (CT) images at baseline (A), 1 month later (B), 3 months later (C), and 2.5 years later (D). Panel (B) shows that the bilateral adrenal masses *(arrows)* had decreased in size and attenuation since the prior scan. The right adrenal mass measured 2.3 × 2.1 cm and the left adrenal mass measured 2.3 × 1.9 cm. The masses had enhancing rims and central portions that did not enhance—appearances consistent with resolving adrenal hemorrhage. Panel (C) shows a dramatic decrease in the size of both adrenal masses *(arrows)* consistent with resolution of bilateral adrenal hemorrhage. There was a residual nodule in the left adrenal that measured 1.3 cm in diameter. Panel (D) shows resolution of the bilateral adrenal masses consistent with resolution of bilateral adrenal hemorrhage. The adrenoform contour of both adrenal glands was normal on this CT.

the adrenal glands, anticoagulation therapy, and coagulopathies such as antiphospholipid-antibody syndrome.

- Although the primary adrenal insufficiency associated with bilateral adrenal hemorrhage is frequently permanent, it is important to periodically reassess for potential recovery of adrenocortical function.

REFERENCES

1. Vella A, Nippoldt TB, Morris JC 3rd. Adrenal hemorrhage: a 25-year experience at the Mayo Clinic. *Mayo Clin Proc.* 2001;76(2):161–168.
2. Head WC, Bynum LJ. Bilateral adrenal hemorrhage: a complication of prophylactic anticoagulation. *Orthopedics.* 1981;4(11):1252–1254.
3. Houlden RL, Janmohamed A. Bilateral adrenal hemorrhage with adrenal insufficiency after dalteparin use post hip athroplasties. *AACE Clin Case Rep.* 2020;6(3):e141–e143.
4. Tan GX, Sutherland T. Adrenal congestion preceding adrenal hemorrhage on CT imaging: a case series. *Abdom Radiol (NY).* 2016;41(2):303–310.

Primary Adrenal Teratoma

Tumors of the adrenal gland that contain macroscopic fat are usually myelolipomas; however, the differential diagnosis includes lipomas, teratomas, angiomyolipomas, and liposarcoma. Herein we present a case of a patient with a large multilobulated lipomatous tumor that proved to be an adrenal teratoma.

Case Report

The patient was a 66-year-old man who had intermittent abdominal pain for about a month, which led to a computed tomography (CT) scan of the abdomen that demonstrated a large right adrenal mass (Fig. 69.1). He had no paroxysmal symptoms. His weight had been stable. He had no signs or symptoms of Cushing syndrome. He had been diagnosed with hypertension 10 years previously. There was no history of hypokalemia. He did have a 30-year history of diabetes mellitus.

His medications included metformin 1000 mg twice daily, glipizide 2.5 mg daily, lisinopril 40 mg daily, and pravastatin 40 mg daily. On physical examination his body mass index was 27.5 kg/m^2, blood pressure 131/78 mmHg, and heart rate 98 beats per minute. He had no stigmata of an adrenal disorder. Heart and lung examinations were normal.

INVESTIGATIONS

The laboratory studies were normal (Table 69.1). There was no biochemical evidence of functioning pheochromocytoma, aldosteronoma, or cortisol secretory autonomy.

TREATMENT

Based on the large size of the adrenal mass, surgical resection was recommended. The right adrenal mass underwent subtotal resection by the laparoscopic approach. A 17.0 × 16.0 × 4.5–cm aggregate of fibrofatty tissue was provided to pathology. The tumor was

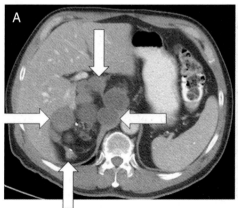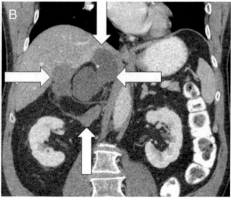

Fig. 69.1 Axial image (A) and coronal image (B) from a contrast-enhanced abdominal computed tomography scan demonstrated a 12.5 × 11.0 × 12.2–cm right adrenal mass *(arrows)*. The mass contained a large amount of macroscopic fat and several round internal loculated areas of fluid density. Several of the loculated areas contained mural calcification.

TABLE 69.1   Laboratory Tests

Biochemical Test	Result	Reference Range
Sodium, mmol/L	143	135–145
Potassium, mmol/L	4.9	3.6–5.2
Fasting plasma glucose, mg/dL	140	70–100
Creatinine, mg/dL	1.1	0.74–1.35
8 AM serum cortisol, mcg/dL	17	7–25
8 AM serum ACTH, pg/mL	38	1060
Plasma metanephrine, nmol/L	<0.2	<0.5
Plasma normetanephrine, nmol/L	0.3	<0.9
Plasma aldosterone, ng/dL	4.0	≤21
Plasma renin activity, ng/mL per hour	4.8	≤0.6–3.0
Prostate specific antigen, ng/mL	1.0	<6.5
24-Hour urine:		
Metanephrine, mcg	105	<400
Normetanephrine, mcg	279	<900
Norepinephrine, mcg	44	<80
Epinephrine, mcg	4.8	<20
Dopamine, mcg	185	<400
Cortisol, mcg	17	3.5–45

ACTH, Corticotropin.

a primary adrenal teratoma composed predominantly of mature prostatic tissue and hair was present on cut section.

OUTCOME AND FOLLOW-UP

The patient was discharged from the hospital the day after surgery. Follow-up abdominal CT scan 1 year later showed a residual 4.6 × 5.1 × 5.2–cm right adrenal bed mass. Four years after surgery the complex cystic mass measured 7.2 × 7.0 × 6.0 cm (Fig. 69.2). Because of its documented growth and marked mass effect and lateral displacement of the suprarenal and intrahepatic inferior vena cava, an open operation was advised. At surgery the mass was adherent to the inferior vena cava, and it was decided to leave a portion of cyst wall on the inferior vena cava. At pathology the 5.5 × 5 × 4–cm specimen was primarily cystic, lined by mucinous epithelium and containing abundant mucin and compatible with recurrent teratoma.

Key Points

- Primary adrenal teratomas are rare neoplasms, and there are limited data on their surgical outcomes and long-term prognosis.
- Most reported cases have been mature cystic teratomas that displayed well-differentiated respiratory, digestive, and squamous epithelia.[1–3]

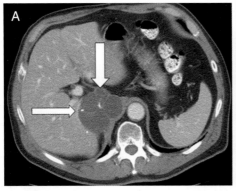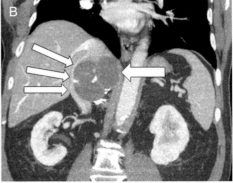

Fig. 69.2 Axial (A) and coronal (B) images from a contrast-enhanced abdominal computed tomography scan obtained 4 years after surgery demonstrated a 7.2 × 7.0 × 6.0–cm complex cystic mass *(large arrows)* with thin enhancing and partially calcified septations in the right adrenalectomy bed consistent with recurrent cystic teratoma. This mass caused marked mass effect and lateral displacement of the suprarenal and intrahepatic inferior vena cava *(small arrows)*.

- Most patients with primary adrenal teratomas reported in the literature presented with abdominal or flank pain with a median tumor diameter of 9.0 cm.[1-3]
- The imaging phenotype of primary adrenal teratoma is that of adrenal mass with macroscopic fat and cystic components with mural calcification.[1]

REFERENCES

1. Khong PL, Lam KY, Ooi CG, Liu MJ, Metreweli C. Mature teratomas of the adrenal gland: imaging features. *Abdom Imaging*. 2002;27(3):347–350.
2. Lam KY, Lo CY. Adrenal lipomatous tumours: a 30 year clinicopathological experience at a single institution. *J Clin Pathol*. 2001;54(9):707–712.
3. Kuo EJ, Sisk AE, Yang Z, Huang J, Yeh MW, Livhits MJ. Adrenal teratoma: a case series and review of the literature. *Endocr Pathol*. 2017;28(2):152–158.

The Adrenal Stone

You will not find much written about "adrenal stones." Although minor calcific deposits in adrenal masses are not unusual, full eggshell and complete calcification of an adrenal mass is rare. The adrenal stone is usually the result of calcification of an old adrenal hemorrhage. It can appear as a full eggshell calcium distribution or complete calcification.[1] Herein we share some examples.

Case Report: Thin Eggshell Calcification

This 62-year-old man had a history of blunt abdominal trauma at the time of a motor vehicle accident 36 years ago. He had no signs or symptoms of adrenal hypo- or hyperfunction. A recent abdominal computed tomography (CT) detected a thin-walled eggshell calcification of a 3.1 cm × 2.8–cm low-attenuation mass arising from the left adrenal gland

(Fig. 70.1). The thin rim calcification was unchanged in size and appearance from a CT scan performed 2 years previously. We suspected that the mass was most likely an old hematoma or perhaps secondary to prior infection. No further evaluation or follow-up was recommended.

Case Report: Thick Eggshell Calcification

This 53-year-old woman had incidentally discovered to have a 3.2-cm peripherally thickly calcified mass lesion of the left adrenal gland (Fig. 70.2). She had no signs or symptoms of adrenal hypo- or hyperfunction. The differential diagnostic considerations included an adrenal cyst complicated by previous infection or hemorrhage, old adrenal hematoma, or previous hemorrhage in a mass lesion. Imaging 12 years later performed for other reasons showed that the left adrenal mass was unchanged in size and character.

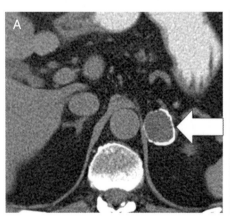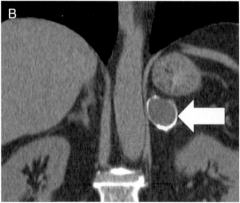

Fig. 70.1 Unenhanced axial (A) and coronal (B) computed tomography (CT) images show thin-walled eggshell calcification of a 3.1 cm × 2.8–cm low-attenuation mass *(arrows)* arising from the left adrenal gland. The thin rim calcification was unchanged in size and appearance when compared to a CT scan performed 2 years previously.

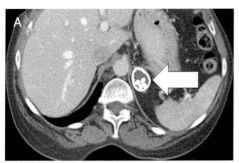
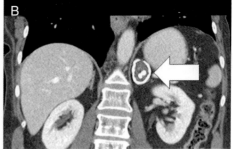

Fig. 70.2 Contrast-enhanced axial (A) and coronal (B) computed tomography images show thick-walled eggshell calcification of a 3.2-cm mass *(arrows)* arising from the left adrenal gland. Several small circular "calcium pebbles" were present within the mass.

Case Report: Adrenal Stone

This 29-year-old man had a CT scan for evaluation of Crohn's disease that incidentally detected a partially calcified 2.6-cm left adrenal mass (Fig. 70.3). He had no signs or symptoms of adrenal hypo- or hyperfunction. The only abdominal trauma he could recall was a snowboarding accident 7 years previously. Serial imaging done for Crohn's disease over the subsequent 3 years showed that the degree of calcification progressively increased, resulting in complete calcification of the mass with an unenhanced CT attenuation

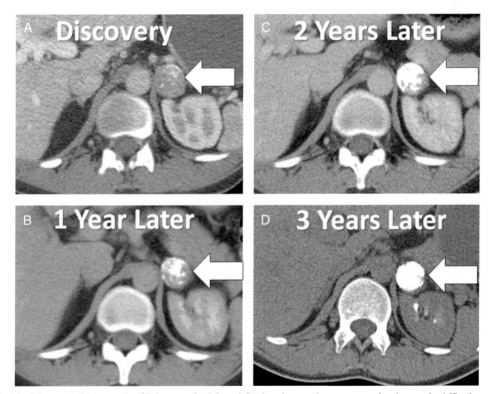

Fig. 70.3 Serial axial computed tomography (CT) images of a 2.6-cm left adrenal mass show a progressive degree of calcification over 3 years. Panel (A) shows a partially calcified left adrenal mass *(arrow)* at the time of detection; the CT attenuation was 109 Hounsfield units (HU). The other three panels show serial imaging over 3 years with increasing degree of calcification. The CT attenuations of the adrenal mass were 174 HU in (B), 251 HU in (C), and 500 HU in (D).

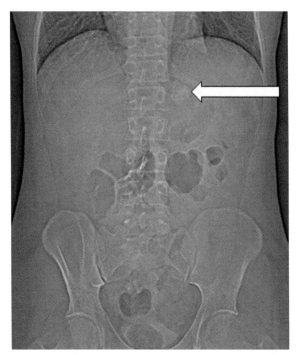

Fig. 70.4 Flat plate roentgenogram of the abdomen from the patient highlighted in Fig. 70.3, which also demonstrates the left adrenal stone.

of 500 Hounsfield units (see Fig. 70.3). It was assumed that this CT scan finding represented progressive calcification of an adrenal hematoma. Adrenal stones can also be visualized on flat plate roentgenogram of the abdomen (Fig. 70.4).

Discussion

Calcification in an adrenal mass is nonspecific.[1–3] However, speckled calcification can be found in neuroblastoma in children, adrenocortical carcinoma, and metastatic disease to the adrenals. Rim calcification can be found in adrenal cysts and adrenal hematomas. Myelolipomas and other benign adrenal lesions may have small calcium deposits. Dystrophic calcification may be seen in adrenal glands with previous involvement of histoplasmosis, tuberculosis, and other infiltrative processes. However, the most common cause of adrenal calcification relates to the natural evolution of adrenal gland hemorrhage—an evolution that may result in progressive calcification and an adrenal stone.

Key Points

- Although speckled calcification can be found in concerning adrenal masses such as adrenocortical carcinoma, eggshell and complete adrenal mass calcification is typically associated with the evolution of adrenal gland hemorrhage.
- The presence and pattern of calcium in an adrenal mass should be correlated with other imaging features (e.g., size, vascularity, homogeneity, enhancement pattern) and adrenal-related signs and symptoms to guide clinical management.

REFERENCES

1. Taguchi T, Inoue K, Shuin T, Terada Y. Giant adrenal calcification. *Intern Med*. 2011;50(16):1781.
2. Hindman N, Israel GM. Adrenal gland and adrenal mass calcification. *Eur Radiol*. 2005;15(6):1163–1167.
3. Kenney PJ, Stanley RJ. Calcified adrenal masses. *Urol Radiol*. 1987;9(1):9–15.

Simple Adrenal Cyst

Cystic adrenal masses are uncommon and may be discovered incidentally or may be symptomatic.[1,2] Adrenal cysts are classified as pseudocysts, endothelial cysts, epithelial cysts, and parasitic cysts. Pseudocysts (typically the result of hemorrhage into an adrenal neoplasm) are the most common clinically recognized form of adrenal cyst (see Case 43). Cystic adrenal neoplasms must be differentiated from simple adrenal cysts—findings on computed tomography (CT) and magnetic resonance imaging (MRI) are key in making this distinction. Herein we share a case of a patient with an incidentally discovered simple adrenal cyst.

Case Report

The patient was a 72-year-old woman referred for evaluation of an incidentally discovered left adrenal cyst. The patient had noticed left upper quadrant fullness for a few years. An abdominal CT scan was obtained and showed a well-circumscribed, thin-walled cystic mass (6.0 × 6.7 × 9 cm) in the left suprarenal region (Fig. 71.1). The CT images were consistent with a primary benign adrenal cyst. There was no prior abdominal imaging for comparison. The patient's sister had been recently diagnosed with pancreatic carcinoma, and our patient was concerned that her left adrenal cyst could be related. She was very active—playing tennis and mowing the lawn. She had a history of normal blood pressure. She had no symptoms related to the apparent adrenal cyst except for the left upper quadrant fullness. The patient took no regular medications. On physical examination she appeared well. Her body mass index was 27.4 kg/m², blood pressure 145/64 mmHg, and heart rate 66 beats per minute. Examination of the abdomen showed no visible asymmetry and the cyst was not palpable.

The patient commented that she could do everything she wanted to do and that the sense of fullness was not troubling her to the degree that she would want an operation. Her main wish was to be reassured that this cystic process did not represent a malignancy and would not predispose to other health issues.

INVESTIGATIONS

The laboratory studies were normal (Table 71.1). Normal plasma fractionated metanephrine levels excluded a functioning pheochromocytoma. Because of the borderline blood pressure, measurements of aldosterone and renin were obtained to be sure that potential adrenal cyst-related renal compression was not causing secondary hyperaldosteronism.

TREATMENT

We discussed with the patient that although the cyst could be related to the pancreas or the kidney, our imaging studies (see Fig. 71.1C and D) were consistent with a benign simple adrenal cyst that had been present for many years. We discussed that treatment options included observation, aspiration, or surgical removal. We advised observation with follow-up abdominal ultrasound in 1 year or sooner if symptoms should develop.

OUTCOME AND FOLLOW-UP

Abdominal ultrasound 1 year later showed a stable size of the adrenal cyst. An annual recheck for several years was advised.

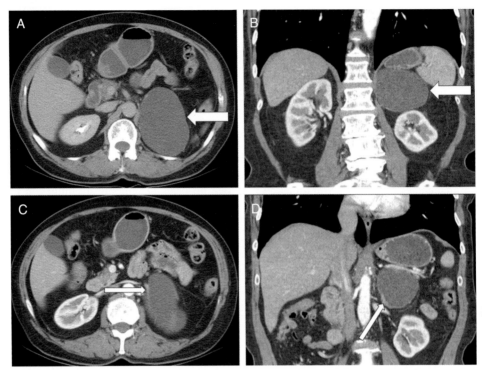

Fig. 71.1 Axial (A, C) and coronal (B, D) images from a contrast-enhanced CT scan. A well-circumscribed, thin-walled cystic mass *(large arrows)* in the left adrenal gland measured 6.0 cm in cephalocaudal dimension × 6.7 in transverse dimension × 9.0 cm in anterior-posterior dimension. A rim of the left adrenal gland *(small arrows* in C, D) was intimately associated with the medial aspect of the cyst. No tumor rind, calcification, or mural nodule was seen. The left kidney was slightly displaced inferiorly. The right adrenal gland appeared normal.

TABLE 71.1 Laboratory Tests		
Biochemical Test	**Result**	**Reference Range**
Sodium, mmol/L	135	135–145
Potassium, mmol/L	3.7	3.6–5.2
Creatinine, mg/dL	0.6	0.6–1.1
Aldosterone, ng/dL	<4.0	≤21 ng/dL
Plasma renin activity ng/mL per hour	<0.6	≤0.6–3
Plasma metanephrine, nmol/L	<0.2	<0.5
Plasma normetanephrine, nmol/L	0.45	<0.9

Key Points

- The distinction between a true cystic lesion and a cystic adrenal neoplasm is important and requires a thorough evaluation.

- A total of 41 cases of macroscopically cystic adrenal lesions among patients who underwent surgery at the Mayo Clinic were identified over a 25-year period.[2] Of the 41 cases, 32 were pseudocysts, 8 were endothelial cysts, and 1 was an epithelial cyst. Of the 32 pseudocysts, 6 were associated with adrenal neoplasms, including 2 adrenal cortical carcinomas, 2 adrenal cortical adenomas, and 2 pheochromocytomas.[2]
- Exclude pheochromocytoma in all patients with an adrenal cyst (see Case 43).

REFERENCES

1. Chien HP, Chang YS, Hsu PS, et al. Adrenal cystic lesions: a clinicopathological analysis of 25 cases with proposed histogenesis and review of the literature. *Endocr Pathol.* 2008;19(4):274–281.
2. Erickson LA, Lloyd RV, Hartman R, Thompson G. Cystic adrenal neoplasms. *Cancer.* 2004;101(7):1537–1544.

Adrenal Cystic Lymphangioma

Cystic lymphangiomas are rare benign vascular tumors that arise from lymphatic endothelial cells and usually are located in the neck or axilla. Adrenal cystic lymphangiomas are rare benign vascular lesions that usually remain asymptomatic throughout life.[1] Although in the past adrenal cystic lymphangiomas were found primarily at autopsy, over the past three decades they are detected more frequently during life because of the widespread use of computed imaging. Herein we share such a case of a patient with an incidentally discovered adrenal cystic lymphangioma.

Case Report

The patient was a 24-year-old woman referred for evaluation of an incidentally discovered left adrenal mass. An episode of persistent diarrhea led to an abdominal computed tomography (CT) scan on which a cystic 5.2 × 4.5 × 5.0–cm left adrenal mass with peripheral calcifications was found (Fig. 72.1). The cystic process appeared to arise from the adrenal gland. The patient was healthy and took no regular medications. There was no history of back trauma or flank discomfort. She was at ideal body weight and had regular menstrual cycles and no hirsutism. She had never been treated with anticoagulants and did not take aspirin.

INVESTIGATIONS

The laboratory studies were normal (Table 72.1). The normal fractionated plasma metanephrines and normal 24-hour urine fractionated metanephrine and catecholamine levels excluded the possibility of a functioning cystic pheochromocytoma.

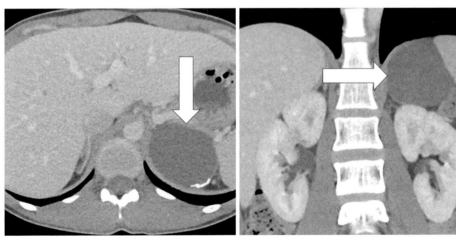

Fig. 72.1 Axial image *(left)* and coronal image *(right)* from contrast-enhanced computed tomography (CT) scan. In the left upper retroperitoneum there was a 6.0 × 5.3 × 5.7–cm nonenhancing cystic lesion *(arrows)*. The unenhanced CT attenuation was 20.1 Hounsfield units. There was a small amount of peripheral wall calcification. No septations or solid components were seen. The lesion abutted the posterior stomach, spleen, and tail of the pancreas without evidence of invasion.

TABLE 72.1   Laboratory Tests

Biochemical Test	Result	Reference Range
Sodium, mmol/L	140	135–145
Potassium, mmol/L	4.6	3.6–5.2
Fasting plasma glucose, mg/dL	84	70–100
Creatinine, mg/dL	0.6	0.6–1.1
DHEA-S, mcg/dL	293	44–332
Plasma metanephrine, nmol/L	<0.2	<0.5
Plasma normetanephrine, nmol/L	0.26	<0.9
24-Hourr urine:		
Metanephrine, mcg	154	<400
Normetanephrine, mcg	284	<900
Norepinephrine, mcg	78	<80
Epinephrine, mcg	19	<20
Dopamine, mcg	394	<400

DHEA-S, Dehydroepiandrosterone sulfate.

TREATMENT

Because of her relatively young age and large size of the left adrenal mass, we advised laparoscopic resection. It proved to be a typical adrenal cystic lymphangioma.

OUTCOME AND FOLLOW-UP

The patient recovered well from surgery and, to exclude persistent disease, she was advised to have a follow-up abdominal CT scan in 1 year.

Key Points

- Adrenal cystic lymphangiomas are rare, benign vascular lesions that usually remain asymptomatic throughout life.[1,2]
- In a series of nine adrenal cystic lymphangiomas (six women and three men), the mean age at time of diagnosis was 42 years (range, 28–56 years). The average size was 4.9 cm (range, 2.0–13.5 cm). Four (44%) of the nine lesions presented with abdominal, flank, or back pain. No evidence of recurrence after resection or development of a contralateral lesion was encountered in any of the patients.[3]

REFERENCES

1. Papotti M, Rosai J, Tsang WYW, Volante M. Benign vascular tumours. In: Lloyd RV, Osamura RY, Kloppel G, Rosai J, eds. *WHO classification of tumours of endocrine organs.* Lyon: International Agency for Research on Cancer (IARC) Press; 2017:129.
2. Koperski Ł, Pihowicz P, Anysz-Grodzicka A, Górnicka B. Cystic lymphangiomatous lesions of the adrenal gland: a clinicopathological study of 37 cases including previously unreported cysts with papillary endothelial proliferation. *Pathol Res Pract.* 2019;215(6):152385.
3. Ellis CL, Banerjee P, Carney E, Sharma R, Netto GJ. Adrenal lymphangioma: clinicopathologic and immunohistochemical characteristics of a rare lesion. *Hum Pathol.* 2011;42(7): 1013–1018.

Adrenal Hemangioma

Lipid-poor adrenal masses raise concerns about the underlying pathology, especially in young people. Herein we present a case of a lipid-poor adrenal mass in a 22-year-old woman that proved to be a benign adrenal hemangioma.

Case Report

The patient was a 22-year-old woman who was found to have a 2.5-cm left adrenal mass incidentally discovered on a chest computed tomography (CT) that was obtained to evaluate pneumonitis. On a follow-up abdominal CT scan 1 year later it measured 2.5 × 2.5 cm with an unenhanced CT attenuation of 29 Hounsfield units (HU) and 61% contrast washout at 15 minutes (Fig. 73.1). She had no paroxysmal symptoms and there was no history of hypertension. Her weight had been stable. She had no signs or symptoms of Cushing syndrome. There was no history of hypokalemia. Her only regular medication was an oral contraceptive pill. On physical examination her body mass index was 33.5 kg/m², blood pressure 122/91 mmHg, and heart rate 94 beats per minute. She had no stigmata of an adrenal disorder. Heart and lung examinations were normal.

INVESTIGATIONS

The laboratory studies were normal (Table 73.1). There was no biochemical evidence for functioning pheochromocytoma or cortisol secretory autonomy.

TREATMENT

Based on the suspicious imaging phenotype on the CT scan and the patient's young age, surgical resection was recommended. The left adrenal gland was removed by the laparoscopic approach. Although initial findings on frozen section suggested pheochromocytoma, the subsequent histologic and immunohistochemical studies demonstrated the tumor to be an adrenal medullary anastomosing hemangioma (Fig. 73.2).

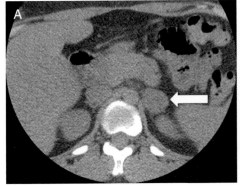 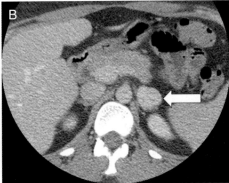

Fig. 73.1 Axial images from unenhanced (A) and contrast-enhanced (B) abdominal computed tomography (CT) scan. A 2.5 × 2.5–cm left adrenal mass *(arrows)* had an unenhanced CT attenuation of 29 Hounsfield units. After contrast administration there was 61% contrast washout at 15 minutes.

TABLE 73.1   Laboratory Tests

Biochemical Test	Result	Reference range
Sodium, mmol/L	140	135–145
Potassium, mmol/L	4.3	3.6–5.2
Fasting plasma glucose, mg/dL	91	70–100
Creatinine, mg/dL	0.9	0.6–1.1
1-mg overnight DST cortisol, mcg/dL	0.7	<1.8
Plasma metanephrine, nmol/L	<0.2	<0.5
Plasma normetanephrine, nmol/L	0.5	<0.9

DST, dexamethasone suppression test.

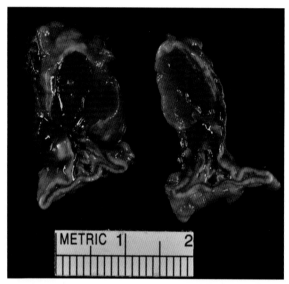

Fig. 73.2 Gross pathology photograph of bisected adrenal mass. The adrenal gland weighed 9.0 g (normal, 4–5 g) and contained a 2.6 cm × 2.0 cm × 1.3–cm red soft mass that did not extend beyond the adrenal gland. The initial findings on frozen section favored a pheochromocytoma. However, histologic and immunohistochemistry (IHC) studies demonstrated the tumor to be an adrenal medullary anastomosing hemangioma. IHC showed that CD31 and CD34 highlighted the endothelial cell populations, which were dominate in the mass. There was no evidence of epithelial differentiation as demonstrated by IHC stains for cytokeratin, OSCAR, CAM5.2, inhibin, and Melan A, which were all negative. No neuroendocrine cell populations were found based on lack of IHC staining for chromogranin, S-100, and synaptophysin. There was no evidence of stromal cell populations based on lack of IHC staining for HMB45 and smooth muscle actin.

OUTCOME AND FOLLOW-UP

The patient was discharged from the hospital the day after surgery. She was reassured with regard to the benign nature of her adrenal tumor, and no specific follow-up was advised.

Key Points

- Anastomosing adrenal hemangiomas are exceedingly rare and are not included in the encyclopedic 2017 WHO classification of tumors of endocrine organs.
- Anastomosing adrenal hemangiomas can have imaging features consistent with pheochromocytoma and angiosarcoma.[1-3]
- Because of their benign nature and lack of any syndromic associations, anastomosing adrenal hemangiomas require no follow-up after surgical resection.

REFERENCES

1. Zhou J, Yang X, Zhou L, Zhao M, Wang C. Anastomosing hemangioma incidentally found in kidney or adrenal gland: study of 10 cases and review of literature. *Urol J*. 2020;17(6):650–656.
2. O'Neill AC, Craig JW, Silverman SG, Alencar RO. Anastomosing hemangiomas: locations of occurrence, imaging features, and diagnosis with percutaneous biopsy. *Abdom Radiol* (NY). 2016;41(7):1325–1332.
3. Patel SR, Abimbola O, Bhamber T, Weida C, Roy O. Incidental finding of bilateral renal and adrenal anastomosing hemangiomas: a rare case report. *Urol Case Rep*. 2019;27:100912.

Adrenal Ganglioneuroma

Adrenal ganglioneuroma is a rare benign tumor that is characterized by ganglion cells individually distributed in Schwannian stroma.[1] Adrenal ganglioneuroma is found in approximately 2% of adrenalectomies.[2] The unique imaging characteristics of this tumor can lead to a presumptive diagnosis, which is potentially important because when small, adrenal ganglioneuromas may not need to be resected. Herein we present a case of a young patient with a 5-cm adrenal mass that was suspected to be an adrenal ganglioneuroma based on imaging.

Case Report

This 28-year-old woman was seen in endocrine consultation for the incidental discovery of a 5-cm right adrenal mass on computed tomography (CT) performed for pelvic pain. The CT findings were unique, with the mass having a triangular shape, uniform ground-glass density, well-defined tumor edges, indeterminate unenhanced CT attenuation, and relative lack of vascularity with contrast administration (Fig. 74.1). She had no signs or symptoms of an adrenal disorder. She had normal blood pressure and stable body weight. She had been taking no regular medications. She had never been treated with anticoagulants and did not take aspirin.

INVESTIGATIONS

The laboratory studies were normal with the exception of the mild elevation in plasma normetanephrine (Table 74.1). The false-positive rate of plasma normetanephrine is 15%, and because of the rarity of pheochromocytoma, 97% of patients with increased plasma normetanephrine on the Mayo Clinic campus do not have a pheochromocytoma.[3]

Mild elevations in plasma normetanephrine always need to be interpreted with the clinical context in mind. In this case, the uniform density and lack of vascularity on CT made pheochromocytoma extremely unlikely.

TREATMENT

We advised the patient that, based on the CT imaging characteristics, we suspected she had a benign ganglioneuroma. However, in a shared decision-making discussion with the patient it was decided—based on the size of the mass and her young age—to proceed with laparoscopic right adrenalectomy. Preoperative adrenergic blockade was not administered. The adrenal gland weighed 49 g (normal, 4–5 g). The tumor was located in the medulla and measured 7.6 × 4.9 × 2.4 cm (Fig. 74.2).

OUTCOME AND FOLLOW-UP

The patient recovered well from surgery and was advised to have a follow-up abdominal CT scan in 1 year.

Discussion

There are not many large case series of adrenal ganglioneuroma.[4] In a retrospective study of the Mayo Clinic experience with adrenal ganglioneuroma we diagnosed 45 patients with adrenal ganglioneuroma from 1995 to 2019—3% of all adrenalectomies over that time period.[5] There was a slight female predominance (n = 25, 55%), and the median age at diagnosis was 44 years (range, 6–87 years). Most tumors were discovered incidentally (n = 34, 75%). The median tumor size was 4.5 cm (range, 1.5–12.5 cm). Twenty patients (44%) had a composite tumor of adrenal ganglioneuroma and pheochromocytoma. The prognosis

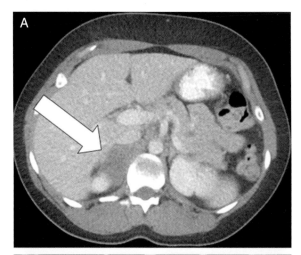

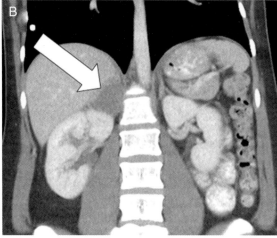

Fig. 74.1 Axial image (A) and coronal image (B) from contrast-enhanced computed tomography (CT) scan shows a 5 × 4.5 × 3–cm triangular-shaped homogeneous right adrenal mass *(arrows)*. The unenhanced CT attenuation was 28.4 Hounsfield units (HU). There was limited enhancement with contrast administration (CT attenuations of 45 HU at 70 seconds and 68 HU at 15 minutes after contrast administration).

TABLE 74.1 Laboratory Tests

Biochemical Test	Result	Reference Range
Sodium, mmol/L	137	135–145
Potassium, mmol/L	4.1	3.6–5.2
Fasting plasma glucose, mg/dL	66	70–100
Creatinine, mg/dL	0.7	0.6–1.1
Plasma metanephrine, nmol/L	0.38	<0.5
Plasma normetanephrine, nmol/L	1.2	<0.9
1-mg overnight DST cortisol, mcg/dL	1.1	<1.8
24-Hour urine:		
Metanephrine, mcg	194	<400
Normetanephrine, mcg	472	<900
Norepinephrine, mcg	69	<80
Epinephrine, mcg	14	<20
Dopamine, mcg	313	<400

DST, Dexamethasone suppression test.

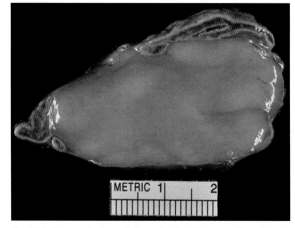

Fig. 74.2 Gross pathology photograph of cut tumor section shows a 7.6 × 4.9 × 2.4–cm firm white mass located in the medulla, which did extend beyond the adrenal gland. Histologic features were diagnostic of ganglioneuroma.

was excellent in all cases, with no tumor recurrence reported on long-term follow-up.

Key Points

- Adrenal ganglioneuroma is a benign adrenal lesion found in approximately 2%–3% of adrenalectomies.
- Findings on cross-sectional computed imaging can be diagnostic and include triangular/oblong shape, homogeneous ground-glass appearance, well-defined edges, unenhanced CT attenuation of <40 Hounsfield units, relative lack of enhancement with contrast administration, homogeneous hypointense adrenal mass on T1-weighted magnetic resonance imaging (MRI), and a heterogeneous hyperintense mass on T2-weighted MRI.
- When small, adrenal ganglioneuromas may be followed with serial imaging to confirm the image-based diagnosis.

- When laboratory studies document catecholamine hypersecretion, a composite pheochromocytoma-ganglioneuroma should be suspected and resection is indicated.

REFERENCES

1. Shimada H, DeLellis RA, Tissier F. Neuroblastic tumours of the adrenal gland. In: Lloyd RV, Osamura RY, Kloppel G, Rosai J, eds. *WHO classification of tumours of endocrine organs*. Lyon: International Agency for Research on Cancer (IARC) Press; 2017:196–203.

2. Lee JH, Chai YJ, Kim TH, et al. Clinicopathological features of ganglioneuroma originating from the adrenal glands. *World J Surg*. 2016;40(12):2970–2975.

3. Sawka AM, Jaeschke R, Singh RJ, Young WF, Jr. A comparison of biochemical tests for pheochromocytoma: measurement of fractionated plasma metanephrines compared with the combination of 24-hour urinary metanephrines and catecholamines. *J Clin Endocrinol Metab*. 2003;88(2):553–558.

4. Fan H, Li HZ, Ji ZG, Shi BB, Zhang YS. [Diagnosis and treatment of adrenal ganglioneuroma: a report of 80 cases]. *Zhonghua Wai Ke Za Zhi*. 2017;55(12):938–941.

5. Dages KN, Kohlenberg JD, Young WF Jr, et al. Presentation and outcomes of adrenal ganglioneuromas: a cohort study and a systematic review of literature. *Clin Endocrinol (Oxf)*. 2021;95(1):47–57.

42-Year-Old Woman With a Large Composite Adrenal Mass

Composite adrenal tumors occur in approximately 4% of adrenal tumors. Imaging characteristics may be suggestive of different tumor etiologies or present as one heterogeneous adrenal mass. Assessment of malignancy potential and hormonal excess should be performed in all adrenal tumors, and treatment should be guided by imaging characteristics and biochemical workup.

Case Report

The patient was a 42-year-old woman who presented for evaluation of an incidentally discovered left adrenal mass on a computed tomography (CT) scan performed for abdominal pain after hernia repair surgery. Medical history was positive for depression. She denied hypertension, diabetes mellitus type 2, or history of malignancy. She did note new symptoms over the preceding 5 months, including night sweats (multiple times per night), weight gain of 20 pounds, fatigue, worsening depressive symptoms, and episodes characterized by anxiety and hyperventilation. On physical examination, her blood pressure was 127/85 mmHg, body mass index 31 kg/m^2, and heart rate 82 beats per minute. She demonstrated mild supraclavicular pads and abdominal obesity but no striae, skin thinning, or proximal myopathy.

INVESTIGATIONS

Review of an outside CT of the abdomen revealed a heterogeneous 3.4 × 2.3–cm left adrenal mass with two components, one measuring –8 Hounsfield units and the other measuring 22 Hounsfield units on unenhanced CT (Fig. 75.1). No prior imaging was available for comparison. Hormonal workup included evaluation for catecholamine excess and autonomous cortisol secretion (Table 75.1). Workup for catecholamine excess was negative, with normal 24-hour urine metanephrine and normetanephrine levels. However, the overnight 1-mg dexamethasone suppression test was abnormal. In addition, low serum concentrations of corticotropin (ACTH) and dehydroepiandrosterone sulfate further corroborated the diagnosis of autonomous cortisol secretion. Adrenalectomy was recommended.

TREATMENT

The patient was treated with laparoscopic adrenalectomy and initiated on glucocorticoid replacement therapy. Macroscopically, two components were demonstrated: a 2.5-cm red-brown, soft mass located in the medulla and a 4.4-cm yellow, firm mass located in the cortex (Fig. 75.2). Further histopathologic analysis confirmed a 2.5-cm pheochromocytoma and a synchronous 4.4-cm adrenocortical adenoma. Given the diagnosis of pheochromocytoma, genetic evaluation was recommended (deferred by the patient). The patient recovered from adrenal insufficiency 14 months later.

Discussion

Composite adrenal tumors have been reported in 4% of patients undergoing adrenalectomy for pheochromocytoma.[1] In our case, pheochromocytoma was initially suspected based on symptoms of spells reported by the patient and imaging consistent with a pheochromocytoma. As workup for catecholamine excess was negative, pheochromocytoma was dismissed from the differential diagnosis. Diagnosis of ACTH-independent mild Cushing syndrome was made, thought to be the result of a large lipid-poor adenoma. Biochemically "silent" pheochromocytomas represent 4% of patients

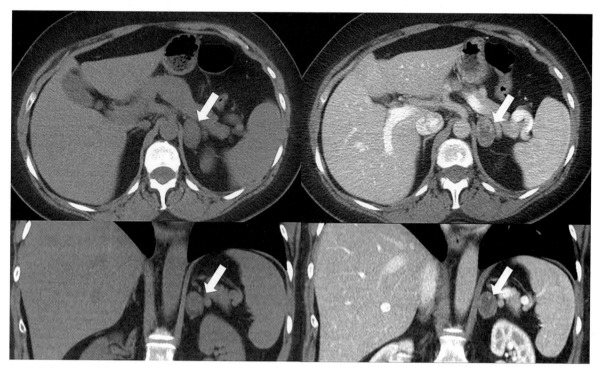

Fig. 75.1 Axial *(top)* and coronal *(bottom)* images from a baseline unenhanced *(left)* and enhanced *(right)* computed tomography (CT) scan showed a 3.4 × 2.3 cm left adrenal mass. The mass is heterogeneous, with two components on unenhanced CT, one with an attenuation of 22 Hounsfield units (HU), and another measuring −8 HU.

TABLE 75.1	Laboratory Tests	
Biochemical Test	**Result**	**Reference Range**
Cortisol after overnight 1-mg DST, mcg/dL	5.9	<1.8
Cortisol, mcg/dL	10	7–21
ACTH, pg/mL	<5	7.2–63
DHEA-S, mcg/dL	27	18–244
Aldosterone, ng/dL	Not performed	<21
Plasma renin activity, ng/mL per hour	Not performed	2.9–10.8
24-Hour urine metanephrines, mcg/24 h	71	<400
24-Hour urine normetanephrines, mcg/24 h	200	<900

ACTH, Corticotropin; *DHEA-S,* dehydroepiandrosterone sulfate; *DST,* dexamethasone suppression test.

undergoing adrenalectomy for pheochromocytoma.[2] Interestingly, a third of patients with biochemically "silent" pheochromocytomas did report symptoms suggestive of catecholamine excess.[2] It is unclear whether symptoms in our patient were related to pheochromocytoma. Germline mutation testing should be discussed with all patients with pheochromocytoma.

Key Points

- Biochemically silent pheochromocytomas occur in approximately 4% of surgically removed pheochromocytomas.
- Composite adrenal tumors (such as adenomas and pheochromocytomas) may occur in a minority of patients.
- Workup should follow the guidelines and determine (1) the risk of malignancy and (2) the presence of adrenal hormone excess. Therapy should be guided by the results of the workup.
- Germline mutation testing should be discussed with all patients with pheochromocytoma.

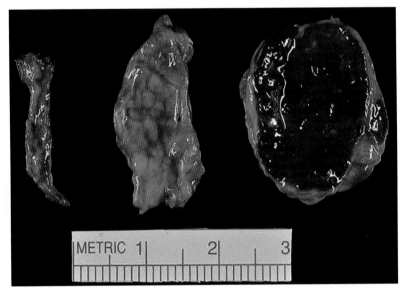

Fig. 75.2 Macroscopic pathology from the left adrenalectomy demonstrates a pheochromocytoma *(right)*, adenoma *(middle)*, and normal adrenal tissue *(left)*.

REFERENCES

1. Hasassri ME, Pandian TK, Bobr AA, et al. Pheochromocytoma with synchronous ipsilateral adrenal cortical adenoma. *World J Surg.* 2017;41(12):3147–3153.

2. Gruber LM, Hartman RP, Thompson GB, et al. Pheochromocytoma characteristics and behavior differ depending on method of discovery. *J Clin Endocrinol Metab.* 2019;104(5):1386–1393.

Primary Adrenal Leiomyosarcoma

Lipid-poor adrenal masses raise concerns about the underlying pathology. Herein we present a case of a patient with a lipid-poor adrenal mass that proved to be a rare adrenal leiomyosarcoma.

Case Report

The patient was a 72-year-old man who was incidentally discovered to have a 2-cm left adrenal mass on an abdominal computed tomography (CT) scan that was obtained to evaluate abdominal pain (Fig. 76.1). His physician advised follow-up CT scan 6 months later. However, the follow-up abdominal CT scan was not performed until 1.5 years later, when the left adrenal mass measured 5.1 × 3.2 × 5.1 cm with an unenhanced CT attenuation of 32.3 Hounsfield units (HU) (see Fig. 76.1). He had no paroxysmal symptoms. He did have a 30-year history of hypertension, which was controlled with a four-drug program. Type 2 diabetes mellitus had been diagnosed 6 years previously. His weight had been stable. He had no signs or symptoms of Cushing syndrome. There was no history of hypokalemia. His medications included amlodipine, 10 mg daily; lisinopril, 20 mg daily; metoprolol, 50 mg daily; hydrochlorothiazide, 12.5 mg daily; and metformin, 850 mg twice daily. On physical examination his body mass index was 41.8 kg/m^2, blood pressure 125/72 mmHg, and heart rate 69 beats per minute. He had no stigmata of an adrenal disorder. Heart and lung examinations were normal.

INVESTIGATIONS

The laboratory studies were normal (Table 76.1). There was no biochemical evidence of functioning pheochromocytoma, cortisol secretory autonomy, or primary aldosteronism. A F-18 fluorodeoxyglucose (FDG) positron emission tomography scan showed a FDG-avid left adrenal mass and no other areas of abnormal uptake (Fig. 76.2).

TREATMENT

The patient underwent an open left adrenalectomy. The tumor proved to be a dedifferentiated leiomyosarcoma forming a 7.6 × 3.6 × 3.1–cm adrenal mass (Fig. 76.3).

OUTCOME AND FOLLOW-UP

The patient was followed with serial imaging. Two years postoperatively, metastatic disease was detected in the liver and pulmonary hilar lymph nodes, both of which were treated with radiation therapy and systemic therapy was initiated.

Discussion

First described in 1981, primary adrenal leiomyosarcoma is a rare nonfunctioning neoplasm that derives from the smooth muscle wall of the adrenal vein or its branches.[1] With fewer than 50 patients described in the world literature, a large series is considered 2–3 cases.[2,3] In a review of 40 cases reported in the English-language literature, the age at diagnosis ranged from 14 to 78 years (80% of patients were diagnosed at older than 40 years of age).[2] At the time of surgery more than 80% of primary adrenal leiomyosarcomas were ≥4 cm in the largest lesional diameter, most being discovered incidentally on imaging done for other reasons.[2] On CT scan, these tumors are lipid poor, irregularly shaped, and inhomogeneous. The diagnosis of adrenal leiomyosarcoma is based on histopathologic and immunohistochemical findings, as demonstrated in the case presented herein. The prognosis is poor because of the

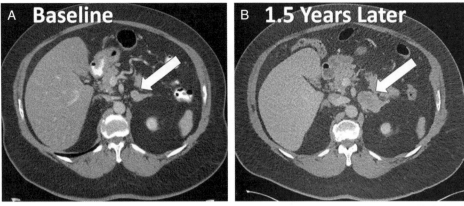

Fig. 76.1 Axial images from enhanced abdominal computed tomography (CT) scans at baseline (A) and 1.5 years later (B). At baseline, the left adrenal mass measured 2.0 cm × 1.3 cm × g 1.9 cm *(arrow)*, and unenhanced images were not obtained. On the follow-up scan the left adrenal mass measured 5.1 cm × 3.2 cm × 5.1 cm, and the unenhanced CT attenuation was 32.3 Hounsfield units.

TABLE 76.1 Laboratory Tests		
Biochemical Test	**Result**	**Reference Range**
Sodium, mmol/L	138	135–145
Potassium, mmol/L	4.4	3.6–5.2
Fasting plasma glucose, mg/dL	115	70–100
Creatinine, mg/dL	0.9	0.8–1.3
Aldosterone, ng/dL	8.1	≤21 ng/dL
Plasma renin activity ng/mL per hour	6.8	≤0.6–3
DHEA-S, mcg/dL	199	25–131
1-mg overnight DST, cortisol mcg/dL	<1.0	<1.8
Plasma metanephrine, nmol/L	<0.2	<0.5
Plasma normetanephrine, nmol/L	0.56	<0.9

DHEA-S, Dehydroepiandrosterone sulfate; *DST,* dexamethasone suppression test.

high risk of metastatic disease at the time of discovery or on follow-up.[2] The longest reported metastasis-free survival after adrenalectomy was 3 years,[3] whereas the longest reported survival in a patient with known metastatic disease was 4.4 years.[4] Metastatic disease is typically found in liver, lymph nodes, lung, and bone.[2] Early detection and an oncologic operation offer the best chance of prolonging life.

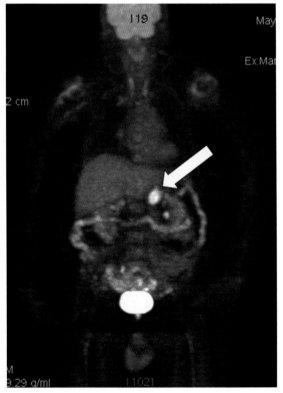

Fig. 76.2 F-18 fluorodeoxyglucose (FDG) positron emission tomography scan showed an FDG-avid (11.6 standard unit value) left adrenal mass and no other areas of abnormal uptake.

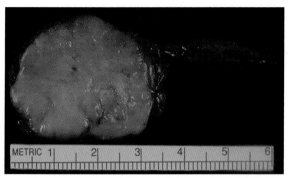

Fig. 76.3 Gross pathology photograph of bisected white-to-pale colored left adrenal mass. The tumor proved to be a dedifferentiated leiomyosarcoma forming a 7.6 × 3.6 × 3.1–cm adrenal mass. All margins were negative for sarcoma. Immunoperoxidase stains were positive for smooth muscle actin and lacked staining for desmin, inhibin, MiTF-1, and HMB45.

Key Points

- Primary adrenal leiomyosarcoma is a high-grade proliferating mesenchymal tumor that is exceedingly rare and not included in the encyclopedic 2017 WHO Classification of Tumours of Endocrine Organs.[5]
- On CT imaging, these tumors are lipid poor, irregularly shaped, and inhomogeneous.

- The diagnosis of primary adrenal leiomyosarcoma is based on histopathologic and immunohistochemical findings.
- The prognosis for patients with primary adrenal leiomyosarcoma is poor because of the high risk of metastatic disease at the time of discovery or on follow-up.
- Early detection and an oncologic operation offer the best chance of prolonging life in a patient with primary adrenal leiomyosarcoma, supporting the concept of aggressive management of lipid-poor adrenal masses.

REFERENCES

1. Choi SH, Liu K. Leiomyosarcoma of the adrenal gland and its angiographic features: a case report. *J Surg Oncol.* 1981;16(2):145–148.
2. Jabarkhel F, Puttonen H, Hansson L, Muth A, Ragnarsson O. Primary adrenal leiomyosarcoma: clinical, radiological, and histopathological characteristics. *J Endocr Soc.* 2020;4(6): bvaa055.
3. Quildrian S, Califano I, Carrizo F, Daffinoti A, Calónico N. Primary adrenal leiomyosarcoma treated by laparoscopic adrenalectomy. *Endocrinol Nutr.* 2015;62(9):472–473.
4. Tomasich FD, Luz Mde A, Kato M, et al. [Primary adrenal leiomyosarcoma]. *Arq Bras Endocrinol Metabol.* 2008;52(9):1510–1514.
5. Lloyd RV, Osamura RY, Kloppel G, Rosai J. *WHO Classification of Tumours of Endocrine Organs* 4th ed. IARC, Lyon, 2017.

Primary Adrenal Lymphoma

Primary adrenal lymphoma is rare and typically presents in older men with progressive signs and symptoms of adrenal insufficiency, weight loss, and abdominal pain.[1,2] Computed cross-sectional imaging usually reveals large (up to 18 cm in diameter) lipid-poor adrenoform bilateral adrenal masses. On magnetic resonance imaging (MRI), the lesions are hypointense in T1-weighted images and hyperintense in T2-weighted images. F-18 fluorodeoxyglucose (FDG) positron emission tomography (PET)-computed tomography (CT) typically shows high FDG avidity and it may reveal extraadrenal locations of disease. Adrenalectomy is not indicated. Chemotherapy is the treatment of choice. Herein we present a case of a patient with primary adrenal lymphoma.

Case Report

The patient was a 57-year-old man who had been previously healthy and running 3 miles per day. He took no regular medications. He had traveled to Europe 3 weeks previously and for 48 hours he had fairly intense abdominal pain. As the abdominal pain resolved, it became more of a pleuritic posterior back and chest discomfort that persisted—leading to a chest CT scan that detected bilateral adrenal masses. The subsequent abdominal CT showed bilateral oblong adrenoform 11-cm adrenal masses (Fig. 77.1). The CT appearance was that of an infiltrating process such as lymphoma or infection. His pleuritic chest pain was 3 out of 10 in severity during the day and 10 out of 10 in severity at night. He had lost 5 pounds because of poor appetite that was associated with the pain. He had no fevers. He had limited laboratory studies before referral and they included: morning serum cortisol concentration of 12.4 mcg/dL (normal, 7–25 mcg/dL), morning serum corticotropin (ACTH) concentration of 92 pg/mL (normal, 10–60 pg/mL), and 1-mg overnight dexamethasone suppression test with a next day cortisol concentration of 1.34 mcg/dL (normal, <1.8 mcg/dL).

INVESTIGATIONS

The laboratory studies are listed in Table 77.1. All adrenal gland–related testing was normal except for a mild elevation in serum ACTH concentration. Hypercalcemia was associated with low blood concentration of parathyroid hormone and elevated 1,25-dihydroxyvitamin D. The imaging findings and hypercalcemia were consistent with lymphoma. CT-guided right adrenal mass biopsy was performed and showed findings consistent with diffuse large B-cell lymphoma. The FDG-PET-CT scan showed the large bilateral adrenal masses to have very intense FDG uptake compatible with malignancy (Fig. 77.2). No other sites of involvement were identified by FDG-PET-CT, including the spleen and lymph nodes.

TREATMENT

Because of the massive adrenal gland involvement, mild elevation in serum ACTH concentration, and recognizing the dynamic nature of the adrenal lymphoma impact on adrenocortical function, we initiated safety net dosages of hydrocortisone (10 mg twice daily) and fludrocortisone (0.05 mg daily). He was also advised to initiate a low-calcium diet to treat the hypercalcemia. The patient was seen in consultation by a hematologist on the sixth day of his Mayo Clinic evaluation. The hematologist commented that the elevated serum lactate dehydrogenase concentration and low serum 25-hydroxyvitamin D level were adverse prognostic factors. However, favorable prognostic factors were normal serum immunoglobulin free light chains and

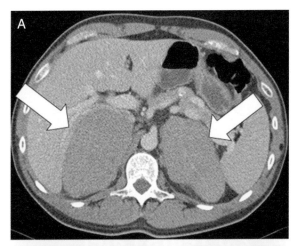

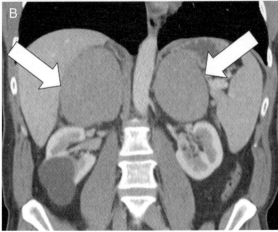

Fig. 77.1 Axial (A), coronal (B), images from contrast-enhanced abdominal computed tomography (CT) scan showed bilateral adrenoform and homogeneous adrenal masses *(arrows)*. The right adrenal mass measured 11 × 9 × 6.5 cm and had an unenhanced CT attenuation of 42 Hounsfield units (HU). The left adrenal mass was very similar, although slightly smaller, and the unenhanced CT attenuation was 42.5 HU. The CT appearance was that of an infiltrating process such as lymphoma or infection.

TABLE 77.1   Laboratory Tests

Biochemical Test	Result	Reference Range
Sodium, mmol/L	140	135–145
Potassium, mmol/L	4.2	3.6–5.2
Creatinine, mg/dL	1.3	0.8–1.3
Calcium, mg/dL	11.3	8.9–10.1
Phosphorus, mg/dL	3.2	2.5–4.5
1,25-Dihydroxy-vitamin D, pg/mL	84	18–64
25-Hydroxy-vitamin D, ng/mL	18	20–50
Parathyroid hormone, pg/mL	12	15–65
8 AM serum cortisol, mcg/dL	12	7–25
8 AM serum ACTH, pg/mL	10.0	10–60
Aldosterone, ng/dL	<4	≤21
Plasma renin activity, ng/mL per hour	1.2	≤0.6–3
Metanephrine, nmol/L	<0.2	<0.5
Normetanephrine, nmol/L	0.35	<0.9
Lactate dehydrogenase, U/L	668	122–222
24-Hour urine:		
Calcium, mg	385	25–300
Cortisol, mcg	8.9	3.5–45

ACTH, Corticotropin.

no evidence of bone marrow involvement on bone marrow biopsy. The head MRI scan showed no central nervous system involvement. The treatment plan was for R-CHOP (rituximab, cyclophosphamide, doxorubicin, and vincristine) for two cycles and then an FDG-PET-CT scan before cycle 3. If the FDG-PET-CT scan showed efficacy of treatment, then the plan was to proceed with cycles 3–6 of R-CHOP. The treatment goal was for the FDG-PET-CT to show no tumor involvement after cycle 6 of R-CHOP.

OUTCOME AND FOLLOW-UP

The FDG-PET-CT scan completed after two cycles of R-CHOP showed marked interval treatment response with resolution of the intense abnormal FDG uptake in the large bilateral adrenal masses (Fig. 77.3). The small amount of residual adrenal soft tissue that was present was non-FDG avid. He developed complete alopecia and had decreased exercise tolerance, although still managing to run-walk about 2.5 miles every day. The pleuritic back pain resolved. On the

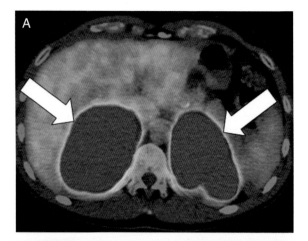

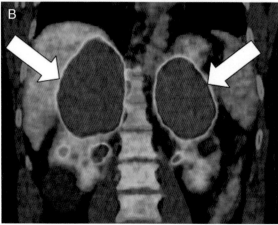

Fig. 77.2 Axial (A) and coronal (B) images from an F-18 fluorodeoxyglucose (FDG) positron emission tomography-(PET)-computed tomography (CT) scan demonstrated that the large bilateral adrenal masses shown in Fig. 77.1 were intensely FDG avid *(arrows)*, a finding compatible with malignancy. No other sites of involvement were identified by FDG-PET-CT, including the spleen and lymph nodes.

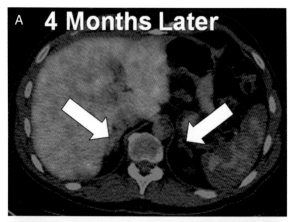

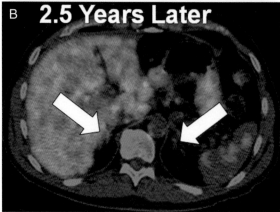

Fig. 77.3 (A) Axial image from an F-18 fluorodeoxyglucose (FDG) positron emission tomography-(PET)-computed tomography (CT) scan completed after two cycles of rituximab, cyclophosphamide, doxorubicin, and vincristine (and 4 months post-diagnosis) showed marked interval treatment response with resolution of the intense abnormal FDG uptake in the large bilateral adrenal masses. The small amount of residual adrenal soft tissue *(arrows)* that was present was non-FDG avid. (B) Axial image from FDG-PET-CT scan completed 2.5 years after his diagnosis showed no evidence of recurrent lymphoma.

low-calcium diet his serum calcium concentration was normal at 9.4 mg/dL.

He went on to complete six cycles of R-CHOP. We reassessed adrenal gland function after cycle 6 of R-CHOP. At 24 hours after his last dose of hydrocortisone, his serum cortisol concentration was normal (12 mcg/dL) and serum ACTH concentration was normal (27 pg/mL). We omitted his afternoon dose of hydrocortisone for 2 weeks and then discontinued it altogether. Serum electrolytes remained normal and the fludrocortisone was also

discontinued. The FDG-PET-CT scan 2.5 years later showed no abnormal uptake (see Fig. 77.3).

Key Points

- Primary adrenal lymphoma is rare and typically presents in older men with progressive signs and symptoms of adrenal insufficiency, weight loss, and abdominal pain.[1,2]
- Primary adrenal lymphoma is easily detected on CT or MRI as bilateral large lipid-poor adrenoform adrenal masses.

- FDG-PET-CT typically shows high FDG avidity and may reveal extraadrenal locations of primary adrenal lymphoma.
- Chemotherapy with R-CHOP is the treatment of choice for primary adrenal lymphoma.

REFERENCES

1. Rashidi A, Fisher SI. Primary adrenal lymphoma: a systematic review. *Ann Hematol*. 2013;92(12):1583–1593.

2. Laurent C, Casasnovas O, Martin L, et al. Adrenal lymphoma: presentation, management and prognosis. *QJM*. 2017;110(2):103–109.

39-Year-Old Man With a Large Adrenal Mass

Neuroblastomas are heterogeneous neuroblastic tumors that occur almost exclusively in childhood. Most neuroblastomas occur in the abdomen, usually in the adrenal gland. Catecholamine secretion may occur in approximately 70% of cases. Patient age at diagnosis, stage of disease, and cytogenetics have prognostic implications

Case Report

The patient was a 39-year-old man who initially presented with abdominal discomfort and symptoms of radiculopathy. In addition, he reported occasional spells with anxiety and episodic elevated blood pressure. Initially, he was treated with physical therapy to improve his symptoms of radiculopathy. However, because of incomplete improvement, spine imaging was recommended. Unexpectedly, magnetic resonance imaging (MRI) of the spine demonstrated metastatic bone disease, and further imaging revealed a large adrenal mass (Fig. 78.1).

INVESTIGATIONS

Workup for catecholamine excess was pursued and demonstrated elevated urinary normetanephrine and dopamine (Table 78.1). A preliminary diagnosis of pheochromocytoma with bone metastases was considered, and open left adrenalectomy was recommended. Appropriate preparation with α- and β-adrenergic blockade was initiated before adrenalectomy. During surgery, in addition to the left adrenal mass, multiple lymph nodes were removed. Surprisingly, pathologic diagnosis was neuroblastoma with lymph node metastases.

Discussion

Neuroblastomas arise from anywhere in the sympathetic nervous system, with the adrenal gland most commonly affected (~40%).[1,2] Neuroblastomas occur almost exclusively in children; thus the diagnosis at the age of our patient is unusual.[3] Neuroblastoma frequently metastasizes to lymph nodes, bone, and liver. Catecholamine secretion can occur in more than half

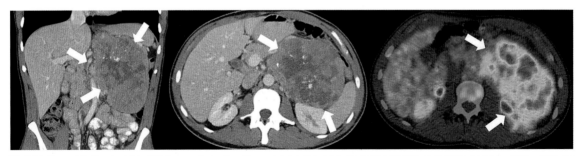

Fig. 78.1 Coronal *(left)* and axial *(middle)* images from a baseline contrast-enhanced computed tomography scan showed a 12.0 × 13.2 × 18.0–cm left adrenal mass with patchy calcifications. The mass was heterogeneously F-18 fluorodeoxyglucose avid, with maximum standard unit value ranging between 5.7 and 13.9 *(right)*. The mass compressed the left kidney.

TABLE 78.1   Laboratory Tests

Biochemical Test	Result	Reference Range
Cortisol after overnight 1-mg DST, mcg/dL	Not performed	<1.8
Cortisol, mcg/dL	12	7–21
ACTH, pg/mL	Not performed	7.2–63
DHEA-S, mcg/dL	172	65–344
Aldosterone, ng/dL	13	<21
Plasma renin activity, ng/mL per hour	Not performed	2.9–10.8
24-Hour urine metanephrine, mcg/24 h	126	<400
24-Hour urine normetanephrine, mcg/24 h	1582	<900
24-Hour urine epinephrine, mcg/24 h	3	<21
24-Hour urine norepinephrine, mcg/24 h	72	15–80
24-Hour urine dopamine, mcg/24 h	1016	65–400

ACTH, Corticotropin; DHEA-S, dehydroepiandrosterone sulfate; DST, dexamethasone suppression test.

of neuroblastomas, as neuroblastoma cells have the enzymes required for catecholamine secretion and metabolism.[4] Patients are at high risk for disease progression and mortality if diagnosed at an older age, present with metastatic disease, or with unfavorable markers such as *MYCN* amplification (duplicate copies of the *MYCN* gene).[5] In these patients, although improved survival outcomes are achieved with multimodality therapies, prolonged survival is still very low.[2]

TREATMENT

Cytogenetic evaluation was recommended, and pathogenic variants in *ALK F11741* and *ATRXQ219* were found. In addition, a *CREBBPQ 1330 frameshift*22

alteration was found. After careful discussion in the multidisciplinary team, therapy with cyclophosphamide and topotecan was initiated first. Subsequently, because of progressive disease, the patient was treated with a number of treatment modalities including multiple cytotoxics, I-131 metaiodobenzylguanidine therapy, and radiotherapy, with variable response. Eventually, the disease progressed, and the patient died 4 years after the initial diagnosis.

Key Points

- Neuroblastoma is an unusual diagnosis in adulthood and may present with catecholamine excess.
- A multidisciplinary approach involving the endocrinologist, surgeon, pathologist, and oncologist is needed to ensure the best management.
- Multimodality therapies are usually required in high-risk disease.

REFERENCES

1. Cohn SL, Pearson AD, London WB, et al. The International Neuroblastoma Risk Group (INRG) classification system: an INRG Task Force report. *J Clin Oncol.* 2009;27(2):289–297.
2. DuBois SG, Kalika Y, Lukens JN, et al. Metastatic sites in stage IV and IVS neuroblastoma correlate with age, tumor biology, and survival. *J Pediatr Hematol Oncol.* 1999;21(3):181–189.
3. Ebbehoj A, Li D, Kaur RJ, et al. Epidemiology of adrenal tumors in Olmsted County, Minnesota, USA: a population-based study. *Lancet Diabetes Endocrinol.* 2020;8(11):894–902.
4. Mahoney NR, Liu GT, Menacker SJ, Wilson MC, Hogarty MD, Maris JM. Pediatric Horner syndrome: etiologies and roles of imaging and urine studies to detect neuroblastoma and other responsible mass lesions. *Am J Ophthalmol.* 2006;142(4):651–659.
5. Bagatell R, Beck-Popovic M, London WB, et al. Significance of MYCN amplification in international neuroblastoma staging system stage 1 and 2 neuroblastoma: a report from the International Neuroblastoma Risk Group database. *J Clin Oncol.* 2009;27(3):365–370.

59-Year-Old Man With Enlarging Bilateral Adrenal Masses

Bilateral adrenal metastases should be suspected in any case of the rapidly enlarging indeterminate bilateral adrenal masses, even in the absence of a known extraadrenal malignancy. Although otherwise rarely needed in the workup of adrenal tumors, adrenal biopsy is indicated when adrenal metastasis is strongly suspected, and only after exclusion of pheochromocytoma.

Case Report

The patient was a 59-year-old man with history of well-controlled hypertension and obesity. He presented for evaluation of bilateral adrenal masses discovered incidentally on abdominal imaging performed in the emergency department for work-up of abdominal pain. He reported weight gain of 40 pounds over 2 years that he attributed to quitting smoking (50 pack-year history). He had a skin lesion removed 3 years prior that was reportedly benign. He worked as a farmer. He took lisinopril 5 mg daily for hypertension. Review of systems was positive only for chronic cough, and abdominal pain was no longer present. Physical examination was unrevealing, without features of Cushing syndrome.

INVESTIGATIONS

On review of unenhanced computed tomography (CT) from 4 months ago, large bilateral masses were noted with indeterminate imaging characteristics (Fig. 79.1). The baseline laboratory test results are shown in Table 79.1. The serum corticotropin and dehydroepiandrosterone sulfate concentrations were within normal ranges, and cortisol suppressed normally with an overnight 1-mg dexamethasone

suppression test. Workup for primary aldosteronism and catecholamine excess was negative (see Table 79.1).

A follow-up CT was obtained and demonstrated that both adrenal masses enlarged considerably (~3 cm in 4 months) (Fig. 79.2). A chest radiograph was subsequently obtained and did not reveal abnormalities. Because of high suspicion of extraadrenal malignancy (and after excluding pheochromocytoma), the decision was made to proceed with adrenal biopsy that revealed the adrenal masses to be metastatic melanoma.

Discussion

Bilateral adrenal tumors occur in approximately 15% of all patients.[1,2] Bilateral tumors are most likely to represent bilateral adenomas, bilateral adrenal metastases, or lymphoma and rarely bilateral pheochromocytomas or myelolipomas.[1,2] In patients with large adrenal tumors, bilaterality is strongly associated with adrenal metastatic disease.[1,2]

In this case, size of bilateral masses, indeterminate imaging characteristics (unenhanced CT attenuation >20 Hounsfield units [HU]), and significant enlargement over a short period of time suggested bilateral malignant adrenal masses—most likely metastases or lymphoma.[3] It was important to exclude bilateral functioning pheochromocytoma, as was done in this case. However, although the size and imaging characteristics could be consistent with pheochromocytomas, rapid growth is unusual, because the natural history of pheochromocytomas is a slow enlargement over years. Bilateral adenomas were unlikely in the current case. At least 15% of all adenomas may demonstrate unenhanced CT attenuation of >20 HU; however, a growth rate of 3 cm over a period of only

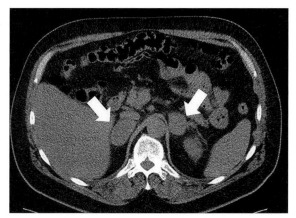

Fig. 79.1 Axial image from a baseline unenhanced computed tomography (CT) scan showed bilateral indeterminate adrenal masses *(arrows)*. The right adrenal mass measured 4.5 × 2.2 cm and had an unenhanced CT attenuation of 25 Hounsfield units (HU). The left adrenal mass measured 3.8 × 2.8 cm and had an unenhanced CT attenuation of 27 HU.

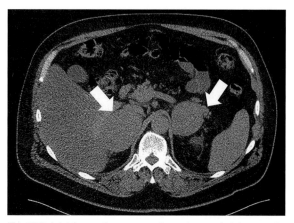

Fig. 79.2 Axial image from an unenhanced computed tomography scan performed 4 months after the baseline imaging demonstrated enlarged bilateral adrenal masses *(arrows)*. The right adrenal mass measured 7.5 × 4.3 cm (27 Hounsfield units [HU]), and the left adrenal mass measured 5.8 × 5.1 cm (28 HU).

4 months would be extremely unusual for adrenal adenomas.[1]

Adrenal metastases may be incidentally discovered (as was in this case) in up to 36%–48% of cases.[2,4] Adrenal metastases most commonly originate from cancers of the lung, genitourinary, and gastrointestinal origins, followed by melanomas and lymphomas.[4–6] At the time of diagnosis, 24% of patients with adrenal metastases present with bilateral adrenal involvement.[4] Patients initially diagnosed with unilateral adrenal metastasis are at high risk for development of contralateral adrenal metastasis during follow-up, which may have implications in monitoring for primary adrenal insufficiency.[4]

TREATMENT

Once melanoma was confirmed on adrenal biopsy, the patient was evaluated by the melanoma oncology team and treated with chemotherapy. At 16 months of follow-up, the patient had stable disease. He was clinically and biochemically monitored for adrenal insufficiency throughout his follow-up, and his adrenal function was normal.

Key Points

- Bilateral adrenal tumors are found in 15% of patients with adrenal adenomas, up to 25% of patients with adrenal metastases, and 10% of patients with pheochromocytomas.
- Large tumor size, indeterminate adrenal imaging (unenhanced CT attenuation >20 HU), and rapid tumor growth indicate that bilateral adrenal masses are likely malignant.
- Adrenal metastases are diagnosed incidentally in one-third to one-half of all cases.
- Most adrenal metastases originate from lung, genitourinary, and gastrointestinal malignancies.
- Patients with bilateral metastases should be clinically and/or biochemically monitored for adrenal insufficiency.

TABLE 79.1	Laboratory Tests	
Biochemical Test	**Result**	**Reference Range**
1-mg overnight DST	1.4	<1.8
ACTH, pg/mL	24	7.2–63
DHEA-S, mcg/dL	196	20–299
Aldosterone, ng/dL	7	<21
Plasma renin activity, ng/mL per hour	2.3	2.9–10.8
Plasma metanephrine, nmol/L	0.42	<0.5
Plasma normetanephrine, nmol/L	0.34	<0.9

ACTH, Corticotropin; *DHEA-S,* dehydroepiandrosterone sulfate; *DST,* dexamethasone suppression test.

REFERENCES

1. Ebbehoj A, Li D, Kaur RJ, et al. Epidemiology of adrenal tumors in Olmsted County, Minnesota, USA: a population-based study. *Lancet Diabetes Endocrinol.* 2020;8(11):894–902.

2. Iniguez-Ariza NM, Kohlenberg JD, Delivanis DA, et al. Clinical, biochemical, and radiological characteristics of a single-center retrospective cohort of 705 large adrenal tumors. *Mayo Clin Proc Innov Qual Outcomes.* 2018;2(1):30–39.

3. Dinnes J, Bancos I, Ferrante di Ruffano L, et al. Management of endocrine disease: imaging for the diagnosis of malignancy in incidentally discovered adrenal masses: a systematic review and meta-analysis. *Eur J Endocrinol.* 2016;175(2):R51–R64.

4. Mao JJ, Dages KN, Suresh M, Bancos I. Presentation, disease progression and outcomes of adrenal gland metastases. *Clin Endocrinol (Oxf).* 2020;93(5):546–554.

5. Bancos I, Tamhane S, Shah M, et al. Diagnosis of endocrine disease: the diagnostic performance of adrenal biopsy: a systematic review and meta-analysis. *Eur J Endocrinol.* 2016;175(2):R65–R80.

6. Delivanis DA, Bancos I, Atwell TD, et al. Diagnostic performance of unenhanced computed tomography and (18) F-fluorodeoxyglucose positron emission tomography in indeterminate adrenal tumours. *Clin Endocrinol (Oxf).* 2018;88(1):30–36.

65-Year-Old Man With Primary Adrenal Insufficiency

Primary adrenal insufficiency is most commonly due to autoimmune adrenalitis.[1] Much less frequently, primary adrenal insufficiency may occur due to destruction of the adrenal cortex as a result of infection (e.g., tuberculosis, fungal infection), systemic disorders (e.g., sarcoidosis, histiocytosis), or cancer (e.g., adrenal metastases, lymphoma).[1,2] An infiltrative process should be suspected in patients with primary adrenal insufficiency who have abnormal adrenal imaging.

Case Report

The patient was a 65-year-old man who was referred to our adrenal clinic for newly diagnosed primary adrenal insufficiency. He provided a history of fatigue, muscle aches, decreased appetite, mild nausea, and weight loss of around 5–6 pounds over several months. He was hospitalized locally when his blood pressure was found to be low and his electrolytes were abnormal with a serum sodium concentration of 124 mEq/L and serum potassium concentrations that were above normal limits (i.e., >5.2 mEq/L). At that time, primary adrenal insufficiency was suspected, and workup in the hospital revealed a morning serum cortisol concentration of 2.5 mcg/dL (normal, 7–25 mcg/dL) and a serum corticotropin concentration of 316 pg/mL (normal, 10–60 pg/mL). The patient was initiated on hydrocortisone and fludrocortisone replacement and had noticed a remarkable improvement in his initial symptoms. At the time of evaluation in our clinic, his medications included hydrocortisone, fludrocortisone, and amlodipine. Review of systems was positive for occasional night sweats, which had improved since hydrocortisone initiation. On physical examination, his vital signs were normal and

the only positive finding was vitiligo. He reported no family history of autoimmune disorders.

INVESTIGATIONS

The laboratory tests obtained on presentation to the adrenal clinic confirmed primary adrenal insufficiency (Table 80.1). Autoimmune primary adrenal insufficiency was suspected, and measurement of 21-hydroxylase antibodies was performed to confirm this diagnosis. However, when the 21-hydroxylase antibodies were found undetectable, abdominal imaging was obtained to look for other etiologies of primary adrenal insufficiency. On review of unenhanced and contrast-enhanced computed tomography (CT), bilateral masses were noted with indeterminate imaging characteristics (Figs. 80.1–80.3). The 1.9-cm left adrenal mass had a CT attenuation of 29 Hounsfield units (HU) on unenhanced CT and was slightly heterogeneous on enhanced CT. The 5.1-cm right adrenal mass had a CT attenuation of 26 HU on unenhanced CT and heterogeneity on enhanced CT. Both adrenal masses demonstrated irregular borders. Additional workup performed for catecholamine excess was negative (plasma metanephrine, <0.2 nmol/L [normal,

TABLE 80.1 Laboratory Tests		
Biochemical Test	Result	Reference Range
Cortisol, mcg/dL	<1	7–25
ACTH, pg/mL	550	7.2–63
DHEA-S, mcg/dL	29	25–131
Plasma renin activity, ng/mL per hour (while patient is treated with fludrocortisone)	0.6	2.9–10.8
21-Hydroxylase antibodies, U/mL	<1	<1

ACTH, Corticotropin; *DHEA-S,* dehydroepiandrosterone sulfate.

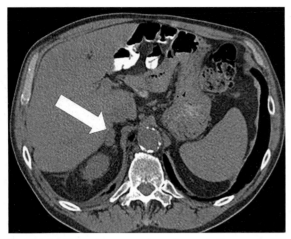

Fig. 80.1 Axial image from an unenhanced computed tomography (CT) scan demonstrated a 1.9 × 1.1–cm right adrenal mass *(arrow)* with an unenhanced CT attenuation of 29 Hounsfield units. The left adrenal mass is not visible on this image.

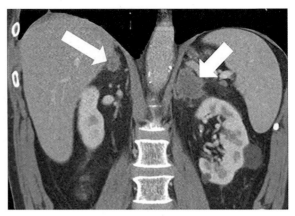

Fig. 80.3 Coronal image from an enhanced computed tomography scan demonstrated bilateral adrenal masses *(arrows)* (1.9 × 1.1–cm right adrenal mass and 5.1 × 4.3–cm left adrenal mass). Both adrenal masses were heterogeneous and demonstrate irregular borders.

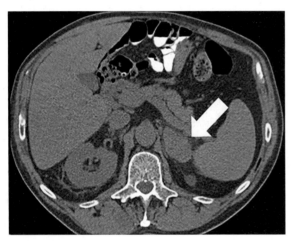

Fig. 80.2 Axial image from an unenhanced computed tomography (CT) scan demonstrated a left 5.1 × 4.3–cm adrenal mass *(arrow)* with an unenhanced CT attenuation of 26 Hounsfield units. The right adrenal mass is not visible on this image.

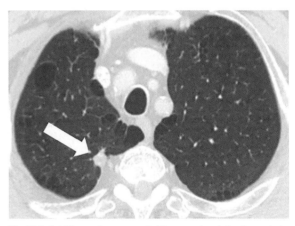

Fig. 80.4 Axial image from computed tomography of chest revealed a 9-mm nodule *(arrow)* in the right apex posteriorly.

<0.5 nmol/L]; plasma normetanephrine, 0.65 nmol/L [normal, <0.9 nmol/L]). As the patient did not have a known extraadrenal malignancy, it was decided to proceed with the adrenal biopsy of the larger adrenal mass. Cytology confirmed malignancy, with a diagnosis of a poorly differentiated non–small cell carcinoma with focal squamous and glandular formation. Immunohistochemical studies showed neoplastic cells were positive for TTF1, CK7, and CK903 and negative for CK20, inhibin, Melan A, and CDX2. The immunohistochemical profile was consistent with a lung primary malignancy. A chest CT scan was obtained and revealed a 9-mm nodule in the right apex posteriorly (Fig. 80.4).

Discussion

Primary adrenal insufficiency as a result of the destruction of adrenal cortex by adrenal metastases was recently reported to occur in 12.4% of all patients with bilateral adrenal metastases and in 20% of patients with large bilateral adrenal metastases (tumor size >4 cm).[3] Primary adrenal insufficiency in the setting of metastatic disease to the adrenal glands is most common in patients with lymphoma, non–small cell lung carcinoma, or renal cell carcinoma.[2,3] However, adrenal insufficiency is likely underrecognized because many patients are tested for adrenal insufficiency only after presenting with clear signs or symptoms. Moreover, a minority of patients with adrenal metastases are evaluated by endocrinologists.[3] As bilateral adrenal metastases occur in 25% of patients at the time of initial diagnosis and almost half of patients during follow-up,[3] case detection strategies for primary adrenal insufficiency should be considered in all patients with bilateral adrenal metastases.

TREATMENT

Once metastatic lung non–small cell carcinoma was diagnosed, patients initiate chemotherapy. Unfortunately, his disease progressed and he passed away 18 months later.

Key Points

- Primary adrenal insufficiency resulting from the destruction of adrenal cortex by adrenal metastases occurs in 12% of patients with bilateral metastases.
- Primary adrenal insufficiency occurs in 20% of patients with bilateral metastases >4 cm.
- Patients with bilateral metastases should be clinically and/or biochemically monitored for adrenal insufficiency.

REFERENCES

1. Bancos I, Hahner S, Tomlinson J, Arlt W. Diagnosis and management of adrenal insufficiency. *Lancet Diabetes Endocrinol.* 2015;3(3):216–226.
2. Herndon J, Nadeau AM, Davidge-Pitts CJ, Young WF, Bancos I. Primary adrenal insufficiency due to bilateral infiltrative disease. *Endocrine.* 2018;62(3):721–728.
3. Mao JJ, Dages KN, Suresh M, Bancos I. Presentation, disease progression and outcomes of adrenal gland metastases. *Clin Endocrinol (Oxf).* 2020;93(5):546–554.

47-Year-Old Man With Primary Adrenal Insufficiency

An infiltrative adrenal process due to a systemic disorder, such as sarcoidosis or histiocytosis, is very rare. Primary adrenal insufficiency occurs when the majority of the adrenal cortex is destroyed, resulting in glucocorticoid deficiency, and, frequently, mineralocorticoid deficiency. Patients may present with either symptoms of the underlying systemic disorder or symptoms of adrenal insufficiency. Therapy is targeted toward treatment of adrenal insufficiency with glucocorticoid and mineralocorticoid therapy and treatment of the underlying systemic disorder.

Case Report

The patient was a 47-year-old man who initially presented with fatigue, weakness, lightheadedness, and abdominal pain. A computed tomography (CT) scan of the abdomen revealed infiltration of perinephric space and adrenal glands (Fig. 81.1). Because of ongoing symptoms, as well as imaging findings, the patient was referred to our institution for evaluation of the etiology of noted infiltrative process. On evaluation in our clinic, the patient continued to be troubled by fatigue and weakness, but also had night sweats and persistent abdominal pain. His physical examination was unrevealing. His comorbidities included diabetes mellitus type 2 treated with metformin and hypertension treated with lisinopril.

INVESTIGATIONS

Workup for adrenal insufficiency was performed and confirmed primary adrenal insufficiency (Table 81.1). A CT-guided biopsy of the right kidney, right adrenal gland, and right retroperitoneum was performed, and histopathology

revealed fibromyxoid proliferation and chronic inflammatory infiltrate. A subsequent nuclear medicine bone scan revealed increased uptake in the lower extremities compatible with the diagnosis of Erdheim-Chester disease (non–Langerhans cell histiocytosis).

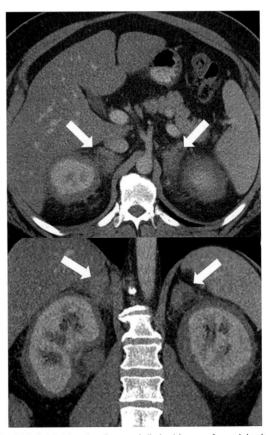

Fig. 81.1 Axial *(above)* and coronal *(below)* images from abdominal computed tomography scan demonstrated an infiltrative process surrounding the kidneys and adrenal glands *(arrows* indicate adrenal infiltration).

TABLE 81.1 Laboratory Tests		
Biochemical Test	Result	Reference Range
Cortisol, mcg/dL	6	7–25
ACTH, pg/mL	70	7.2–63
Plasma renin activity, ng/mL per hour	6	2.9–10.8

ACTH, Corticotropin; *DHEA-S,* dehydroepiandrosterone sulfate.

Discussion

Erdheim-Chester disease is a rare non–Langerhans cell histiocytosis characterized by infiltration of histiocytes in multiple organs. In a study of 64 patients, endocrine manifestations included diabetes insipidus in 33%, anterior pituitary dysfunction in 91%, and primary hypogonadism in 53%.[1] Although adrenal infiltration was demonstrated in 39% of the patients on CT, only one case of primary adrenal insufficiency was observed.[1] Adrenal histiocytosis, along with other infiltrative processes, such as sarcoidosis, tuberculosis, histoplasmosis, cryptococcus infection, and adrenal metastases, should be suspected in any patient with primary adrenal insufficiency and bilateral adrenal masses.[2] The diagnosis of Erdheim-Chester disease involving the adrenal glands is usually made through adrenal biopsy.[3] Treatment of the underlying disorder depends on the etiology. Treatment of primary adrenal insufficiency is similar, with glucocorticoid and mineralocorticoid replacement therapy.[4] Recovery from primary adrenal insufficiency is poorly investigated but is unlikely due to the irreversibility of the adrenal cortex destruction. Patients should be counseled on sick day rules and use of injectable glucocorticoid.[4]

TREATMENT

Hydrocortisone therapy was initiated, leading to improvement of fatigue and weakness. His electrolytes were normal, and he was not orthostatic; thus fludrocortisone was not initiated. The patient was treated with cyclophosphamide and his disease was stable during the 9 months of available follow-up.

Key Points

- Erdheim-Chester disease is a rare non–Langerhans cell histiocytosis characterized by infiltration of histiocytes in multiple organs, including the adrenal and pituitary glands.
- As pituitary infiltration in Erdheim-Chester is frequent, both secondary and primary adrenal insufficiency may occur in patients with this form of histiocytosis. Appropriate case detection strategies should be in place.

REFERENCES

1. Courtillot C, Laugier Robiolle S, Cohen Aubart F, et al. Endocrine manifestations in a monocentric cohort of 64 patients with Erdheim-Chester disease. *J Clin Endocrinol Metab.* 2016;101(1):305–313.
2. Herndon J, Nadeau AM, Davidge-Pitts CJ, Young WF, Bancos I. Primary adrenal insufficiency due to bilateral infiltrative disease. *Endocrine.* 2018;62(3):721–728.
3. Bancos I, Tamhane S, Shah M, et al. Diagnosis of endocrine disease: the diagnostic performance of adrenal biopsy: a systematic review and meta-analysis. *Eur J Endocrinol.* 2016;175(2):R65–R80.
4. Bancos I, Hahner S, Tomlinson J, Arlt W. Diagnosis and management of adrenal insufficiency. *Lancet Diabetes Endocrinol.* 2015;3(3):216–226.

Bilateral Adrenal Myelolipoma: Think of Congenital Adrenal Hyperplasia

Adrenal myelolipomas are benign, hormonally inactive neoplasms composed of myeloid elements and mature adipose tissue in varying proportions. Unilateral adrenal myelolipomas are uncommon (see Case 65), and bilateral adrenal myelolipomas are even more uncommon and usually associated with chronic corticotropin (ACTH) hypersecretion. The most common clinical setting of bilateral adrenal myelolipomas is untreated or poorly treated congenital adrenal hyperplasia (CAH).[1] Herein we share such a case and additional examples of the findings on computed tomography (CT).

Case Report

The patient was a 26-year-old man referred for evaluation of incidentally discovered bilateral adrenal masses. The patient had an episode of acute gastroenteritis that led to the CT scan (Fig. 82.1). The contrast-enhanced abdominal CT scan showed multiple large bilateral adrenal macroscopic fat-containing masses and marked cortical hyperplasia, imaging findings that were diagnostic of untreated CAH. The patient recalled being treated with hydrocortisone when a young child. However, this treatment was stopped at 14 years of age. On physical examination his body mass index was 27.8 kg/m^2 and his blood pressure and heart rate were normal. The patient appeared well and was not hyperpigmented.

INVESTIGATIONS

The laboratory studies were consistent with CAH with 61-fold and 15-fold elevations above the upper limits of the reference ranges for 17-hydroxyprogesterone and androstenedione, respectively (Table 82.1).

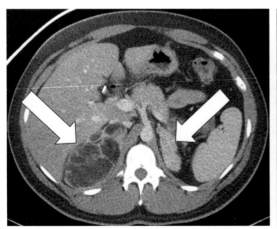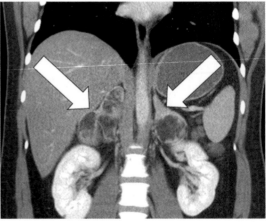

Fig. 82.1 Contrast-enhanced abdominal computed tomography scan axial *(left)* and coronal *(right)* images showed four macroscopic fat-containing masses (6.5 × 7.6 cm, 4.3 × 4.2 cm, 5.1 × 3.2 cm, and 1 cm) replacing both the medial and lateral limbs of the right adrenal gland *(arrows)*. Marked cortical hyperplasia was evident in the left adrenal gland on the axial image. The left adrenal gland also had two macroscopic fat-containing masses (5.1 × 4.4 cm and 2.8 × 2.6 cm). These imaging findings were consistent with cortical hyperplasia and bilateral myelolipomas resulting from untreated congenital adrenal hyperplasia.

TABLE 82.1 Laboratory Tests

Biochemical Test	Result	Reference Range
Sodium, mmol/L	137	135–145
Potassium, mmol/L	4.2	3.6–5.2
Creatinine, mg/dL	0.9	0.8–1.3
17-Hydroxyprogesterone, ng/dL	13,400	<220
Androstenedione, ng/dL	2,250	<150
DHEA-S, mcg/dL	206	89–457
Total testosterone, ng/dL	736	240–950
Bioavailable testosterone, ng/dL	523	83–257
ACTH, pg/mL	445	10–60

ACTH, Corticotropin; *DHEA-S,* dehydroepiandrosterone sulfate.

Sequence analysis of *CYP21A2* identified a homozygous pathogenic variant (g.655A/C>G).

TREATMENT

The adrenal gland enlargement was asymptomatic and surgery was not indicated. The patient was informed of his *CYP21A2*-deficient CAH and the need for glucocorticoid replacement therapy.

OUTCOME AND FOLLOW-UP

Treatment with dexamethasone 0.25 mg at bedtime resulted in a normal serum androstenedione concentration of 188 ng/dL. The goal for serum androstenedione in this setting is a level that is high-normal or mildly elevated above the upper limit of the reference range. In this way overtreatment with glucocorticoids and iatrogenic Cushing syndrome can be avoided.

Discussion

We recently published a retrospective study of 305 consecutive patients with adrenal myelolipomas.[2] The myelolipomas were bilateral in 16 (5.3%) patients.[2] In a recent systematic review the prevalence of adrenal tumors in CAH was 29.3%.[3] The prevalence of myelolipomas in patients with verified *CYP21A2* mutations was 8.6%. In those patients with myelolipomas, 93.5% had undiagnosed or poorly managed CAH.[3] When myelolipomas develop in this setting, the adrenal gland appearance on CT scan is diagnostic of undiagnosed or poorly managed CAH (Figs. 82.2 and 82.3).

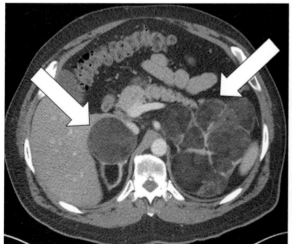 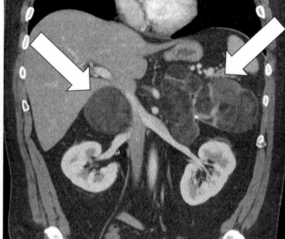

Fig. 82.2 Chronic noncompliance with glucocorticoid replacement therapy for 21-hydroxylase deficiency congenital adrenal hyperplasia (CAH) can have a classic and diagnostic appearance on a computed tomography (CT) scan. Although different patients, the images shown here and in Figs. 82.1 and 82.3 highlight the same findings. The axial image (on left) and coronal image (on right) are from a contrast-enhanced abdominal CT scan from a 48-year-old man with chronic poor compliance with glucocorticoid replacement therapy to treat 21-hydroxylase deficiency CAH. His serum 17-hydroxyprogesterone concentration was documented as high as 29,200 ng/dL (normal, <220 ng/dL), serum androstenedione concentration was as high as 3.250 ng/dL (normal, <150 ng/dL), and corticotropin as high as 972 pg/mL (normal, <60 pg/mL). The bilateral macroscopic fat-containing adrenal masses *(arrows)* measured 6.7 × 5.9 cm on the *right* and 14.2 × 12.1 cm on the *left.*

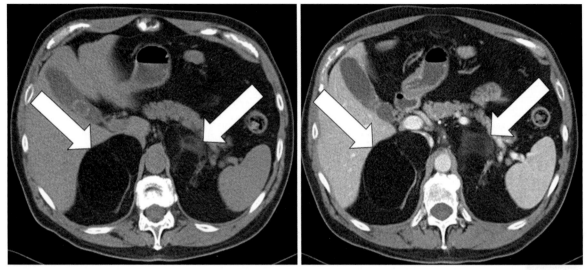

Fig. 82.3 Chronic noncompliance with glucocorticoid replacement therapy for 21-hydroxylase deficiency congenital adrenal hyperplasia (CAH) can have a classic and diagnostic appearance on computed tomography (CT) scan. Although in different patients, the images shown here and in Figs. 82.1 and 82.2 show the same findings. These axial images are from an unenhanced *(left)* and contrast-enhanced *(right)* abdominal CT scan from a 62-year-old man with chronic poor compliance with glucocorticoid replacement therapy to treat 21-hydroxylase deficiency CAH. His serum 17-hydroxyprogeserone concentration was elevated at 6204 ng/dL (normal, <220 ng/dL). The CT images showed the right adrenal mass to measure 10 cm × 6 cm × 10 cm and the left adrenal mass measured 6 cm × 5 cm × 6.5 cm. The unenhanced CT attenuation was −124 Hounsfield units, confirming macroscopic fat and bilateral adrenal myelolipomas.

Key Points

- The finding of macroscopic fat in an adrenal mass is consistent with adrenal myelolipoma.
- All patients with adrenal myelolipomas should be screened for congenital adrenal hyperplasia by measuring serum 17-hydroxyprogesterone, especially in the setting of bilateral adrenal myelolipomas.

REFERENCES

1. Nermoen I, Rørvik J, Holmedal SH, Hykkerud DL, Fougner KJ, Svartberg J, Husebye ES, Løvås K. High frequency of adrenal myelolipomas and testicular adrenal rest tumours in adult Norwegian patients with classical congenital adrenal hyperplasia because of 21-hydroxylase deficiency. *Clin Endocrinol (Oxf)*. 2011;75(6):753–759.
2. Hamidi O, Raman R, Lazik N, et al. Clinical course of adrenal myelolipoma: a long-term longitudinal follow-up study. *Clin Endocrinol (Oxf)*. 2020;93(1):11–18.
3. Nermoen I, Falhammar H. Prevalence and characteristics of adrenal tumors and myelolipomas in congenital adrenal hyperplasia: a systematic review and meta-analysis. *Endocr Pract*. 2020;26(11):1351–1365.

A Unilateral Lipid-Poor Adrenal Mass: An Atypical Presentation of Adrenal Histoplasmosis

Lipid-poor adrenal masses are the landmines of adrenal disorders. Although lipid-poor adrenal masses may be benign nonfunctional cortical adenomas, it can be difficult to make the distinction from more concerning diagnoses such as small adrenocortical carcinoma (ACC) (see Cases 6 and 23) or prebiochemical pheochromocytoma (see Case 36). Choosing nonsurgical management can carry clinically significant risk. Unless metastatic disease or infection is strongly suspected, adrenal biopsy should be avoided. There are atypical presentations of nearly all adrenal disorders, and caring for these patients can be a humbling experience. Herein we present such a case.

Case Report

The patient was a 59-year-old man referred for an evaluation of an incidentally discovered right adrenal mass. He had been hypertensive for 15 years and was treated with a β-adrenergic blocker, thiazide diuretic, and a calcium channel blocker. His home blood pressure measurements averaged 150s/60s mm Hg. There was no history of hypokalemia. He had used tobacco in the past (60 pack-years) and 1 year ago had a contrast-enhanced pulmonary computed tomography (CT) scan to follow up lung nodules, and this detected a new 2.5-cm right adrenal mass. The referral to Mayo Clinic was to follow up on that incidental finding. The patient had no signs or symptoms of pheochromocytoma beyond sustained hypertension. He had no signs or symptoms of malignancy or infection (e.g., no fever, cough, or weight loss). On physical examination his body mass index was 28.9 kg/m², blood pressure 136/73 mmHg, and heart rate 77 beats per minute. He had no stigmata of Cushing syndrome.

INVESTIGATIONS

The baseline laboratory test results are shown in Table 83.1. With the exception of fasting hyperglycemia, the laboratory tests were normal. A dedicated adrenal CT scan was performed. The isolated right adrenal

TABLE 83.1 Laboratory Tests		
Biochemical Test	Result	Reference Range
Sodium, mmol/L	147	135–145
Potassium, mmol/L	3.8	3.6–5.2
Fasting plasma glucose, mg/dL	147	70–100
Creatinine, mg/dL	1.3	0.9–1.3
1-mg overnight DST next day serum cortisol, mcg/dL	1.8	<1.8
Aldosterone, ng/dL	22	≤21
Plasma renin activity, ng/mL per hour	1.4	≤0.6–3
Plasma metanephrine, nmol/L	0.28	<0.5
Plasma normetanephrine, nmol/L	0.5	<0.9
24-Hour urine:		
Metanephrine, mcg	166	<400
Normetanephrine, mcg	533	<900
Norepinephrine, mcg	51	<80
Epinephrine, mcg	2.8	<20
Dopamine, mcg	350	<400

DST, Dexamethasone suppression test.

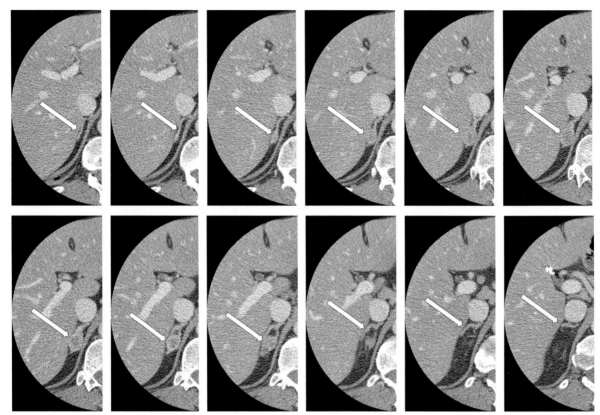

Fig. 83.1 Serial axial images (cranial to caudal, *left* to *right*) of the right adrenal gland *(arrows)* from a contrast-enhanced abdominal computed tomography (CT) scan. The right adrenal mass measured 2.7 cm × 1.7 cm. The unenhanced CT attenuation was 39 Hounsfield units. The mass enhanced with contrast administration. Dynamic and 10-minute delayed imaging of the contrast-enhanced phase of the examination showed that there was less than 50% contrast washout at 10 minutes.

mass measured 2.7 cm × 1.7 cm (Fig. 83.1). The unenhanced CT attenuation was 39 Hounsfield units. The mass enhanced with contrast administration and had slow contrast washout. The remainder of the right adrenal gland appeared normal. The left adrenal gland appeared normal on CT (Fig. 83.2). The chest CT scan performed elsewhere was not available for comparison. The outside reports indicated that bilateral pulmonary nodules were first detected 6 years previously when he had pleuritic right chest pain. The chest radiograph at that time showed a right pleural effusion—a biopsy was nondiagnostic. The chest CT scan from 1 year ago reported bilateral pulmonary nodules and some mediastinal lymphadenopathy.

TREATMENT

The finding of a new lipid-poor and vascular adrenal mass was concerning for a prebiochemical pheochromocytoma, early adrenocortical carcinoma, or metastatic disease (although a primary tumor elsewhere has not been diagnosed in this patient). We recommended a CT scan of the chest and to see a pulmonologist in consultation. If a suspicious pulmonary lesion was evident, then a CT-guided lung or adrenal biopsy could be considered. If there is no obvious pulmonary abnormality at that point, then laparoscopic right adrenalectomy would be a reasonable next step. He chose to return home and complete his evaluation locally.

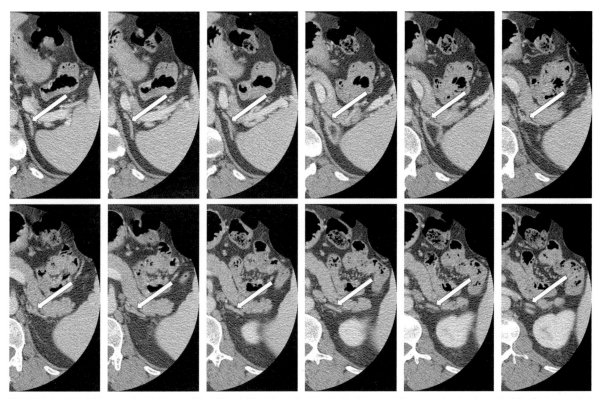

Fig. 83.2 Serial axial images (cranial to caudal, *left* to *right*) of the left adrenal gland *(arrows)* from a contrast-enhanced abdominal computed tomography scan. The left adrenal gland appeared normal on all cuts.

OUTCOME AND FOLLOW-UP

The patient underwent right laparoscopic adrenal-ectomy at a medical center closer to his home. The tissue samples were sent to Mayo Clinic for review. The adrenal gland was hyperplastic and weighed 26 g (normal, 4–5 g). A distinct adenoma or tumor was not identified, and most of the changes present were related to the necrotizing granulomatous inflam-mation with *Histoplasma capsulatum* identified on Grocott-Gomori's methenamine silver (GMS) stain. Thus the reason for the right adrenal gland nodule on CT scan was histoplasmosis. Communication from the patient's local endocrinologist 2 years later documented that follow-up adrenal imaging showed no abnormalities in the contralateral left adrenal gland and that the pulmonary lesions had resolved. The findings on a cosyntropin stimulation test were normal.

Discussion

Histoplasmosis capsulatum is a species of dimorphic fungus endemic to the Midwest and southern regions of the United States. Exposure is due to inhalation of the fungus from soil or caves that contain bat or bird droppings. Patients may develop a wide spectrum of symptoms—from asymptomatic to acute or chronic pulmonary symptoms. Disseminated infection may involve lungs, liver, spleen, bone marrow, central nervous system, and the adrenal glands. In a series of 111 patients at Mayo Clinic, 78 patients had dissemi-nated histoplasmosis and 55 patients had *Histoplasma capsulatum* fungemia.[1] The mean age of patients was 55 years, 66% were male, and 59% of patients were immunocompromised. Fever was the most frequently reported symptom (63%), followed by respiratory complaints (43%) and weight loss (37%). When the adrenal glands are involved, it is typically bilateral, and patients may present with symptoms of primary adrenal insufficiency.[2,3] The presentation of histoplasmosis-related adrenal gland involvement as a unilateral adrenal nodule has been rarely reported.[4]

Key Points

- If you have not been humbled in the evaluation and treatment of a patient with an incidentally discovered adrenal mass, you have not seen enough patients with adrenal incidentalomas . . . yet!
- Lipid-poor adrenal masses are the landmines of adrenal disorders. Although lipid-poor adrenal masses may be benign nonfunctional cortical adenomas, it can be difficult to make the distinction from more concerning diagnoses such as small adrenocortical carcinoma or prebiochemical pheochromocytoma. Choosing nonsurgical management in this setting can carry clinically significant risk. Unless metastatic disease or infection is strongly suspected, adrenal biopsy should be avoided.
- There are atypical presentations of nearly all adrenal disorders. For example, when there is adrenal involvement from histoplasmosis, it is nearly always bilateral.

REFERENCES

1. Assi MA, Sandid MS, Baddour LM, Roberts GD, Walker RC. Systemic histoplasmosis: a 15-year retrospective institutional review of 111 patients. *Medicine* (Baltimore). 2007;86(3):162–169.

2. Roxas MCA, Sandoval MAS, Salamat MS, Matias PJ, Cabal NP, Bartolo SS. Bilateral adrenal histoplasmosis presenting as adrenal insufficiency in an immunocompetent host in the Philippines. *BMJ Case Rep*. 2020;13(5):e234935.

3. Herndon J, Nadeau AM, Davidge-Pitts CJ, Young WF, Bancos I. Primary adrenal insufficiency due to bilateral infiltrative disease. *Endocrine*. 2018;62(3):721–728.

4. May D, Khaled D, Gills J. Unilateral adrenal histoplasmosis. *Urol Case Rep*. 2018;19:54–56.

Bilateral Macronodular Adrenal Hyperplasia in the Setting of Multiple Endocrine Neoplasia Type 1

Bilateral macronodular adrenal hyperplasia (BMAH) is typically a computed tomography (CT)-based diagnosis. Patients with multiple endocrine neoplasia type 1 (MEN-1) may present with normal-appearing adrenal glands, solitary adrenal adenomas, or BMAH. When adrenal nodularity is detected in a patient with MEN-1, it is important to determine if it is associated glucocorticoid secretory autonomy—either clinically evident Cushing syndrome or subclinical Cushing syndrome (also referred to as "mild autonomous cortisol excess"). When BMAH is associated with glucocorticoid secretory autonomy, adrenal venous sampling is not needed because, by definition, the disorder is bilateral. Dependent on the degree of symptomatology and comorbidities, management options include observation, unilateral adrenalectomy of the larger adrenal gland, or bilateral adrenalectomy. If the patient has subclinical Cushing syndrome (mild autonomous cortisol excess), then there is the opportunity to resect the larger adrenal gland to debulk the disease. Herein we share such a case.

Case Report

Six years before consultation at Mayo Clinic this 63-year-old woman was diagnosed with MEN-1 (based on multigland hyperparathyroidism and a family history of MEN-1). The visit to Mayo Clinic was triggered by the finding of BMAH on the abdominal CT scan that was performed to assess her pancreas (Fig. 84.1). Adrenal nodularity was noted on a CT scan 7 years previously, but no evaluation was performed. Although she did not have overt clinical Cushing syndrome, she did have excessive bruising, mild facial plethora, type 2 diabetes mellitus treated with two oral agents (metformin and glipizide), and hypertension treated with two drugs (lisinopril and metoprolol). In addition, she was recently found to have osteopenia. On physical examination her body mass index was 29.3 kg/m^2, blood pressure 148/86 mmHg, and heart rate 63 beats per minute. She did not appear clinically cushingoid. She did not have hirsutism or purple red striae. Her skin turgor was normal. Proximal muscle weakness was not evident.

INVESTIGATIONS

The laboratory test results are shown in Table 84.1. The diagnosis of glucocorticoid secretory autonomy was based on the following: low serum corticotropin (ACTH) concentration; low-normal serum dehydroepiandrosterone sulfate (DHEA-S) concentration; mild elevation in 24-hour urinary free cortisol excretion and lack of complete suppression in serum cortisol with an overnight 8-mg dexamethasone suppression test (DST) (Table 84.1).

The patient was informed that both adrenal glands were autonomously producing cortisol. She understood that because she had subclinical Cushing syndrome (mild autonomous cortisol excess), rather than overt Cushing syndrome, we had the opportunity to treat her with a debulking operation by resecting her larger right adrenal gland.

TREATMENT

With perioperative glucocorticoid coverage (100 mg hydrocortisone administered intravenously on call to the operating room and again 8 hours later), the

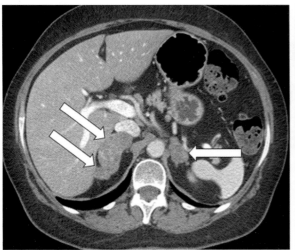 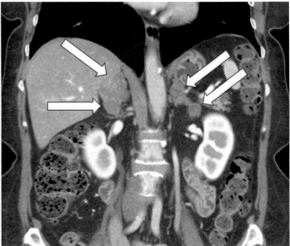

Fig. 84.1 Axial *(left)* and coronal *(right)* images of the adrenal glands on a contrast-unenhanced abdominal computed tomography (CT) scan. Bilateral multinodular adrenal glands are shown *(arrows)*. The largest nodule in the right adrenal gland was 3.9 cm in diameter and had an unenhanced CT attenuation of −0.8 Hounsfield units (HU). The largest nodule in the left adrenal gland was 2.1 cm in diameter and had an unenhanced CT attenuation of 8 HU.

TABLE 84.1	Laboratory Tests		
Biochemical Test	**Results Baseline**	**Results 4 Years After Surgery**	**Reference Range**
Sodium, mmol/L	140		135–145
Potassium, mmol/L	5.3		3.6–5.2
Creatinine, mg/dL	0.7		0.6–1.1
Aldosterone, ng/dL	5.2		≤21 ng/dL
Plasma renin activity, ng/mL per hour	1.2		≤0.6–3
8 AM serum cortisol, mcg/dL	6.8	11.0	7–25
DHEA-S, mcg/dL	38.0	38.7	16–195
ACTH, pg/mL	<5	11.0	10–60
1-mg overnight DST, mcg/dL	7.0		<1.8
8-mg overnight DST, mcg/dL	6.1		<1.0
24-Hour urine cortisol, mcg	52, 33		<45

ACTH, Corticotropin; *DHEA-S,* dehydroepiandrosterone sulfate; *DST,* dexamethasone suppression test.

patient underwent laparoscopic right adrenalectomy. The right adrenal gland weighed 35.4 g (normal, 4–5 g). The specimen was diffusely nodular with a thin rim of normal tissue. The patient was discharged from the hospital on 10 mg of hydrocortisone twice daily with the instructions to decrease the dosage to 15 mg every morning at 2 weeks postoperatively.

OUTCOME AND FOLLOW-UP

The patient's morning serum cortisol concentrations were 8.7 mcg/dL and 9.3 mcg/dL (normal, 7–25 mcg/dL) at 1 and 4 months after surgery, respectively. Hydrocortisone was discontinued 4 months postoperatively. The laboratory data obtained 4 years after surgery are shown in Table 84.1. Despite the adrenal debulking procedure, the patient did not notice any changes in body weight, blood pressure control, or glycemic control after unilateral adrenalectomy. She remained on the same antihypertensive and antihyperglycemic agents. It was determined that the clinical findings did not support a completion adrenalectomy and annual reevaluation was advised. Our hope was that the debulking surgery, although not associated with any objective benefit in her case, did "set the clock back" on her need for complete bilateral adrenalectomy.

Key Points

- Approximately 30%–40% of patients with MEN-1 develop an adrenal gland lesions.[1–5]
- When Cushing syndrome develops in patients with MEN-1, it is usually due to an ACTH-secreting pituitary tumor; however, in approximately 20% of the cases it is adrenal dependent.[6]
- Patients with MEN-1 are at risk to develop adrenocortical hyperfunction from either adrenal adenoma, BMAH, or adrenocortical cancer (see Case 32). The adrenal glands should be routinely inspected at the time of computed cross-sectional abdominal imaging when it is performed to assess the status of pancreatic neuroendocrine tumors.
- The 8-mg overnight DST has a role to confirm absolutely glucocorticoid secretory autonomy in patients with an abnormal 1-mg overnight DST. A normal serum cortisol concentration after 8 mg of dexamethasone is undetectable.
- If a patient with MEN-1 has subclinical Cushing syndrome (mild autonomous cortisol excess) in the setting of BMAH, a debulking operation by resecting the larger adrenal gland is a reasonable first operation—recognizing that completion adrenalectomy may be needed in the future.[7]

REFERENCES

1. Burgess JR, Harle RA, Tucker P, Parameswaran V, Davies P, Greenaway TM, Shepherd JJ. Adrenal lesions in a large kindred with multiple endocrine neoplasia type 1. *Arch Surg*. 1996;131(7):699–702.

2. Langer P, Cupisti K, Bartsch DK, et al. Adrenal involvement in multiple endocrine neoplasia type 1. *World J Surg*. 2002;26:891–896.

3. Waldmann J, Bartsch DK, Kann PH, Fendrich V, Rothmund M, Langer P. Adrenal involvement in multiple endocrine neoplasia type 1: results of 7 years prospective screening. *Langenbecks Arch Surg*. 2007;392:437–443.

4. Whitley SA, Moyes VJ, Park KM, et al. The appearance of the adrenal glands on computed tomography in multiple endocrine neoplasia type 1. *Eur J Endocrinol*. 2008;159:819–824.

5. Barzon L, Pasquali C, Grigoletto C, Pedrazzoli S, Boscaro M, Fallo F. Multiple endocrine neoplasia type 1 and adrenal lesions. *J Urol*. 2001;166:24–27.

6. Simonds WF, Varghese S, Marx SJ, Nieman LK. Cushing's syndrome in multiple endocrine neoplasia type 1. *Clin Endocrinol (Oxf)*. 2012;76(3):379–386.

7. Yoshida M, Hiroi M, Imai T, et al. A case of ACTH-independent macronodular adrenal hyperplasia associated with multiple endocrine neoplasia type 1. *Endocr J*. 2011;58(4):269–277.

Pseudo-Adrenal Masses

It is not an uncommon scenario for a patient to be referred to an endocrinologist for an adrenal mass that proves to not be an adrenal mass. Surgically resected nonadrenal masses that were initially diagnosed as an adrenal disease represent about 3.5% of all adrenal surgeries.[1] The differential diagnosis includes: retroperitoneal tumors that may be malignant (e.g., kidney tumors, lymphoma, sarcoma), benign vascular and lymph-related anomalies (e.g., cystic lymphangioma, angiomyolipoma), other retroperitoneal tumors (e.g., ganglioneuroma, paraganglioma), and normal anatomic structures that are mistaken for adrenal tissue (e.g., gastric diverticulum). Herein we share several cases to highlight this clinical scenario.

Case Report: Malignant Renal Epithelioid Angiomyolipoma

The patient was a 31-year-old woman who presented with daily epigastric discomfort that responded to treatment with a proton pump inhibitor. However,

an ultrasound of the abdomen detected an 8-cm right retroperitoneal mass. Computed tomography (CT) and magnetic resonance imaging (MRI) scans of the abdomen showed a 6.5 × 4–cm mixed-density right retroperitoneal mass of either renal, adrenal, or hepatic origin (Fig. 85.1). Immunohistochemistry on a CT-guided biopsy was positive for synaptophysin, S-100 epithelial membrane antigen, and vimentin, whereas the chromogranin stain was negative. The pathologist thought that the likely tissue of origin was adrenocortical and unlikely to be renal—the report read: "adrenocortical neoplasm with oncocytic features." She was referred to endocrinology for evaluation of an adrenal mass. She showed signs or symptoms of adrenocortical or medullary hormone excess. Her blood pressure was normal and she had no change in body weight. The 24-hour urine studies were normal for cortisol, fractionated metanephrine levels, and fractionated catecholamines. She underwent a flank incision with a right radical nephrectomy and right adrenalectomy. Pathology documented a 9.2 × 8 × 3–cm malignant

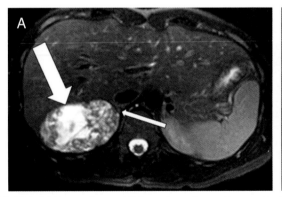
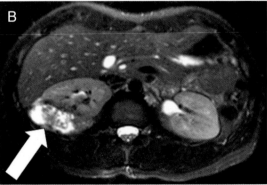

Fig. 85.1 Axial images from gadolinium-enhanced magnetic resonance imaging scan. (A) A 7.3-cm retroperitoneal heterogeneous mass *(large arrow)* is seen along with a normal-appearing adrenal gland limb just medial and ventral *(small arrow)* to the large mass. (B) A more caudal image shows that the mass *(arrow)* appears to arise from the upper pole of the right kidney.

renal epithelioid angiomyolipoma—a malignant mesenchymal neoplasm, characterized by proliferating epithelioid cells. The adrenal gland was anatomically normal. Epithelioid renal angiomyolipoma is a rare malignant variant of angiomyolipoma.[2] There was no evidence for recurrent disease on periodic abdominal cross-sectional imaging completed over the subsequent 14 years.

Case Report: Retroperitoneal Lymphangioma

The patient was a 58-year-old man who had a slowly growing incidentally discovered cystic left retroperitoneal mass (Fig. 85.2). Seven years previously, it measured 2.3 × 1.8 cm in diameter. It measured 6.7 × 6.6 cm on the most recent CT scan (see Fig. 85.2). The mass was located along the lateral wing of the left adrenal gland. It was clearly distinct from the left kidney, pancreas, and surrounding vascular structures. There was no apparent solid component or an enhancing ring to the cystic mass. The patient had no signs or symptoms of pheochromocytoma. He had been troubled by a left flank discomfort over the past year. He graded the pain at 6–7 out of 10 in severity and he felt it every day. Plasma fractionated metanephrine levels were normal. In view of his flank discomfort and the slow enlargement over 7 years, surgical resection was advised. At laparoscopic surgery, the cystic mass abutted the adrenal gland but did not involve the adrenal gland. At pathology the mass proved to be a lymphangioma. An abdominal CT scan completed 6 months postoperatively showed no evidence of persistent lymphangioma. His flank pain resolved after surgery. Lymphangioma is a rare benign proliferation of lymph vessels, which results in fluid-filled cysts as a result of the blockage of lymphatic flow.[3] Surgical resection should be considered if there is associated pain or documented enlargement.

Case Report: Gastric Diverticulum

The patient was a 64-year-old woman referred for evaluation of an incidentally discovered left adrenal mass. The mass measured 1.6 cm in diameter and had an unenhanced CT attenuation of 20.4 Hounsfield units (Fig. 85.3). However, on careful inspection, it was apparent that the small mass was located superior to the left adrenal gland and consistent with a small gastric diverticulum arising from the gastric cardia (see Fig. 85.3). The patient was reassured and no endocrine workup was recommended. Eleven years later a CT scan was performed to investigate abdominal pain, and the gastric diverticulum was slightly larger, contained air, and on the coronal image was clearly separate from the left adrenal gland (Fig. 85.3).

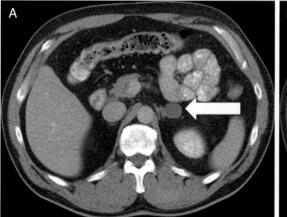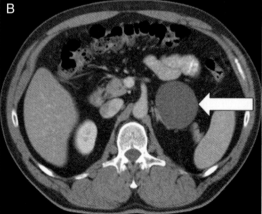

Fig. 85.2 Axial images from contrast-enhanced computed tomography (CT) scans. (A) 2.3 × 1.8–cm retroperitoneal cystic mass *(arrow)* abutting the lateral limb of the left adrenal. Unenhanced CT attenuation was 18.3 Hounsfield units. (B) Seven years later the unilocular cystic lesion *(arrow)* measured 6.7 × 6.6 cm. There was no abnormal soft tissue nodularity or enhancement. The cyst was directly adjacent to the left kidney, pancreatic tail, splenic vein, left renal vein, and fourth portion of the duodenum and did not appear to arise directly or invade these structures.

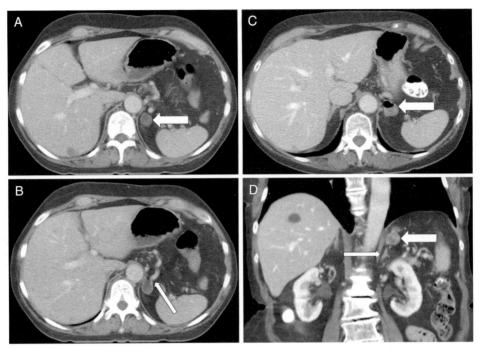

Fig. 85.3 Axial images from a contrast-enhanced computed tomography scan at the time of discovery of the left retroperitoneal mass. (A) A 1.6-cm round mass *(arrow)* with an unenhanced CT attenuation of 20.4 Hounsfield units. (B) The connection *(arrow)* of the mass to the stomach—a finding consistent with a small gastric diverticulum. (C) and (D) Images from a contrast-enhanced CT scan obtained 11 years later. (C) An axial image shows that the gastric diverticulum *(arrow)* was slightly larger and contained air. (D) The coronal image shows that the gastric diverticulum *(large arrow)* was clearly separate from the left adrenal gland *(small arrow)*.

Case Report: Renal Lymphangiomyoma in the Setting of Pulmonary Lymphangioleiomyomatosis

This 17-year-old woman initially presented with recurrent pneumothorax, and video-assisted thora-coscopic (VATS) biopsy demonstrated pulmonary lymphangioleiomyomatosis. However, the chest CT scan incidentally detected a 4.5-cm "left adrenal mass" (Fig. 85.4). Adrenal function testing was normal. CT-guided biopsy showed renal lymphangiomyoma. Observation was advised. However, she presented 6 months later with severe left flank pain as a result of hemorrhage into the renal lymphangiomyoma. It was treated with embolization of the superior left renal artery that represented 95% of the blood supply to the mass. Subsequent serial abdominal CT scans showed shrinkage and stability of the residual mass over the subsequent 18 years (see Fig. 85.4). Because

of recurrent pneumothorax, her pulmonary lymphan-gioleiomyomatosis was treated with rapamycin.

Case Report: Splenic Artery Aneurysm

An abdominal CT scan was performed for this 63-year-old man for non–adrenal gland related reasons, and an incidentally discovered "adrenal mass" led to endo-crine referral. As shown in Fig. 85.5, the left suprare-nal mass did not appear consistent with adrenal tissue. Angiography confirmed this suspicion by document-ing a 4-cm symmetric renal artery aneurysm (see Fig. 85.5). Because of the risk of rupture, this patient underwent splenic artery ligation and splenectomy.

Key Points

- Immunohistochemistry findings on CT-guided needle biopsies of adrenal or pseudo-adrenal

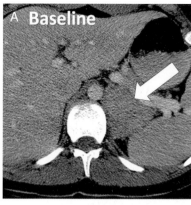 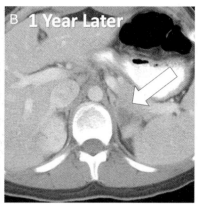 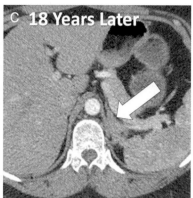

Fig. 85.4 Serial axial computed tomography (CT) images show the 4.5-cm triangular-shaped lipid-poor (47.5 Hounsfield units) left suprarenal mass *(arrow)* at the time of discovery (A), 6 months after arterial ablation therapy (B), and 18 years after the discovery image (C).

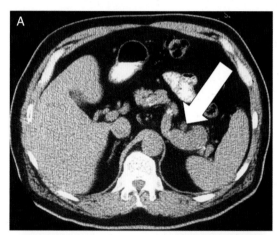

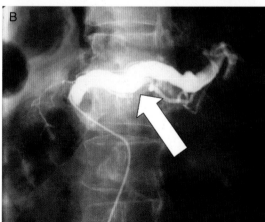

Fig. 85.5 (A) The axial computed tomography (CT) image shows a gourd-shaped left suprarenal mass *(arrow)*. This finding was initially interpreted as an adrenal mass. However, as shown with the coronal arteriogram image (B), the CT finding was actually due to an asymmetric splenic artery aneurysm.

masses should serve as a guide to the underlying pathology but may not be diagnostic.

- The clinician should be aware that surgically resected nonadrenal masses that were initially diagnosed as an adrenal disease represent about 3.5% of all adrenal surgeries. The differential diagnosis for an adrenal mass includes retroperitoneal tumors that may be malignant (e.g., kidney tumors, lymphoma, sarcoma), benign vascular and lymph-related anomalies (e.g., cystic lymphangioma, angiomyolipoma), other retroperitoneal tumors (e.g., ganglioneuroma, paraganglioma), and normal anatomic structures that are mistaken for adrenal tissue (e.g., gastric diverticulum, splenic artery aneurysm).

REFERENCES

1. Frey S, Caillard C, Toulgoat F, Drui D, Hamy A, Mirallié É. Non-adrenal tumors of the adrenal area; what are the pitfalls? *J Visc Surg.* 2020;157(3):217–230.

2. Brimo F, Robinson B, Guo C, Zhou M, Latour M, Epstein JI. Renal epithelioid angiomyolipoma with atypia: a series of 40 cases with emphasis on clinicopathologic prognostic indicators of malignancy. *Am J Surg Pathol.* 2010;34(5):715–722.

3. Makni A, Chebbi F, Fetirich F, et al. Surgical management of intra-abdominal cystic lymphangioma: report of 20 cases. *World J Surg.* 2012;36(5):1037–1043.

Adrenal and Ovarian Hyperandrogenism

In adulthood, clinical manifestations of hyperandrogenism affect mostly women, with symptoms of hirsutism, acne, oily skin, alopecia, and, in severe forms, virilization of genitalia. Hyperandrogenism can be endogenous (adrenal or ovarian) or exogenous as a result of administration of DHEA or testosterone (Box H.1). The most common causes of *postmenopausal* hyperandrogenism include ovarian hyperthecosis, ovarian or adrenal tumor, or nonclassic congenital adrenal hyperplasia. The most common causes of *premenopausal* hyperandrogenism include polycystic ovarian syndrome, nonclassic congenital adrenal hyperplasia, and adrenal or ovarian tumors.

Approach to a patient with hyperandrogenism includes *careful history* of symptoms and their progression, age at onset, duration, menstrual history (in women), medications, ethnicity, and family history.[1] *Physical examination* assesses for hirsutism, acne, presence of symptoms suggestive of cortisol excess, and pelvic examination.

Biochemical workup includes measurements of androgens (total testosterone, androstenedione, dehydroepiandrosterone sulfate [DHEA-S]) and 17-hydroxyprogesterone (for diagnosis of congenital adrenal hyperplasia). Dexamethasone suppression testing can be used to distinguish between neoplastic and nonneoplastic hyperandrogenism (see Case 88).

If neoplastic hyperandrogenism is suspected, *pelvic ultrasonography* is indicated to evaluate for ovarian morphology (though absence of the tumor

BOX H.1 CONDITIONS ASSOCIATED WITH HYPERANDROGENISM

Adrenal	
Corticotropin-Dependent	***Corticotropin-Independent***
Corticotropin-dependent Cushing syndrome	Androgen-secreting adrenal cortical carcinoma
CYP21A2 deficiency	Androgen-secreting adrenal adenoma (very rare)
CYP11B1 deficiency	Bilateral macronodular adrenal hyperplasia (rare)
11-β-Hydroxysteroid dehydrogenase type 1 deficiency	
Glucocorticoid receptor resistance syndrome	

Ovarian
Polycystic ovarian syndrome
Ovarian hyperthecosis
Ovarian tumor
Iatrogenic
Dehydroepiandrosterone
Testosterone

on ultrasonography does not rule out its presence). *Adrenal imaging* with an unenhanced computed tomography is indicated to evaluate for presence of adrenal tumors.

A *combined ovarian and adrenal venous sampling* is occasionally employed to locate the source of hyperandrogenism in women with uninformative imaging findings. This is frequently the case in postmenopausal hyperandrogenism when locating the source of hyperandrogenism can represent a diagnostic challenge, and imaging studies may be misleading.[1–3]

The evaluation should be guided by the chronicity of signs and symptoms and the degree of androgen excess.[1,2,4] When there is an abrupt onset of marked signs and symptoms and marked increases in serum testosterone concentrations, it is important to assess the patient with a full androgen profile and imaging studies of the ovaries and adrenal glands. On the other hand, if the signs and symptoms related to androgen excess are chronic and mild, and androgen measurements are only mildly increased, imaging may not be needed.

REFERENCES

1. Martin KA, Anderson RR, Chang RJ, et al. Evaluation and treatment of hirsutism in premenopausal women: an Endocrine Society clinical practice guideline. *J Clin Endocrinol Metab*. 2018;103(4):1233–1257.
2. Mamoojee Y, Ganguri M, Taylor N, Quinton R. Clinical case seminar: postmenopausal androgen excess-challenges in diagnostic work-up and management of ovarian thecosis. *Clin Endocrinol (Oxf)*. 2018;88(1):13–20.
3. Yance VRV, Marcondes JAM, Rocha MP, et al. Discriminating between virilizing ovary tumors and ovary hyperthecosis in postmenopausal women: clinical data, hormonal profiles and image studies. *Eur J Endocrinol*. 2017;177(1):93–102.
4. Di Dalmazi G. Hyperandrogenism and adrenocortical tumors. *Front Horm Res*. 2019;53:92–99.

A Huge Adrenal Myelolipoma in a Patient With a Suboptimally Controlled Congenital Adrenal Hyperplasia

Adrenal tumors in patients with congenital adrenal hyperplasia (CAH) are common, affecting 25%–30% of patients, and are associated with suboptimal control of CAH. Here we present a case of a patient with CAH who had huge myelolipoma.[1]

Case Report

The patient was a 52-year-old man with history of 21-hydroxylase deficiency diagnosed at 2 months of age during workup for failure to thrive. He had a sporadic follow-up for known CAH. Several months before current presentation, he was incidentally found to have a large adrenal mass that was visualized on a computed tomography (CT) scan performed for evaluation of coronary calcium. Adrenal mass biopsy was performed under the direction of his local health care providers and demonstrated possible myelolipoma versus liposarcoma. Open adrenalectomy was scheduled, but the patient chose to pursue a second opinion on treatment and presented to our institution.

His review of systems was negative for signs of Cushing syndrome. He described occasional episodes of lightheadedness. He also reported abdominal discomfort and abnormalities in gastrointestinal transit. In addition to CAH, his medical history was positive for hypertension. His medications included hydrocortisone (15 mg on waking and 5 mg in the afternoon) and telmisartan. He was not taking fludrocortisone. On physical examination, his body mass index was 45.9 kg/m^2, blood pressure 126/74 mmHg, and heart rate 79 beats per minute. He had no features of Cushing syndrome and no edema on examination.

INVESTIGATIONS

Laboratory test results are shown in Table 86.1. Serum androstenedione concentration was markedly elevated, and serum dehydroepiandrosterone sulfate (DHEA-S) concentration was slightly elevated, suggestive of suboptimal control of CAH. His renin plasma activity was elevated. CT images obtained elsewhere were reviewed and demonstrated a heterogeneous left 22.5 × 19.1 × 14.7–cm adrenal mass with areas of macroscopic fat and multiple 2–3 cm fat-containing right adrenal nodules (Fig. 86.1A).

TABLE 86.1 Laboratory Tests			
Biochemical Test	Baseline	12 Months Later	Reference Range
17-Hydroxyprogesterone, ng/dL	14,700		<220
DHEA-S, mcg/dL	446	209	20–299
Androstenedione, ng/dL	6150	1290	40–150
Total testosterone, ng/dL	592	147	240–950
Bioavailable testosterone, ng/dL	326	44	50–190
Plasma renin activity, ng/mL per hour	69	18	<0.6–3.0

DHEA-S, Dehydroepiandrosterone sulfate.

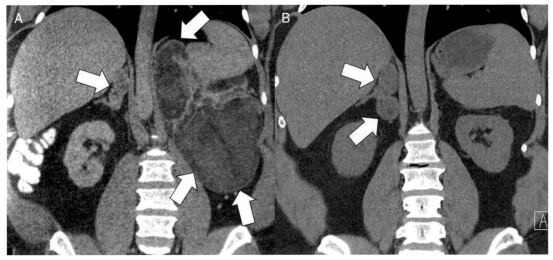

Fig. 86.1 Coronal images from an abdominal computed tomography (CT) scan at the time of presentation (A) and 12 months after left adrenalectomy (B). (A) Contrast-enhanced CT image shows a heterogeneous left 22.5 × 19.1 × 14.7–cm adrenal mass with areas of macroscopic fat and multiple 2–3 cm fat-containing right adrenal nodules (*arrows*). (B) Unenhanced CT image shows absent left adrenal gland, and multiple right adrenal masses that had increased in size, now measuring 3.7 cm, 5.2 cm, and 1.2 cm (*arrows*).

TREATMENT

The patient was treated with open left adrenalectomy without complications. Perioperative glucocorticoid coverage was provided. Pathologic analysis demonstrated a left adrenal myelolipoma measuring 31.0 × 21.3 × 11.6 cm and weighing 4335 g (Fig. 86.2).

FOLLOW-UP

His glucocorticoid replacement regimen was changed to hydrocortisone 10 mg on waking, 10 mg at noon, and 2.5 mg of prednisone in the evening. In addition, fludrocortisone 50 mcg daily was added. Several months later, the patient reported feeling better on the new regimen but was able to come for follow-up only 12 months after adrenalectomy. His laboratory tests showed improvement in androstenedione and normalization of DHEA-S, but control of CAH was still suboptimal (see Table 86.1). Unenhanced CT demonstrated that multiple right adrenal nodules increased in size by 1–3 cm (see Fig. 86.1B). Compliance with medications was confirmed and the glucocorticoid regimen was modified with a plan to reassess in 3 months.

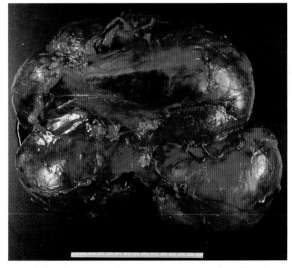

Fig. 86.2 Gross pathology photograph showing the intact 31.0 × 21.3 × 11.6–cm left adrenal mass that weighed 4335 g. At pathologic analysis the mass consisted of adipose tissue, hematopoietic cells, and epithelial cells of possible adrenocortical origin.

Discussion

Adrenal myelolipoma is usually diagnosed at a median size of 2 cm, and 15% of patients have large myelolipoma (>6 cm).[2] In a series of 305 patients with myelolipoma, the largest measured 18 cm.[2] Symptoms of mass effect, accelerated growth, and hemorrhagic changes are usual indications for adrenalectomy in patients with myelolipoma. Few patients with myelolipomas are tested for CAH, even when large or bilateral.[2]

The prevalence of any adrenal mass in CAH is 29%, and the prevalence of myelolipoma in CAH is 7.4–8.6%.[1] Myelolipomas almost always occur in patients with undiagnosed or suboptimally managed CAH.[1] Men with CAH are more likely to develop adrenal masses compared to women, possibly because of a higher likelihood of suboptimally controlled CAH.[1]

Key Points

- The diagnosis of CAH should be considered in any patient with myelolipoma, especially when large or bilateral.
- Diagnosis of adrenal mass in a patient with known CAH may indicate suboptimal control of CAH; compliance should be reassessed and the glucocorticoid regimen modified if necessary.

REFERENCES

1. Nermoen I, Falhammar H. Prevalence and characteristics of adrenal tumors and myelolipomas in congenital adrenal hyperplasia: a systematic review and meta-analysis. *Endocr Pract*. 2020;26(11):1351–1365.

2. Hamidi O, Raman R, Lazik N, et al. Clinical course of adrenal myelolipoma: a long-term longitudinal follow-up study. *Clin Endocrinol (Oxf)*. 2020;93(1):11–18.

Balancing Glucocorticoid and Androgen Excess in Congenital Adrenal Hyperplasia

The most common type of congenital adrenal hyperplasia (CAH) is 21-hydroxylase deficiency, which occurs in 1 in 10,000 live births.[1] The goals of therapy in CAH include (1) replacement therapy for glucocorticoid and mineralocorticoid deficiency and (2) controlling androgen excess. Here we present a case of classic salt-losing CAH to illustrate the basic principles of CAH management.

Case Report

The patient was a 24-year-old man with history of 21-hydroxylase deficiency who was referred to establish follow-up in the adult endocrine clinic.

PREVIOUS HISTORY

He was diagnosed with 21-hydroxylase deficiency at 10 days of age. At that time, he was hospitalized due to vomiting and weight loss. On admission, he was noted to be hyponatremic (serum sodium concentration, 121 mEq/L) and hyperkalemic (serum potassium concentration, 7.1 mEq/L). Adrenal crisis from primary adrenal insufficiency caused by 21-hydroxylase deficiency was suspected and confirmed with significantly elevated serum 17-hydroxyprogesterone concentrations. Glucocorticoid and mineralocorticoid replacement therapy was initiated (exact doses unknown). He had good follow-up for CAH during childhood. His height was maintained at the 25th–50th percentiles. Initially he was treated with hydrocortisone three times a day, later on with prednisone, and then with dexamethasone to ensure a better control. In addition, he was taking fludrocortisone 150 mcg per day.

CURRENT EVALUATION

The patient reported fatigue and muscle weakness, weight gain, and striae over his abdomen and hip area. He noticed occasional edema in lower extremities. Medications included dexamethasone 0.75 mg at night and fludrocortisone 150 mcg daily. Compliance was excellent. On physical examination, his body mass index was 32.38 kg/m^2, blood pressure 145/102 mmHg, and heart rate 79 beats per minute. He had abdominal obesity, mild dorsocervical pad, mild supraclavicular pads, and bright purple striae over his abdomen and hips. His skin was not thin, and there were no visible bruises. He had mild bilateral lower extremity edema.

INVESTIGATIONS

Laboratory test results are shown in Table 87.1. The serum androstenedione concentration was low and the serum concentration of 17-hydroxyprogesterone was normal. Bone mineral density revealed low bone mass with a T score of –2.8 at the level of spine and T score of –1.7 at the level of hips. Ultrasound of testes was performed to evaluate for presence of testicular adrenal rest tumors (TARTs) and was normal. Biochemical workup demonstrated a normal fasting glucose but abnormal lipid profile (total cholesterol of 220 mg/dL, normal range, <200).

TREATMENT AND FOLLOW-UP

Dexamethasone was replaced by hydrocortisone at a total daily dose of 30 mg, 15 mg in the morning, 10 mg in afternoon, and 5 mg in the evening. Three months later he reported a 22-pound weight loss and feeling more energetic. In addition, dyslipidemia improved

TABLE 87.1 Laboratory Tests			
	Baseline	Follow-up	
Biochemical Test	Dexamethasone 0.75 mg Daily Fludrocortisone 150 mcg Daily	Hydrocortisone 30 mg Daily Fludrocortisone 100 mcg Daily	Reference Range
17-Hydroxyprogesterone, ng/dL	205	2390	<220
DHEA-S, mcg/dL	—	76	89–457
Androstenedione, ng/dL	29	116	40–150
Total testosterone, ng/dL	—	288	240–950
Bioavailable testosterone, ng/dL	—	127	50–190
Plasma renin activity, ng/mL per hour	0.8	2.7	<0.6–3.0

DHEA-S, Dehydroepiandrosterone sulfate.

(total cholesterol decreased from 220 mg/dL to 168 mg/dL, normal range, <200). Hormonal workup demonstrated elevated serum 17-hydroxyprogesterone concentration but normal serum concentrations of androstenedione and testosterone (see Table 87.1).

Bone mineral density was repeated 2 years later and revealed an 8.8% improvement in bone mineral density at the level of spine.

Discussion

Goals of therapy in an adult with CAH shift from optimization of growth and pubertal development to overall health and quality of life.[2] Adults with CAH present with a high prevalence of obesity, metabolic syndrome, cardiovascular morbidity, and low bone mass–findings suggestive of excessive exposure to glucocorticoids.[3,4] Thus it is important to reevaluate the glucocorticoid therapy in any adult with CAH. Glucocorticoid therapy has a dual role: (1) to provide a physiologic replacement therapy to treat adrenal insufficiency and (2) to control androgen excess and its consequences. Measurement of 17-hydroxyprogesterone is not helpful to guide glucocorticoid therapy; 17-hydroxyprogesterone in the normal ranges indicates over treatment with glucocorticoids. Hydrocortisone should be tried first, either twice a day or more commonly three times a day, with each meal. Using hydrocortisone minimizes the risk of iatrogenic Cushing syndrome and metabolic consequences related to glucocorticoid excess.

However, the short half-life of hydrocortisone does not always provide an optimal suppression of corticotropin (ACTH) when administered in the evening. In these cases, adding a small dose of prednisone in the evening could be tried. Dexamethasone treatment should be the last resort, and only after other interventions failed. Dexamethasone has a long half-life and a high potency, frequently leading to iatrogenic Cushing syndrome even when used at doses <0.5 mg/day.[5]

Fludrocortisone therapy is typically used at dose of 50 mcg to 200 mcg daily, and adjusted based on clinical examination (blood pressure, absence of orthostasis) and biochemical workup (normal potassium and renin plasma activity).

Key Points

- Management of CAH in an adult targets optimization of overall health and quality of life.
- Glucocorticoid therapy in CAH has dual role: (1) to provide a physiologic replacement for adrenal insufficiency and (2) to control androgen excess and its consequences.
- Adults with CAH should be evaluated for glucocorticoid excess clinically (physical examination), imaging (bone density), and biochemically (androgens, glycosylated hemoglobin, and lipid panel).
- Serum 17-hydroxyprogesterone concentrations in the normal range indicates overtreatment with glucocorticoids.

REFERENCES

1. Merke DP, Auchus RJ. Congenital adrenal hyperplasia due to 21-hydroxylase deficiency. *N Engl J Med*. 2020;383(13):1248–1261.

2. Auchus RJ. Management considerations for the adult with congenital adrenal hyperplasia. *Mol Cell Endocrinol*. 2015;408:190–197.

3. Riehl G, Reisch N, Roehle R, Claahsen van der Grinten H, Falhammar H, Quinkler M. Bone mineral density and fractures in congenital adrenal hyperplasia: findings from the dsd-LIFE study. *Clin Endocrinol (Oxf)*. 2020;92(4):284–294.

4. Falhammar H, Filipsson Nystrom H, Wedell A, Thoren M. Cardiovascular risk, metabolic profile, and body composition in adult males with congenital adrenal hyperplasia due to 21-hydroxylase deficiency. *Eur J Endocrinol*. 2011;164(2):285–293.

5. Whittle E, Falhammar H. Glucocorticoid regimens in the treatment of congenital adrenal hyperplasia: a systematic review and meta-analysis. *J Endocr Soc*. 2019;3(6):1227–1245.

Dehydroepiandrosterone Sulfate:
The "Love It" or "Hate It" Hormone

Endocrinologists have a "love-hate relationship" with the measurement of dehydroepiandrosterone sulfate (DHEA-S). Measurement of serum DHEA-S concentration is very useful when it is either very low or very high in a patient with an adrenal mass. When the serum DHEA-S is suppressed in a patient with an adrenal mass, it suggests chronic suppression of pituitary corticotropin (ACTH) secretion: a finding consistent with either subclinical glucocorticoid secretory autonomy or adrenal-dependent Cushing syndrome. On the other hand, when the serum DHEA-S concentration is high in a patient with an adrenal mass, it is suggestive of an androgen-secreting adrenal tumor and frequently adrenocortical carcinoma; again, it is a useful biomarker in this setting. However, in the United States the most common reason clinicians measure serum DHEA-S is for a premenopausal woman with hirsutism—the serum DHEA-S concentration is frequently mildly to moderately elevated above the upper limit of the reference range. An elevated serum DHEA-S concentration in a premenopausal woman frequently leads to imaging studies of the adrenal glands and ovaries because of the concern about a neoplastic source—something only rarely found. Herein we share one approach to the clinical conundrum of increased serum DHEA-S concentrations in premenopausal women.

Case Report

The patient was a 25-year-old woman who had progressively increasing facial hair over the past 10 years. She had tried laser therapy but found the effects not optimal. Menarche was at age 11 years, and her menstrual cycles had always

been irregular. She had acne in her teenage years, but much less so now. She had no temporal scalp hair recession or increased hair on her breasts, abdomen, and back. She had no change in libido. Three months before referral, serum concentrations of DHEA-S and total testosterone were measured and found to be elevated at 565 mcg/dL (normal, 83–377 mcg/dL) and 76 ng/dL (normal, 8–60 ng/dL), respectively. The elevated DHEA-S was further evaluated with computed tomography (CT) scan of the abdomen (which showed normal-appearing adrenal glands) and transvaginal ovarian ultrasound (which showed normal sized ovaries with several cysts present). She was moderately overweight but had no recent weight gain. She had no signs or symptoms of Cushing syndrome. There was no history of hypertension or hypokalemia. She was taking no regular medications. On physical examination, her body mass index was 32.7 kg/m^2, blood pressure 118/76 mmHg, and heart rate 84 beats per minute. She had marked hirsutism on her chin and cheeks. The degree of hirsutism elsewhere was minimal to mild. Her Ferriman-Gallwey score was 11 (normal, <8; maximum = 36). She had no signs of scalp hair loss. External genitalia examination showed a normal appearing clitoris. There were no signs of glucocorticoid excess.

INVESTIGATIONS

Laboratory test results are shown in Table 88.1. The serum DHEA-S concentration remained elevated at 526 mcg/dL (normal, 83–377 mcg/dL). There was minimal elevation in serum testosterone. To determine if the source of DHEA-S hypersecretion was neoplastic, we completed a 7-day dexamethasone suppression test (DST): dexamethasone 0.5 mg at bedtime daily for 7 days and on the morning of day 8 serum DHEA-S

TABLE 88.1 **Laboratory Tests**		
Biochemical Test	**Result**	**Reference Range**
Sodium, mEq/L	140	135–145
Potassium, mEq/L	4.2	3.6–5.2
Creatinine, mg/dL	0.8	0.6–1.1
Total testosterone, ng/dL	72	8–60
Bioavailable testosterone, ng/dL	3.8	0.8–4.0
DHEA-S, mcg/dL	605	83–377
Androstenedione, ng/dL	122	30–200
LH, IU/L	9.0	1.9–14.6[a]
FSH, IU/L	5.2	2.9–14.6[a]
8 AM serum ACTH, pg/mL	20	10–60
8 AM serum cortisol, mcg/dL	14	7–25
4 PM serum cortisol, mcg/dL	7.2	2–14
Midnight salivary cortisol, ng/dL	<50	<100
24-Hour urine: Cortisol, mcg	18	3.5–45

[a]Follicular phase reference ranges are shown. *ACTH,* Corticotropin; *DHEA-S,* dehydroepiandrosterone sulfate; *FSH,* follicle-stimulating hormone; *LH,* luteinizing hormone.

was measured. With the 7-day DST, the serum DHEA-S concentration normalized to 103 mg/dL.

TREATMENT

The patient was reassured that she most likely had polycystic ovarian syndrome and that the elevation in DHEA-S was not caused by a tumor. Treatment options to manage her irregular menses and hirsutism were discussed.

OUTCOME AND FOLLOW-UP

The patient decided to start treatment with an oral contraceptive pill,[1] which resulted in regular menstrual cycles and normalization of serum testosterone concentration. The serum DHEA-S concentration (480 mcg/dL) decreased with this treatment but not into the normal range. Over the next 6 months, her degree of hirsutism improved to a mild degree and she then chose to start treatment with spironolactone.[1]

Discussion

The most common reason clinicians measure DHEA-S in the United States is not during the evaluation of an adrenal mass but rather in a premenopausal woman with hirsutism—and in that setting the serum DHEA-S concentration is frequently mildly to moderately elevated above the upper limit of the reference range. The reference range for DHEA-S in women changes based on age (Box 88.1). An elevated serum DHEA-S concentration in a premenopausal woman frequently leads to imaging studies of the adrenal glands and ovaries because of the concern about a neoplastic source—something only rarely found. The 1-week DST, described herein, is one approach to exclude a neoplastic source for the excess DHEA-S. It is not clear why these women have increased levels of DHEA-S. When germline genetic testing is performed, they do not have pathogenic variants in 3β-hydroxysteroid dehydrogenase gene (*3β-HSD2*). Mutations in *3β-HSD2* cause a rare form of congenital adrenal hyperplasia associated with deficiency in cortisol, aldosterone, and gonadal steroids, whereas the increased serum DHEA-S concentrations in premenopausal women with hirsutism seems to be due to inefficiency at the 3β-hydroxysteroid dehydrogenase step in steroid biosynthesis. The etiology of this inefficiency is not known. However, as demonstrated in this case, this benign cause of increased serum DHEA-S can be confirmed with the 1-week DST.

BOX 88.1 AGE-DEPENDENT REFERENCE RANGES FOR SERUM DEHYDROEPIANDROSTERONE SULFATE IN WOMEN[a]

Age Range, Years	**Reference Lower Limit, mcg/dL**	**Reference Upper Limit, mcg/dL**
18–30	83	377
31–40	45	295
41–50	27	240
51–60	16	195
61–70	9.7	159
≥71	5.3	124

[a]Reference ranges are reported by the Mayo Clinic Laboratories, https://www.mayocliniclabs.com/index.html

Key Points

- When the serum DHEA-S is suppressed in a patient with an adrenal mass, it suggests chronic suppression of pituitary ACTH secretion—a finding consistent with either subclinical glucocorticoid secretory autonomy or adrenal-dependent Cushing syndrome.
- When the serum DHEA-S concentration is markedly elevated in a patient with an adrenal mass, it is suggestive of an androgen-secreting adrenal tumor and frequently adrenocortical carcinoma and is a very useful biomarker in this setting.

- In premenopausal women with hirsutism, mild to moderate elevations in serum DHEA-S concentration are common and nonspecific. One approach in this setting is to exclude a tumorous source of DHEA hypersecretion with the 7-day DST.

REFERENCE

1. Martin KA, Anderson RR, Chang RJ, Ehrmann DA, Lobo RA, Murad MH, Pugeat MM, Rosenfield RL. Evaluation and treatment of hirsutism in premenopausal women: an endocrine society clinical practice guideline. *J Clin Endocrinol Metab*. 2018;103(4):1233–1257.

Sorting Out the Source of Androgen Excess in a Postmenopausal Woman With an Adrenal and an Ovarian Mass

Postmenopausal androgen hypersecretion may be due to an ovarian tumor, an adrenal tumor, or ovarian hyperthecosis. It is important to assess the patient with a full androgen profile and imaging studies of the ovaries and adrenal glands. When an adrenal tumor is identified in a postmenopausal woman with androgen excess, adrenal and gonadal venous sampling may be needed to localize the source of androgen hypersecretion.

Case Report

This 59-year-old woman was evaluated for weight management and was noted to have hirsutism on physical examination. She had no signs or symptoms of glucocorticoid excess. The patient had a long-standing history of mild facial hirsutism and noticed exacerbation of hirsutism and development of coarse facial features over several years before current presentation. She did not have acne but noticed oily skin. She had to shave daily. Her medical history was significant for rheumatoid arthritis treated with methotrexate and frequent courses of prednisone. She also had chronic depression, treated with duloxetine. Twenty years prior, she had hysterectomy and right oophorectomy (for menorrhagia). She did not have vasomotor symptoms to help estimate the onset of menopause. She was not treated with estrogen.

On physical examination her body mass index was 42.8 kg/m², blood pressure 134/72 mmHg, and heart rate 70 beats per minute. Hirsutism was evident over abdomen, chest, chin, back, and face. Her degree of hirsutism was marked with a modified Ferriman-Gallwey score of 30 (normal, <8; maximum, 36).

INVESTIGATIONS

Laboratory test results are shown in Table 89.1. Testosterone hypersecretion was documented. Transabdominal and endovaginal ultrasound of the pelvis showed a 2.2-cm solid left ovarian mass, also visualized on a pelvic CT (Fig. 89.1, right). Adrenal CT showed a 1.9-cm lipid rich left adrenal adenoma (see Fig. 89.1, left). The question was whether the source of testosterone hypersecretion was adrenal or ovarian. Adrenal and gonadal venous sampling was the next step. Adrenal venous sampling was performed without cosyntropin infusion. Testosterone concentration in the left gonadal vein was 100-fold higher than the testosterone concentration in the inferior vena cava, adrenal vein, and the right gonadal vein (Box 89.1). Testosterone hypersecretion from the left ovarian mass was confirmed.

TREATMENT

The patient underwent left salpingo-oophorectomy. Steroid cell tumor, 2.8 × 2.0 × 1.6 cm was demonstrated.

OUTCOME AND FOLLOW-UP

Two weeks after left oophorectomy the serum total testosterone was measured and was undetectable at <7 ng/dL (normal, 8–60 ng/dL).

TABLE 89.1	Laboratory Tests	
Biochemical Test	**Result**	**Reference Range**
Sodium, mEq/L	137	135–145
Potassium, mEq/L	4.2	3.6–5.2
Creatinine, mg/dL	0.96	0.6–1.1
Total testosterone, ng/dL	510	8–60
Androstenedione, ng/dL	113	30–200
Corticotropin, pg/mL	9.4	7.2–63
DHEA-S, mcg/dL	128	15–157
17-hydroxyprogesterone, ng/dL	119	Postmenopausal: <51
LH, IU/L	18	Postmenopausal: 5.3–65.4
FSH, IU/L	25	Postmenopausal: 16–157
Estradiol, pg/mL	28	Postmenopausal: <10
Aldosterone, ng/dL	9.9	≤21
Renin plasma activity, ng/mL per hour	1.3	0.6–3
1-mg overnight DST cortisol, mcg/dL	2.2	<1.8 mcg/dL
24-Hour urine cortisol, mcg	40	3.5–45

DHEA-S, Dehydroepiandrosterone-sulfate; *DST,* dexamethasone suppression; *FSH,* follicle-stimulating hormone; *LH,* luteinizing hormone.

Discussion

Postmenopausal hyperandrogenism is a diagnostic and therapeutic challenge and imaging studies may be misleading.[1] Androgen hypersecretion may be due to an ovarian tumor, an adrenal tumor, or ovarian hyperthecosis. It is important to assess the patient with a full androgen profile and imaging studies of the ovaries and adrenal glands. When an adrenal tumor is identified in a postmenopausal woman with androgen excess, adrenal and gonadal venous sampling may be needed to localize the source of androgen hypersecretion. In this case, both an adrenal and an ovarian tumor were visible on imaging. As suspected, adrenal and gonadal venous sampling confirmed ovarian origin, and pathology confirmed a steroid cell ovarian neoplasm. Ovarian steroid cell tumors are rare, comprising <0.1% of all ovarian tumors. Majority of ovarian steroid cell tumors occur in young women, but postmenopausal onset has been described.[1,2] Treatment of choice is oophorectomy, and prognosis in general is excellent.

Key Points

- Postmenopausal androgen hypersecretion may be due to an ovarian tumor, an adrenal tumor, or ovarian hyperthecosis.

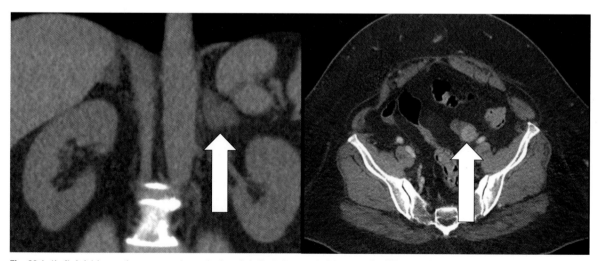

Fig. 89.1 (*Left*) Axial image from an unenhanced adrenal-dedicated computed tomography (CT) scan shows a 1.9 × 1.2–cm left adrenal mass (*arrows*). On unenhanced CT the mass was lipid rich (–9 Hounsfield units [HU]). (*Right*) Coronal image from a contrast-enhanced CT scan demonstrating a 2.2 × 2.7–cm left enhancing solid ovarian mass. The patient had a prior hysterectomy and right salpingo-oophorectomy.

BOX 89.1 ADRENAL AND GONADAL VENOUS SAMPLING

	Right AV	IVC	Left AV	Right Gonadal	Left Gonadal
Testosterone, ng/dL	236	296	250	311	24,700
Cortisol, mcg/dL	16	6	15		

AV, Adrenal vein; *IVC,* inferior vena cava.

- When an adrenal tumor is identified in a post-menopausal woman with androgen excess, adrenal and gonadal venous sampling may be needed to localize the source of androgen hypersecretion.

REFERENCES

1. Durmus Y, Kilic C, Cakir C, et al. Sertoli-Leydig cell tumor of the ovary: analysis of a single institution database and review of the literature. *J Obstet Gynaecol Res.* 2019;45(7):1311–1318.
2. Young RH, Scully RE. Ovarian Sertoli-Leydig cell tumors. a clinicopathological analysis of 207 cases. *Am J Surg Pathol.* 1985;9(8):543–569.

Primary Testosterone-Secreting Adrenocortical Carcinoma in a Premenopausal Woman

Androgen hypersecretion in a premenopausal woman may be due to an ovarian tumor, an adrenal tumor, polycystic ovarian syndrome, or nonclassic congenital adrenal hyperplasia. The expansiveness of the diagnostic evaluation of a woman with androgen excess is dependent on the clinical situation and the degree of androgen hypersecretion. For example, adrenal gland imaging is not needed when the signs and symptoms related to androgen excess are chronic and mild and serum testosterone concentration is mildly increased in a woman with a typical history of polycystic ovarian syndrome. However, with more abrupt onset of marked signs and symptoms and more marked increases in serum testosterone concentrations, it is important to assess the patient with a full androgen profile and imaging studies of the ovaries and adrenal glands. When an adrenal tumor with a suspicious imaging phenotype is identified in a woman with androgen excess, it should be determined if other adrenocortical hormones are also being autonomously secreted. Herein we present a case of a patient with a nearly pure testosterone-secreting adrenocortical carcinoma (ACC).

Case Report

The patient was a 44-year-old woman seen for progressive hirsutism over the prior 2 years. Her self-graded Ferriman-Gallwey score was 25 (normal, <8; maximum = 36). She also had marked androgenic scalp hair loss. The patient had lifelong regular menstrual cycles until 5 months ago, when they became irregular. She has also had treatment-resistant hypertension diagnosed 3 years ago. An abdominal computed tomography (CT) scan, obtained as part of her secondary hypertension evaluation, detected a 2.6 × 2.9 × 2.7–cm left adrenal mass with suspicious imaging characteristics (Fig. 90.1). Although she was overweight, her body weight had been stable. She had no signs or symptoms of Cushing syndrome. There was no history of hypokalemia. Her medications included amlodipine, 5 mg daily; hydrochlorothiazide, 25 mg daily; and spironolactone, 100 mg daily. On physical examination, her body mass index was 36 kg/m², blood pressure 176/104 mmHg, and heart rate 89 beats per minute. She had marked hirsutism and male pattern balding, but she was not virilized.

INVESTIGATIONS

Laboratory test results are shown in Table 90.1. Marked testosterone hypersecretion was documented. Although the midnight salivary cortisol concentration and the 24-hour urinary cortisol excretion were normal, the serum corticotropin concentration was low-normal and a 2-mg overnight dexamethasone suppression test documented glucocorticoid secretory autonomy. These data were consistent with dominant testosterone hypersecretion and mild autonomous cortisol cosecretion. Although the adrenal mass was relatively small, the imaging phenotype on CT scan and the plurihormonal pattern on laboratory testing favored an ACC.

TREATMENT

The patient was treated with perioperative glucocorticoid coverage and underwent laparoscopic left adrenalectomy. The tumor proved to be a

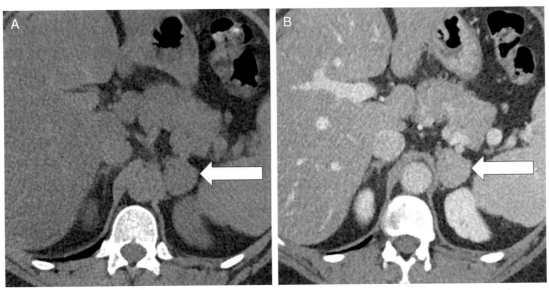

Fig. 90.1 Axial images from an abdominal CT scan demonstrate a 2.6 × 2.9 × 2.7 cm left adrenal mass. (A) Unenhanced CT image shows a lipid poor (31.8 Hounsfield units) adrenal mass (*arrow*). (B) Contrast-enhanced CT image shows moderate contrast enhancement in the adrenal mass (*arrow*).

3.3 × 2.8 × 2.2–cm well-differentiated ACC with oncocytic features (Fig. 90.2). She was discharged from the hospital on 5 mg of prednisone every morning.

OUTCOME AND FOLLOW-UP

Ten days after the left adrenalectomy the serum total testosterone normalized at 9.5 ng/dL (normal, 8–60 ng/dL). One month after surgery the morning serum cortisol concentration was 11 mcg/dL (normal, 7–25 mcg/dL), and treatment with prednisone was discontinued. There was dramatic improvement in her degree of hirsutism over the next 6 months, and regular menstrual cycles returned. She was followed with serial measurement of serum testosterone and CT imaging of the chest, abdomen, and pelvis. At last follow-up, 4 years after surgery, the serum testosterone concentration was normal at 10 ng/dL and CT of the chest, abdomen, and pelvis showed no evidence of tumor recurrence.

Key Points

- Premenopausal androgen hypersecretion may be due to an ovarian tumor, an adrenal tumor, polycystic ovarian syndrome, or nonclassic congenital adrenal hyperplasia. The evaluation should be

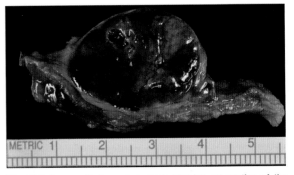

Fig. 90.2 Gross pathology photograph showing cut section of the 3.3 × 2.8 × 2.2–cm well-differentiated ACC that had oncocytic features on microscopy. The adrenal weighed 14 g (normal, 4–5 g). Immunoperoxidase studies showed that the tumor cells were diffusely positive for Melan-A with rare cells staining for calretinin, supporting the diagnosis of a primary adrenal cortical tumor. Ki-67 labeling index was low (<5%), and mitotic activity was not prominent. However, venous invasion and capsular invasion were present, along with nuclear atypia and focal degenerative changes. The oncocytic nature of the tumor in conjunction with venous and capsular invasion led to classification as carcinoma.

guided by the chronicity of signs and symptoms and the degree of androgen excess.[1,2]
- Approximately 50% of patients with ACC present with symptoms and signs of hormone excess.[1]

TABLE 90.1 Laboratory Tests		
Biochemical Test	**Result**	**Reference Range**
Sodium, mEq/L	142	135–145
Potassium, mEq/L	4.6	3.6–5.2
Creatinine, mg/dL	0.8	0.6–1.1
Aldosterone, ng/dL per hour	6.9	<21
Plasma renin activity, ng/Ml per hour	1.6	<0.6–3.0
Total testosterone, ng/dL	412	8–60
Free testosterone, ng/dL	16	0.06–0.095
Bioavailable testosterone, ng/dL	185	<10
DHEA-S, mcg/dL	160	27–240
17-Hydroxyprogesterone, ng/dL	84	<285
8 AM serum ACTH, pg/mL	11	10–60
8 AM serum cortisol, mcg/dL	12	725
Midnight salivary cortisol, ng/dL	<50	<100
2-mg overnight DST cortisol, mcg/dL	9.3	<1.8 mcg/dL
Plasma metanephrine, nmol/L	<0.2	<0.5
Plasma normetanephrine, nmol/L	0.66	<0.9
24-Hour urine:		
Cortisol, mcg	11	3.5–45
Metanephrine, mcg	49	<400
Normetanephrine, mcg	206	<900
Norepinephrine, mcg	25	<80
Epinephrine, mcg	1	<20
Dopamine, mcg	137	<400

ACTH, Corticotropin; *DHEA-S,* dehydroepiandrosterone sulfate; *DST,* dexamethasone suppression test.

When secretory, ACCs most commonly hypersecrete glucocorticoids and adrenal androgens.[3]
• There are exceptional cases of ACC associated with predominant monohormonal hypersecretion as seen in this case and Case 29.

REFERENCES

1. Di Dalmazi G. Hyperandrogenism and adrenocortical tumors. *Front Horm Res.* 2019;53:92–99.
2. Tong A, Jiang J, Wang F, Li C, Zhang Y, Wu X. Pure androgen-producing adrenal tumor: clinical features and pathogenesis. *Endocr Pract.* 2017;23(4):399–407.
3. Else T, Kim AC, Sabolch A, et al. Adrenocortical carcinoma. *Endocr Rev.* 2014;35(2):282–326.

Premenopausal Woman With Testosterone-Secreting Ovarian Tumor

Androgen hypersecretion in a premenopausal woman may be due to an ovarian tumor, an adrenal tumor, polycystic ovarian syndrome, or nonclassic congenital adrenal hyperplasia. The expansiveness of the diagnostic evaluation of a woman with androgen excess is dependent on the clinical situation and the degree of androgen hypersecretion. Herein we present a case of a patient with abrupt onset of marked hirsutism as a result of a testosterone-secreting Sertoli-Leydig cell tumor of the ovary.

Case Report

This 25-year-old woman was doing reasonably well until 18 years of age, when she noticed some increased amount of hair on her chin. Two years ago she noticed the hair was becoming significantly worse on the chin and neck, and then about 1 year ago she noticed onset of hair growth over her entire chest and abdomen, increased dense hair on her forearms, increased hair on the upper arms, and the onset of secondary amenorrhea. She had not noticed any change in scalp hair, the pitch of her voice, libido, skin oiliness, or acne. She did note that it was easier to tone her muscles with weight training. She had normal blood pressure and no signs or symptoms of Cushing syndrome. An evaluation 4 months before referral showed a total testosterone of 349 ng/dL (normal, 8–60 ng/dL) and an ovarian ultrasound that showed prominent-sized ovaries but no mass. On physical examination her body mass index was 23.7 kg/m², blood pressure 115/57 mmHg, and heart rate 58 beats per minute. Her degree of hirsutism was marked with a modified Ferriman-Gallwey score of 28 (normal, <8; maximum 36) (Fig. 91.1). Clitoromegaly was not present. She had no signs or symptoms of Cushing syndrome.

INVESTIGATIONS

Laboratory test results are shown in Table 91.1. Marked testosterone and androstenedione hypersecretion was documented. An abdominal computed tomography (CT) scan showed micronodular changes in both adrenal glands. Transvaginal ultrasound showed the right ovary to be enlarged and a 1.7 cm × 2.4 cm × 2–cm complex cystic area within the right ovary with an appearance consistent with a hemorrhagic corpus luteum cyst, or, in this specific patient, potentially a testosterone-producing ovarian tumor (Fig. 91.2). Venous sampling of the adrenal and gonadal veins was nonlocalizing (Box 91.1). In general, we have had good success with gonadal venous sampling in women

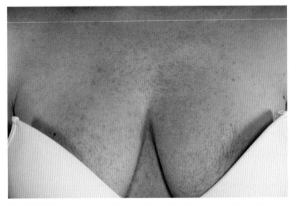

Fig. 91.1 Photograph of patient's chest showing marked hirsutism.

TABLE 91.1   Laboratory Test

Biochemical Test	Result	Reference Range
Sodium, mEq/L	140	135–145
Potassium, mEq/L	4.4	3.6–5.2
Creatinine, mg/dL	0.9	0.7–1.2
Total testosterone, ng/dL	392	8–60
Free testosterone, ng/dL	10.6	0.3–1.9
Bioavailable testosterone, ng/dL	243	0.8–10
Androstenedione, ng/dL	944	30–200
Estradiol, pg/mL	50	Premenopausal: 15–350
LH, IU/L	13.2	Luteal: 0.7–12.9

[a]Blood concentrations of DHEA-S and 17-hydroxyprogesterone were normal.
DHEA-S, Dehydroepiandrosterone-sulfate; *LH,* luteinizing hormone.

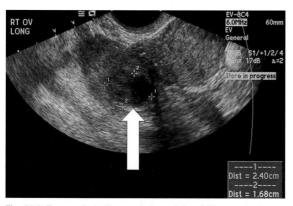

Fig. 91.2 Transvaginal ultrasound showed the right ovary to be enlarged (5 cm × 3 cm × 3.7 cm). There was a 1.7 × 2.4 × 2–cm complex cystic area (*arrow*) within the enlarged right ovary with an appearance consistent with a hemorrhagic corpus luteum cyst, or, in this specific patient, potentially a testosterone-producing ovarian tumor.

BOX 91.1   ADRENAL AND GONADAL VENOUS SAMPLING[a]

	Right AV	IVC	Left AV	Right Gonadal	Left Gonadal
Testosterone, ng/dL	504	223	491	669	316
Cortisol, mcg/dL	660	28	860		

[a]Sequential AVS completed under continuous cosyntropin infusion 50 mcg/h. *AV,* Adrenal vein; *IVC,* inferior vena cava.

with an ovarian source of androgen excess (e.g., see Case 92). However, gonadal venous sampling, just like adrenal venous sampling, lacks 100% accuracy. F-18 fluorodeoxyglucose (FDG) positron emission tomography (PET) showed mild FDG avidity in the right ovary (Fig. 91.3).

TREATMENT

Based on the findings on FDG-PET and ovarian ultrasound, a right salpingo-oophorectomy was performed. The right ovary contained a differentiated Sertoli-Leydig cell tumor (4.2 × 2.7 × 2.3 cm) associated with ovarian stromal hyperplasia (Fig. 91.4). Right pelvic

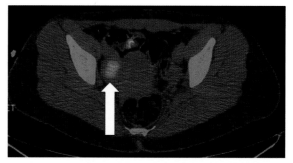

Fig. 91.3 Axial image from F-18 fluorodeoxyglucose (FDG) positron emission tomography showed mild FDG-avidity in right ovary (*arrow*).

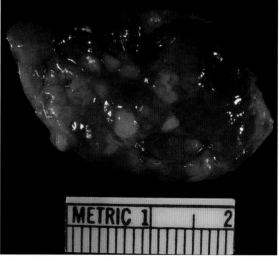

Fig. 91.4 Gross pathology photograph showing cut section of the right ovary containing an intermediately differentiated Sertoli-Leydig cell tumor (4.2 × 2.7 × 2.3 cm) associated with ovarian stromal hyperplasia.

and periaortic lymphadenectomy was performed, and 33 lymph nodes were negative for tumor involvement.

OUTCOME AND FOLLOW-UP

Three days after right salpingo-oophorectomy the serum total testosterone normalized at 11 ng/dL (normal, 8–60 ng/dL). One month after surgery the serum total testosterone was 27 ng/dL. There was dramatic improvement in her degree of hirsutism over the next 6 months, and regular menstrual cycles returned. One year later the serum total testosterone was 19 ng/dL. At last follow-up, 15 years later, her menstrual cycles were regular and she had no symptomatic or biochemical evidence for tumor recurrence.

Discussion

Sertoli-Leydig cell tumors are rare ovarian malignancies with low recurrence rates and are associated with favorable outcomes. Surgical resection with fertility-sparing operations in young patients is the treatment of choice. In an institutional series of 17 patients with Sertoli-Leydig tumors, the median age was 30 years (range, 18–67 years).[1] The patient described herein was the subject of an "Imaging in Endocrinology"

article in the *Journal of Clinical Endocrinology and Metabolism* in 2006.[2]

Key Points

- Premenopausal androgen hypersecretion may be due to an ovarian tumor, an adrenal tumor, polycystic ovarian syndrome, or nonclassic congenital adrenal hyperplasia. The evaluation should be guided by the chronicity of signs and symptoms and the degree of androgen excess.[1,2]
- Sertoli-Leydig cell tumors are rare ovarian malignancies that can be challenging to localize. FDG-PET can be used in the localization of testosterone-secreting neoplasms when CT, ultrasound, and venous sampling studies are inconclusive.

REFERENCES

1. Durmuş Y, Kılıç Ç, Çakır C, et al. Sertoli-Leydig cell tumor of the ovary: analysis of a single institution database and review of the literature. *J Obstet Gynaecol Res.* 2019;45(7):1311–1318.
2. Mattsson C, Stanhope CR, Sam S, Young WF Jr. Image in endocrinology: testosterone-secreting ovarian tumor localized with (fluorine-18)-2-deoxyglucose positron emission tomography. *J Clin Endocrinol Metab.* 2006;91(3):738–739.

Sorting Out the Source of Androgen Excess in a Postmenopausal Woman With an Adrenal Mass

Postmenopausal androgen hypersecretion may be due to an ovarian tumor, an adrenal tumor, or ovarian hyperthecosis. It is important to assess the patient with a full androgen profile and imaging studies of the ovaries and adrenal glands. When an adrenal tumor is identified in a postmenopausal woman with androgen excess, adrenal and gonadal venous sampling may be needed to localize the source of androgen hypersecretion. Herein we present such a case.

Case Report

This 71-year-old woman had an abdominal computed tomography (CT) scan to investigate non-specific abdominal discomfort, and a 3.4-cm right adrenal mass was incidentally discovered (Fig. 92.1). She had no signs or symptoms of glucocorticoid or catecholamine hypersecretion. However, the patient had long-standing hirsutism primarily affecting the extremities and the suprapubic area. Starting 3 years previously, she experienced a steady and progressive increase in her hirsutism—affecting the whole anterior abdomen, anterior chest, chin, upper lip, and her back. She shaved her chin and upper lip every day and her abdomen and chest twice a week. She did not have acne or change in secondary sex characteristics or libido. She had two biologic children. Menopause occurred at 52 years of age, and she was not treated with estrogen or progesterone replacement. She had a 5-year history of hypertension treated with monotherapy (ramipril, 20 mg daily). There was no history of hypokalemia. On physical examination her body mass index was

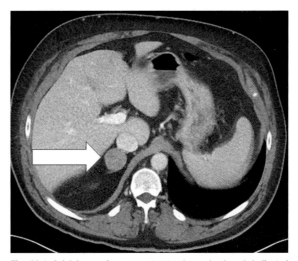

Fig. 92.1 Axial image from a contrast-enhanced adrenal-dedicated computed tomography (CT) scan shows a 3.4 × 2.8–cm oval right adrenal mass (*arrow*). On unenhanced CT the mass was lipid rich (–2.9 Hounsfield units).

31.8 kg/m^2, blood pressure 142/70 mmHg, and heart rate 70 beats per minute. Her degree of hirsutism was marked with a modified Ferriman-Gallwey score of 33 (normal, <8; maximum = 36). Clitoromegaly was present (2.5 cm × 1 cm).

INVESTIGATIONS

Laboratory test results are shown in Table 92.1. Pure testosterone hypersecretion was documented. Transabdominal and endovaginal ultrasound of the pelvis showed a 1.3-cm partially calcified fibroid in the uterine fundus and normal-appearing endometrial stripe, and both ovaries appeared normal. The question was whether the source of testosterone hypersecretion

TABLE 92.1	Laboratory Tests	
Biochemical Test	**Result**	**Reference Range**
Sodium, mEq/L	142	135–145
Potassium, mEq/L	4.9	3.6–5.2
Creatinine, mg/dL	1.2	0.6–1.1
Total testosterone, ng/dL	417	8–60
Free testosterone, ng/dL	60	0.3–1.9
Androstenedione, ng/dL	89	30–200
DHEA-S, mcg/dL	39.5	15–157
17-Hydroxyprogesterone, ng/dL	91	Postmenopausal: <51
LH, IU/L	22.1	Postmenopausal: 5.3–65.4
FSH, IU/L	71.1	Postmenopausal: 16–157
Estradiol, pg/mL	11	Postmenopausal: <10
Aldosterone, ng/dL	7.9	≤21
1-mg overnight DST cortisol, mcg/dL	1.8	<1.8 mcg/dL
24-Hour urine cortisol, mcg	6.1	3.5–45

BSA, Body surface area; *DHEA-S*, dehydroepiandrosterone sulfate; *DST*, dexamethasone suppression test; *FSH*, follicle-stimulating hormone; *LH*, luteinizing hormone.

was adrenal or ovarian. Adrenal and gonadal venous sampling was the next step. Adrenal venous sampling was successful based on adrenal vein-to–inferior vena cava (IVC) cortisol gradients of more to 5-to-1 (Box 92.1). The adrenal vein testosterone concentrations, proportionate to cortisol concentrations, were less than that in the IVC—confirming that the source of excess testosterone was not adrenal in origin. On the other hand, the testosterone concentrations in the right and left gonadal veins were 27-fold and 22-fold

BOX 92.1 ADRENAL AND GONADAL VENOUS SAMPLING[a]

	Right AV	IVC	Left AV	Right Gonadal	Left Gonadal
Testosterone, ng/dL	1070	223	550	6030	5010
Cortisol, mcg/dL	2460	52	391		

[a]Sequential AVS completed under continuous cosyntropin infusion 50 mcg/h. *AV*, Adrenal vein; *IVC*, inferior vena cava.

higher, respectively, than the testosterone concentration in the IVC (see Box 92.1). Bilateral ovarian testosterone hypersecretion was confirmed and consistent with hyperthecosis.

TREATMENT

The patient underwent vaginal hysterectomy and bilateral salpingo-oophorectomy. The uterus had atrophic endometrium and five intramural leiomyoma (ranging in size from 0.3 to 2.1 cm in greatest dimension). The ovaries showed bilateral diffuse stromal hyperplasia (Fig. 92.2).

OUTCOME AND FOLLOW-UP

Three days after bilateral oophorectomy the serum total testosterone normalized at 33 ng/dL (normal, 8–60 ng/dL).

Discussion

Postmenopausal hyperandrogenism is a diagnostic and therapeutic challenge, and imaging studies may be misleading.[1] Androgen hypersecretion may be due to an ovarian tumor (frequently too small to be visualized on transvaginal ultrasound), an adrenal tumor (always visible on CT), or ovarian hyperthecosis (seen as enlarged or normal-appearing ovaries on transvaginal ultrasound). It is important to assess the patient with a full androgen profile and imaging studies of the ovaries and adrenal glands. When an adrenal tumor is identified in a postmenopausal woman with androgen excess, adrenal and gonadal venous sampling may be needed to localize the source of androgen hypersecretion.

Ovarian hyperthecosis is characterized by the abundant ovarian luteinized theca cells that secrete androgens, and it is the most common cause of severe hyperandrogenism in postmenopausal women. Ovarian hyperthecosis may go undetected on ovarian ultrasound. Hysterectomy with bilateral salpingo-oophorectomy is the treatment of choice. In a retrospective study at a tertiary center, 34 postmenopausal women were diagnosed with either virilizing ovarian tumor (38%) or ovarian hyperthecosis (62%).[2] Clinical signs of hyperandrogenism were more prevalent in those with virilizing ovarian tumors than the hyperthecosis group. In addition, the virilizing ovarian

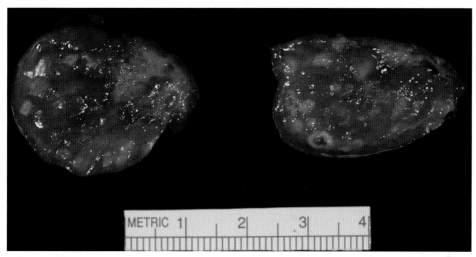

Fig. 92.2 Gross pathology photograph showing cut sections of both ovaries, which demonstrate diffuse stromal hyperplasia.

tumor group had higher testosterone and estradiol levels and lower gonadotropin levels than the hyperthecosis group (although there was marked overlap in the two groups).[2]

Key Points

- Postmenopausal androgen hypersecretion may be due to an ovarian tumor, an adrenal tumor, or ovarian hyperthecosis.
- If adrenal CT is normal in a woman with postmenopausal androgen hypersecretion, she almost certainly has an ovarian source and most frequently bilateral ovarian hyperthecosis.

- When an adrenal tumor is identified in a postmenopausal woman with androgen excess, adrenal and gonadal venous sampling may be needed to localize the source of androgen hypersecretion.

REFERENCES

1. Mamoojee Y, Ganguri M, Taylor N, Quinton R. Clinical case seminar: postmenopausal androgen excess-challenges in diagnostic work-up and management of ovarian thecosis. *Clin Endocrinol (Oxf)*. 2018;88(1):13–20.

2. Yance VRV, Marcondes JAM, Rocha MP, et al. Discriminating between virilizing ovary tumors and ovary hyperthecosis in postmenopausal women: clinical data, hormonal profiles and image studies. *Eur J Endocrinol*. 2017;177(1):93–102.

Testosterone-Secreting Benign Adrenal Adenoma in a Postmenopausal Woman

Androgen hypersecretion in postmenopausal women may be due to an ovarian tumor, an adrenal tumor, ovarian hyperthecosis, or nonclassic congenital adrenal hyperplasia. The expansiveness of the diagnostic evaluation of a woman with androgen excess is dependent on the clinical situation and the degree of androgen hypersecretion. When there is an abrupt onset of marked signs and symptoms and marked increases in serum testosterone concentrations, it is important to assess the patient with a full androgen profile and imaging studies of the ovaries and adrenal glands. When an adrenal tumor with a suspicious imaging phenotype is identified in a woman with androgen excess, it should be determined if other adrenocortical hormones are also being autonomously secreted. Herein we present an unusual case a pure testosterone-secreting adrenal adenoma.

Case Report

The patient was a 52-year-old woman who started noticing increasing facial hair 18 months before referral to Mayo Clinic. She was treated with laser therapy but found she had to repeat the treatment every 3 weeks. Over the past 1 year her symptoms progressed and she noticed new acne, temporal scalp hair recession, and increased hair on her breasts, abdomen, and back. She noticed that when she lifted weights that it took less weightlifting to maintain her muscle bulk and tone. She had also noted increased libido and enlargement of her clitoris. Three months before referral, serum testosterone was measured and found to be markedly elevated at 334 ng/dL (normal, 8–60 ng/dL), and this

led to a computed tomography (CT) scan of the abdomen, which detected a 2.8 × 3.5–cm right adrenal mass (Fig. 93.1). Her medical history was significant for total

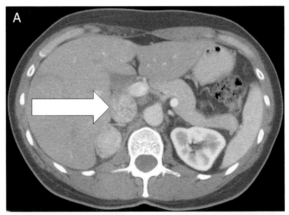

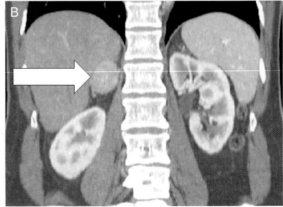

Fig. 93.1 Contrast-enhanced images from an abdominal computed tomography (CT) scan (A, axial plane; B, coronal plane) demonstrate a 2.8 × 3.5–cm heterogeneously enhancing right adrenal gland mass (*arrows*). The unenhanced CT attenuation was 36.6 Hounsfield units.

hysterectomy and bilateral salpingo-oophorectomy 5 years previously for the treatment of uterine fibroids (estrogen replacement therapy was initiated postoperatively). She was at ideal body weight. She had no signs or symptoms of Cushing syndrome. There was no history of hypokalemia. Her medications included piperazine estrone sulfate, 1.5 mg daily, and levothyroxine, 88 mcg daily.

On physical examination, her body mass index was 21.7 kg/m², blood pressure 135/85 mmHg, and heart rate 57 beats per minute. She had marked hirsutism on her chin, abdomen, and pelvis. Her Ferriman-Gallwey score was 17 (normal, <8; maximum = 36). She also had mild androgenic scalp hair loss. External genitalia examination showed a prominent clitoris. There were no signs of glucocorticoid excess.

INVESTIGATIONS

Laboratory test results are shown in Table 93.1. Marked testosterone and androstenedione hypersecretion was documented. The patient had testosterone-associated polycythemia. Measurements of glucocorticoids and mineralocorticoids were normal. Despite the suspicious imaging phenotype on CT scan, the monohormonal hypersecretion favored a benign testosterone-secreting adrenal adenoma.

TREATMENT

The patient underwent laparoscopic right adrenalectomy. The tumor proved to be a 4.2 cm × 3.1 cm × 2.2 cm adrenal adenoma (Fig. 93.2).

TABLE 93.1	Laboratory Tests	
Biochemical Test	Result	Reference Range
Sodium, mEq/L	140	135–145
Potassium, mEq/L	4.9	3.6–5.2
Creatinine, mg/dL	0.9	0.6–1.1
Hemoglobin, g/dL	16.2	12–15.5
Hematocrit, %	47.5	34.9–44.5
Aldosterone, ng/dL	6.1	<21
Plasma renin activity, ng/mL per hour	1.7	<0.6–3.0
Total testosterone, ng/dL	418	8–60
Bioavailable testosterone, ng/dL	75	0.8–4.0
DHEA-S, mcg/dL	214	15–200
Androstenedione, ng/dL	1240	30–200
8 AM serum ACTH, pg/mL	10	10–60
8 AM serum cortisol, mcg/dL	13	7–25
4 PM serum cortisol, mcg/dL	9.1	2–14
Midnight salivary cortisol, ng/dL	78	<100
24-Hour urine:		
Cortisol, mcg	8.4	3.5–45

ACTH, Corticotropin; *DHEA-S*, dehydroepiandrosterone sulfate.

OUTCOME AND FOLLOW-UP

The day after the right adrenalectomy the serum total testosterone normalized at 11 ng/dL (normal, 8–60 ng/dL). To confirm the benign nature of this adrenal mass, she was advised to have serum testosterone checked every

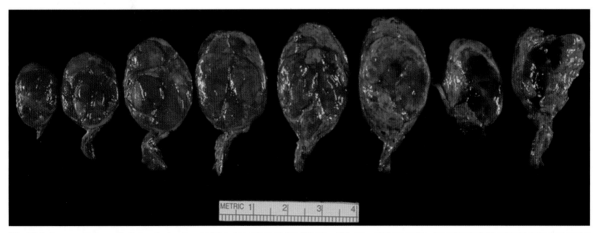

Fig. 93.2 Gross pathology photograph showing serial cut sections of the 4.2 cm × 3.1 cm × 2.2 cm yellow-to-orange right adrenal adenoma and a small portion of normal adrenal gland. The adrenal weighed 18.8 g (normal, 4–5 g).

3 months for 1 year, then every 4 months for 1 year, then every 6 months for 5 years. At last follow-up, 8 years after surgery, the serum testosterone concentration was normal and magnetic resonance imaging of the abdomen showed no evidence of tumor recurrence.

Key Points

- Postmenopausal androgen hypersecretion may be due to an ovarian tumor, an adrenal tumor, ovarian hyperthecosis, or nonclassic congenital adrenal hyperplasia. The evaluation should be guided by the chronicity of signs and symptoms and the degree of androgen excess.[1-3]
- Most androgen-secreting adrenal tumors prove to be adrenocortical carcinoma (ACC). A clue to likely ACC in this setting is plurihormonal hypersecretion (i.e., in addition to androgens, ACCs hypersecrete glucocorticoids and mineralocorticoids).[3] This knowledge led to the development urine steroid metabolomics as a biomarker tool for detecting malignancy in adrenal tumors (see Case 24).[4] A recent study showed that tumor diameter >4 cm, an unenhanced CT tumor attenuation cutoff of >20 Hounsfield units, and urine steroid metabolomics improved the detection of ACC.[5]

REFERENCES

1. Di Dalmazi G. Hyperandrogenism and adrenocortical tumors. *Front Horm Res.* 2019;53:92–99.
2. Tong A, Jiang J, Wang F, Li C, Zhang Y, Wu X. Pure androgen-producing adrenal tumor: clinical features and pathogenesis. *Endocr Pract.* 2017;23(4):399–407.
3. Else T, Kim AC, Sabolch A, et al. Adrenocortical carcinoma. *Endocr Rev.* 2014;35(2):282–326.
4. Arlt W, Biehl M, Taylor AE, et al. Urine steroid metabolomics as a biomarker tool for detecting malignancy in adrenal tumors. *J Clin Endocrinol Metab.* 2011;96(12):3775–3784.
5. Bancos I, Taylor AE, Chortis V, et al. Urine steroid metabolomics for the differential diagnosis of adrenal incidentalomas in the EURINE-ACT study: a prospective test validation study. *Lancet Diabetes Endocrinol.* 2020;8(9):773–781.

Adrenal Disorders in Pregnancy

An underlying theme of this book is that the evaluation and management of adrenal gland–related disorders can be complex and challenging for the clinician. When adrenal disease is diagnosed in the setting of pregnancy, the complexity index increases more than 10-fold.

In Cases 94, 95, and 96 we highlight the diagnosis and management of pheochromocytoma or paraganglioma (PPGL) in the setting of pregnancy. Catecholamine-secreting PPGL in the setting of pregnancy is a high-risk scenario for both mother and fetus.[1] This scenario can be managed successfully with adrenergic blockade and elective cesarean section and delaying resection of the PPGL for several weeks postpartum. Another treatment option for adrenal pheochromocytoma is laparoscopic adrenalectomy during the second trimester. Metastatic pheochromocytoma is not a contraindication to pregnancy, with the exceptions of a high burden of disease or rapidly progressive disease.[1]

In Cases 97, 98, and 99 we discuss the diagnosis and management of glucocorticoid excess, glucocorticoid deficiency, and congenital adrenal hyperplasia in the setting of pregnancy. Each of these disorders is fraught with management pitfalls that require careful navigation.

The diagnostic and treatment challenges of primary aldosteronism (PA) in the setting of pregnancy are highlighted in Case 100. PA in the setting of pregnancy is a high-risk scenario for both mother and fetus.[2] The most frequent complication is superimposed preeclampsia, which, in some cases, leads to preterm delivery. The optimal way to prevent this difficult clinical scenario is a broader awareness of PA by clinicians and patients, which should lead to pre-pregnancy diagnosis and treatment. All woman with hypertension in their reproductive years should have case detection testing for PA, especially before starting a family. Case detection testing for PA in pregnancy is the same as in nonpregnant women. However, captopril, computed tomography, and adrenal venous sampling should be avoided. Patients with PA in the setting of pregnancy can be managed successfully with standard antihypertensive medications and potassium supplementation. Another treatment option is laparoscopic adrenalectomy during the second trimester, assuming that a unilateral adrenal macroadenoma is identified on magnetic resonance imaging.. Treatment with spironolactone should be avoided.

REFERENCES

1. Bancos I, Atkinson E, Eng C, Young WF Jr, Neumann HPH; International Pheochromocytoma and Pregnancy Study Group. Maternal and fetal outcomes in phaeochromocytoma and pregnancy: a multicentre retrospective cohort study and systematic review of literature. *Lancet Diabetes Endocrinol.* 2021;9(1):13–21.
2. Zelinka T, Petrák O, Rosa J, Holaj R, Štrauch B, Widimský J Jr. Primary aldosteronism and pregnancy. *Kidney Blood Press Res.* 2020;45(2):275–285.

Malignant Pheochromocytoma in Pregnancy

As we have highlighted in the other cases, the clinical management of catecholamine-secreting pheochromocytomas or paragangliomas (PPGLs) can be challenging—both diagnostically and therapeutically. However, when PPGL is diagnosed in the setting of pregnancy, the complexity rises more than 10-fold. Herein we share a case of a patient in whom recurrent and malignant pheochromocytoma was diagnosed during pregnancy.

Case Report

This 28-year-old woman was referred to Mayo Clinic during her 13th week of pregnancy for recurrent and malignant pheochromocytoma. She was first seen at Mayo Clinic 8 years previously (at 20 years of age) when she presented with a 1-year history of recurrent paroxysms of nausea, vomiting, headaches, and palpitations. The symptoms proved to be due to a right adrenal pheochromocytoma. The preoperative plasma normetanephrine was 21.2 nmol/L (normal, <0.9) and plasma metanephrine was 18.7 nmol/L (normal, <0.5). The abdominal computed tomography (CT) scan showed a heterogeneous necrotic 6.5-cm right adrenal mass (Fig. 94.1). At open laparotomy the 7.3 × 7.8 × 4.9–cm right adrenal pheochromocytoma was resected without complication or tumor capsule violation (Fig. 94.2). The postoperative plasma fractionated metanephrine levels were normal. Germline genetic testing was discussed, and the patient declined to pursue because of lack of insurance coverage. She had annual biochemical testing to screen for recurrent pheochromocytoma, and it was normal until her last test, which was done 2 years before the current consultation. Spells started

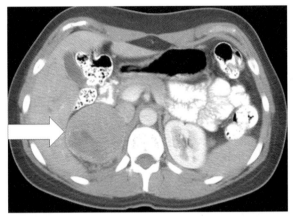

Fig. 94.1 Axial image from a contrast-enhanced computed tomography scan showed a heterogeneous necrotic 6.5-cm right adrenal mass (*arrow*).

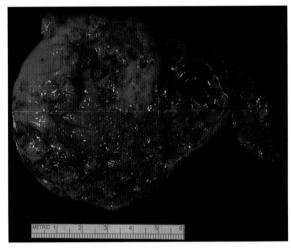

Fig. 94.2 Gross pathology photograph of cut section of the right adrenal that weighed 128 g (normal, 4–5 g) containing a pheochromocytoma that measured 7.3 × 7.8 × 4.9 cm.

6 months before the current presentation—she would wake in the morning with a sense of a rush, pounding in her chest, and "internal shakiness" that would last 5–10 minutes. These symptoms became more marked and frequent after she became pregnant 13 weeks ago. Her only medication was a prenatal vitamin. On physical examination her BMI was 22.1 kg/m², blood pressure 115/72 mmHg, and heart rate 77 beats per minute. The retinal examination was normal, and no Lisch nodules were evident on examination of the iris bilaterally. The thyroid gland was normal to palpation. Examination of the skin was normal with absence of café au lait spots, axillary or inguinal freckling, and subcutaneous neurofibromas.

INVESTIGATIONS

Laboratory studies at Mayo Clinic were diagnostic for an adrenergic catecholamine-secreting tumor (Table 94.1). Magnetic resonance imaging (MRI) of the abdomen without gadolinium showed a soft tissue mass (2.7 cm × 6.3 cm × 5.7 cm) in the retrocaval retroperitoneum in the right adrenalectomy bed (Fig. 94.3).

TREATMENT

Based on multidisciplinary team (endocrinology, surgery, obstetrics, neonatology, and anesthesiology) discussion and informed patient decision making, it was decided to treat her with adrenergic blockade for the duration of her pregnancy and resect the recurrent right adrenal bed pheochromocytoma with an open operative approach postpartum. With initiation of doxazosin 1 mg twice daily, her morning catechol-related

symptoms resolved. At 19 weeks of gestation the plasma fractionated metanephrine levels remained relatively unchanged from her 13-weeks-of-gestation values (see Table 94.1). However, by 30 weeks of gestation, the plasma concentration of metanephrine increased to 18.0 nmol/L (previously 10.0 nmol/L at 13 weeks of gestation and 8.1 nmol/L at 19 weeks of gestation) (see Table 94.1). MRI without gadolinium was obtained to determine if there had been tumor growth—it showed that the right adrenal bed mass was stable in size (Fig. 94.4). With α-adrenergic blockade, blood pressure was maintained at target systolic 100–110 mmHg throughout pregnancy. Heart rate was maintained at target 80 beats per minute with metoprolol 25 mg extended release daily. To optimize α-adrenergic blockade, 10 days before delivery she was switched from doxazosin to phenoxybenzamine 10 mg three times daily. At 37.5 weeks of gestation she had an uneventful cesarean section with delivery of a healthy baby boy—maternal hemodynamics remained stable throughout. Six weeks postpartum she underwent open laparotomy. There were multiple tumor implants discovered in the adrenal bed in the posterior aspect of the liver and gallbladder wall. At pathologic analysis the resected tumor included pericaval recurrent pheochromocytoma (11.2 × 5.7 × 3.8 cm), 2 nodules in the omentum (2.1 cm and 0.6 cm), two masses on the gallbladder margin (1.7 cm and 1.9 cm), perihepatic nodule (0.4 cm), right kidney capsule with multiple small nodules measuring up to 0.2 cm, right diaphragm implants forming multiple nodules between 0.2 and 0.6 cm in diameter, and three

TABLE 94.1 Laboratory Tests

Biochemical Test	Gestational Week				Reference Range
	13 Weeks	19 Weeks	30 Weeks	6 Weeks Postpartum	
Sodium, mmol/L	138				135–145
Potassium, mmol/L	4.4				3.6–5.2
Creatinine, mg/dL	0.6				0.59–1.04
Plasma metanephrine, nmol/L	10	8.1	18	13	<0.5
Plasma normetanephrine, nmol/L	5.3	4.8	7.0	8.6	<0.9
24-Hour urine:					
Metanephrine, mcg	5356				<400
Normetanephrine, mcg	1450				<900

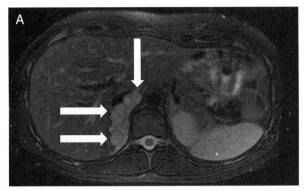
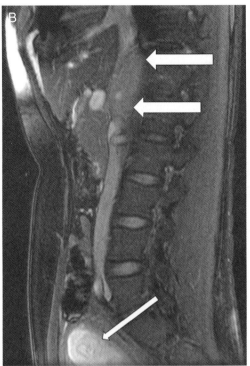

Fig. 94.3 Magnetic resonance imaging of the abdomen without gadolinium completed at 13 weeks of gestation. (A) Axial image showed a soft tissue mass (*arrows*) in the retrocaval retroperitoneum in the right adrenalectomy bed, which was characterized by T2 hyperintensity. It measured 2.2 cm × 6.3 cm in transverse and anterior-posterior dimensions. (B) The sagittal image showed that the right adrenal bed mass (*large arrows*) measured 5.7 cm in craniocaudal dimension. The lesion elevated the inferior vena cava and extended to the aortocaval region posterior to the main portal vein. The left adrenal gland appeared normal. The intrauterine pregnancy (*small arrow*) was incompletely imaged.

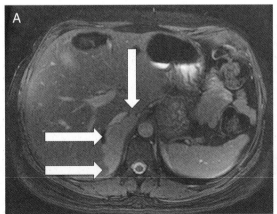
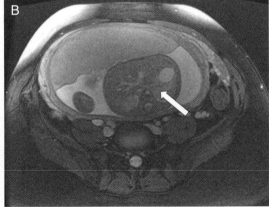

Fig. 94.4 Magnetic resonance imaging (MRI) of the abdomen without gadolinium completed at 30 weeks of gestation. (A) Axial image showed that the lobulated mass (*arrows*) in the right adrenalectomy bed was unchanged in size or appearance compared to the MRI at 13 weeks of gestation. The mass displaced the inferior vena cava (IVC) anteriorly from the level of the diaphragm and extended posteriorly and medially along the IVC to the level of the right renal vein. (B) Axial image through the uterus and fetus showed normal fetal development, and on a happenstance image, the fetal adrenal glands appeared normal (left adrenal gland, denoted by the *arrow*).

perihepatic and pericaval nodules measuring 1.5, 1.5, and 0.7 cm. All visible tumor sites were removed. Postoperatively, the plasma fractionated metanephrine levels were normal and α- and β-adrenergic blockades were discontinued. The patient was informed that she had malignant pheochromocytoma. Her clinical course was that of tumor capsule rupture at the time of her initial surgery. However, because there was no tumor capsule rupture, her pheochromocytoma must have self-seeded the retroperitoneum before resection. She was informed that she would have recurrent disease over time, and close follow-up was advised.

OUTCOME AND FOLLOW-UP

The plasma fractionated metanephrine levels remained normal at 1 year (metanephrine, 0.36 nmol/L; normetanephrine, 0.54 nmol/L) and 2 years (metanephrine, 0.4 nmol/L; normetanephrine, 0.61 nmol/L) after surgery (normal = metanephrine, <0.5 nmol/L; normetanephrine, <0.9 nmol/L). However, at 3 years after surgery the plasma metanephrine concentration was elevated (0.65 nmol/L) and normetanephrine was high-normal (0.82 nmol/L). The gallium 68 (Ga-68) 1,4,7,10-tetraazacyclododecane-1,4,7,10-tetraacetic acid-octreotate (DOTATATE) positron emission tomography (PET)-CT scan showed uptake in a single 0.7 × 0.5–cm lesion between the inferior right hepatic lobe and right kidney. The contrast-enhanced CT scan also showed two additional subcentimeter implants (at hepatic flexure and medial to the inferior right kidney). Her blood pressure was normal and she had no paroxysmal symptoms. She was informed that surgery would not be curative, and observation was advised. Follow-up 1 year later (4 years postpartum) showed a minimal increase in plasma metanephrine (0.7 nmol/L) and normetanephrine remained normal (0.79 nmol/L). Contrast-enhanced CT showed that the three known small retroperitoneal implants were unchanged in size (Fig. 94.5). Germline genetic testing with next-generation sequencing did not identify a pathogenic variant in any of the known pheochromocytoma susceptibility genes. Annual follow-up with biochemical and imaging studies was advised.

Key Points

- Pheochromocytoma in the setting of pregnancy is a high-risk scenario for both mother and fetus.[1]
- Patients with pheochromocytoma in the setting of pregnancy can be managed successfully with adrenergic blockade and elective cesarean section.[1] Another treatment option is laparoscopic adrenalectomy during the second trimester—an option not available for the patient documented herein because of the needed open laparotomy

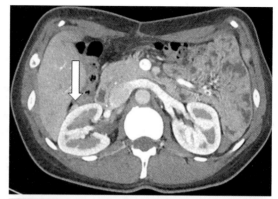
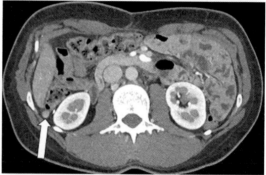
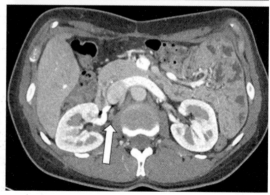

Fig. 94.5 Axial images from a contrast-enhanced computed tomography (CT) scan, completed 4 years postpartum and 12 years after the patient's right adrenalectomy, showed three small right retroperitoneal tumor implants (*arrows*).

and extensive resection of recurrent pheochromocytoma.
- Malignant pheochromocytoma is not a contraindication to pregnancy—with the exceptions of a high burden of disease or rapidly progressive disease.[1]

- Although there is no cure for malignant pheochromocytoma, in most patients the progression of disease is indolent, and the aggressiveness of treatment should be planned to match the aggressiveness of the neoplasm.[2,3]

REFERENCES

1. Bancos I, Atkinson E, Eng C, Young WF Jr, Neumann HPH. International Pheochromocytoma and Pregnancy Study Group. Maternal and fetal outcomes in phaeochromocytoma and pregnancy: a multicentre retrospective cohort study and systematic review of literature. *Lancet Diabetes Endocrinol.* 2021;9(1):13–21.

2. Hamidi O, Young WF Jr, Gruber L, Smestad J, Yan Q, Ponce OJ, Prokop L, Murad MH, Bancos I. Outcomes of patients with metastatic phaeochromocytoma and paraganglioma: a systematic review and meta-analysis. *Clin Endocrinol (Oxf).* 2017;87(5):440–450.

3. Young WF. Metastatic pheochromocytoma: in search of a cure. *Endocrinology.* 2020;161(3):bqz019.

Catecholamine-Secreting Paraganglioma in Pregnancy

As we have highlighted in the other cases, the clinical management of catecholamine-secreting pheochromocytomas or paragangliomas (PPGLs) can be challenging—both diagnostically and therapeutically. However, when PPGL is diagnosed in the setting of pregnancy, the complexity rises more than 10-fold. Herein we share a case of a patient with a large retroperitoneal paraganglioma (PGL) discovered during pregnancy.

Case Report

This 35-year-old woman (gravida 2, para 1) presented to the emergency department during her 28th week of pregnancy with palpitations, severe headache, and lightheadedness. Two years previously she had been diagnosed with "reversible cerebral vasoconstriction syndrome" associated with four thunderclap headaches; she was on chronic treatment with metoprolol 25 mg extended release twice daily. In the emergency department her blood pressure was 190/101 mmHg. The elevated blood pressure rapidly returned to normal without intervention. She was admitted to the hospital for observation. She had episodic surges in blood pressure, which appeared to be associated with positional change (e.g., with sitting up, turning to the side). Monitoring during the episodes revealed a transient drop in blood pressure with a subsequent surge in blood pressure and then bradycardia. Forty-five minutes after she received her evening dose of metoprolol, she had sustained systolic blood pressure in the 220s mmHg for 10 minutes that was associated with fetal heart rate decelerations. The metoprolol was discontinued and her episodes seemed to improve. Pheochromocytoma was suspected. Plasma normetanephrine was markedly elevated

at 22.4 nmol/L (normal, <0.9) and metanephrine was <0.2 nmol/L (normal, <0.5). Abdominal magnetic resonance imaging (MRI) performed during the 29th week of gestation detected a 3.8 cm × 4.9 cm × 6.8 cm PGL at the inferior aspect of the right kidney flanking the aorta and inferior vena cava (Fig. 95.1). The PGL compressed the inferior vena cava and the posterior-superior aspect of the gravid uterus. There is no family history of PPGL. She has had no prior computed abdominal imaging.

TREATMENT

Based on multidisciplinary team (endocrinology, surgery, obstetrics, neonatology, and anesthesiology) discussion and informed patient decision making, it was decided to treat her with adrenergic blockade for the duration of her pregnancy and resect the PGL with an open operative approach postpartum. Because of the body position impact on blood pressure, she was kept at bedrest for the remainder of the pregnancy. Phenoxybenzamine was titrated to 10 mg three times a day and β-adrenergic blockade was added with propranolol 10 mg three times a day. She was maintained on a high-sodium diet with 1-g sodium chloride tablets—two tablets three times a day with food. With this approach, her seated systolic blood pressure ran 80–90 mm Hg in the morning and 100–120 mmHg in the afternoon. Her paroxysmal symptoms resolved. A preplanned cesarean section (C-section) was performed at 36 weeks of gestation. Except for a slight increase in blood pressure at the time of delivery, maternal hemodynamics remained stable throughout the C-section. The baby boy was healthy and required no medical assisted support.

Two weeks postpartum an abdominal MRI with gadolinium redemonstrated the retroperitoneal PGL that was hyperintense on T2-weighted images and

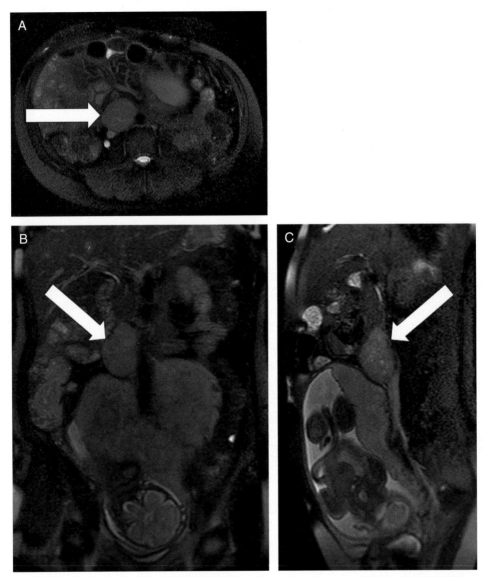

Fig. 95.1 Axial (A), coronal (B), and sagittal (C) magnetic resonance imaging images of the abdomen and pelvis completed at 29 weeks of gestation showed a 3.8 × 4.9 × 6.8–cm right retroperitoneal mass. The mass compressed the inferior vena cava and the posterior-superior aspect of the gravid uterus.

had heterogeneous enhancement. Compared to MRI completed during pregnancy, the mass was slightly larger at 4.3 × 5.6 × 6.9 cm (Fig. 95.2). The gallium 68 (Ga-68) 1,4,7,10-tetraazacyclododecane-1,4,7,10-tetraacetic acid (DOTA)-octreotate (DOTATATE)-positron emission tomography (PET)-CT scan showed that the PGL was intensely tracer avid and there was no

evidence for metastatic disease or additional PGLs (see Fig. 95.2). However, the MRI scan did detect an additional mass along the greater curvature of the stomach near the antrum that measured 2.4 × 2.1 × 1.7 cm (Fig. 95.3). This lesion had no avidity on the Ga-68 DOTATATE PET-CT scan. We suspected that it was most likely a gastrointestinal stromal tumor (GIST), which is

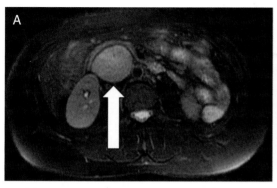
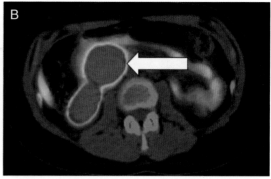

Fig. 95.2 Axial images from gadolinium enhanced magnetic resonance imaging (MRI) scan (A) and Ga-68 1,4,7,10-tetraazacyclododecane-1,4,7,10-tetraacetic acid-octreotate (DOTATATE)-positron emission tomography (PET)-computed tomography (CT) (B) obtained 2 weeks postpartum. The MRI showed the mass (*arrow*) was slightly larger at 4.3 × 5.6 × 6.9 cm. On the Ga-68 DOTATATE-PET-CT the mass (*arrow*) was intensely tracer avid (standard unit value 33.7). There was no evidence of metastatic disease or additional paragangliomas.

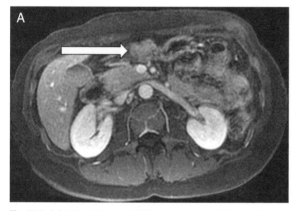

Fig. 95.3 Axial (A) and coronal (B) images from gadolinium enhanced magnetic resonance imaging scan obtained 2 weeks postpartum detected an additional mass (*arrows*) along the greater curvature of the stomach near the antrum that measured 2.4 × 2.1 × 1.7 cm. This mass was not Ga-68 1,4,7,10-tetraazacyclododecane-1,4,7,10-tetraacetic acid-octreotate avid.

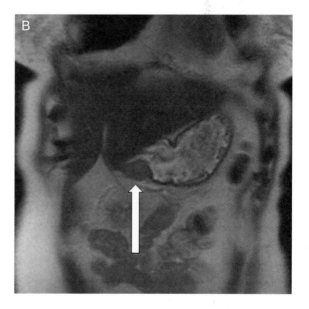

associated with PGLs in the setting of succinate dehydrogenase germline pathogenic variants. Although a germline genetic testing panel for pathogenic variants in PPGL susceptibility genes had been obtained, the results were pending.

Four weeks postpartum she underwent open laparotomy. The PGL was easily separated from the underlying vena cava and there was no evidence of invasion of any surrounding structures. The PGL was resected completely intact (Fig. 95.4). As predicted by MRI, a walnut-sized mass was found extending off the distal

antrum of the stomach (Fig. 95.5). At pathology, this proved to be a GIST.

OUTCOME AND FOLLOW-UP

The germline genetic testing, as expected, detected a *SDHB* pathogenic variant (c.137G>A; p.R46Q). Postoperatively, blood pressure normalized and paroxysmal symptoms resolved. Plasma fractionated metanephrines normalized. Because of the risks for recurrence of the PGL that was resected and the development of additional PGLs, she was advised to have biochemical

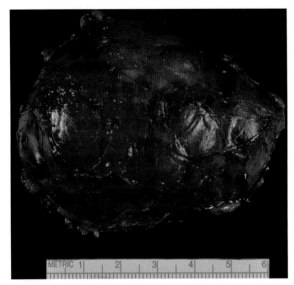

Fig. 95.4 Gross pathology photograph of the retroperitoneal paraganglioma that formed a 7.5-cm mass.

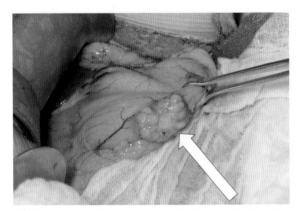

Fig. 95.5 Intraoperative photograph showing the gastrointestinal stromal tumor (GIST) (*arrow*) extending off the distal antrum of the stomach. At pathology, the GIST measured 2.8 × 2.0 × 1.7 cm.

screening with plasma fractionated metanephrine levels annually for life. The plans for surveillance imaging included MRI of the abdomen and pelvis 6 months after surgery and then annually for several years and then, assuming no tumor recurrence, every 2 to 3 years; MRI of the skull base and neck every 2–3 years, MRI of the chest every 5 years, and total body scan with Ga-68 DOTATATE PET-CT every 5 years (approximately 2.5 years after the last chest MRI).

Key Points

- Catecholamine-secreting PGL in the setting of pregnancy is a high-risk scenario for both mother and fetus.[1]
- Patients with catecholamine-secreting PGL in the setting of pregnancy can be managed successfully with adrenergic blockade and elective cesarean section.[1]
- Patients with pathogenic variants in the SDHx subunits are at risk for additional neoplasms, including GISTs and renal cell carcinoma.[2]
- Because of the risk for recurrent PGL and the development of additional PGLs, patients with SDHx pathogenic variants require lifelong biochemical testing and imaging surveillance studies.

REFERENCES

1. Bancos I, Atkinson E, Eng C, Young WF Jr, Neumann HPH; International Pheochromocytoma and Pregnancy Study Group. Maternal and fetal outcomes in phaeochromocytoma and pregnancy: a multicentre retrospective cohort study and systematic review of literature. *Lancet Diabetes Endocrinol.* 2021;9(1):13–21.
2. Neumann HPH, Young WF Jr, Eng C. Pheochromocytoma and paraganglioma. *N Engl J Med.* 2019;381(6):552–565.

The Peripartum Diagnosis of Pheochromocytoma and a Genetic Mystery Solved

As we have highlighted in the other cases, the clinical management of catecholamine-secreting pheochromocytomas or paragangliomas (PPGLs) can be very challenging—both diagnostically and therapeutically. However, when PPGL is diagnosed in the setting of pregnancy, the complexity rises 10-fold. Herein we share a case of a patient in whom the pheochromocytoma was diagnosed peripartum. In addition, a positive family history of pheochromocytoma but negative genetic testing led to an unexpected discovery.

Case Report

This 32-year-old woman had no history of hypertension or diabetes before her recent first pregnancy. She was noted to have hyperglycemia in the first trimester and abnormal liver function tests in the third trimester. The finding of abnormal liver function tests led to a decision to induce labor. During induction, her blood pressure rose to 180/90–100 mmHg. Labor lasted 24 hours, and her blood pressure was elevated throughout and treated with magnesium sulfate. Her baby boy's delivery was complicated by pneumothorax and hypoglycemia, and he was kept in the neonatal intensive care unit for 5 days. Treatment of the mother's hypertension with magnesium sulfate was continued for 24 hours after delivery. However, she developed fast and forceful palpitations, headache, and nausea, and the poorly controlled hypertension persisted. Because of nausea and emesis she was treated with metoclopramide. Shortly after receiving metoclopramide, she had a sense of impending doom and was diffusely diaphoretic. An electrocardiogram showed findings consistent with acute myocardial infarction. She was transferred from the obstetric floor to the coronary care unit, where an echocardiogram showed an ejection fraction of 45% and hypokinesis of the cardiac apex. Troponin I was elevated at 10 ng/mL (normal, <0.04 ng/mL). Coronary angiogram showed normal coronary arteries. Treatment with carvedilol was initiated. While in the coronary care unit, she mentioned that some family members had been diagnosed with pheochromocytoma in the past; this triggered a 24-hour urine collection for fractionated metanephrines and catecholamines, which showed: norepinephrine 1555 mcg (normal, <80 mcg) and normetanephrine 13,000 mcg (normal, <900 mcg). Treatment with phenoxybenzamine was initiated, and computed tomography of the abdomen detected a 4.5-cm right adrenal mass (Fig. 96.1), and she was referred to Mayo Clinic at 5 weeks postpartum. With the addition of phenoxybenzamine (10 mg twice daily), her blood pressure averaged 100/60 mmHg.

Her family history was remarkable. Her paternal grandfather died at age 47 after returning from World War II with hypertension and a known pheochromocytoma. Her paternal aunt had a pheochromocytoma removed at 38 years of age. A cousin (offspring of her paternal aunt) had a pheochromocytoma removed at 18 years of age. In addition, three children of her paternal grandfather's brother had pheochromocytoma. There was no family history of medullary thyroid carcinoma, hyperparathyroidism, cerebellar tumors, spinal cord tumors, retinal angiomas, pancreatic tumors, kidney tumors, neurofibromas, or any other familial

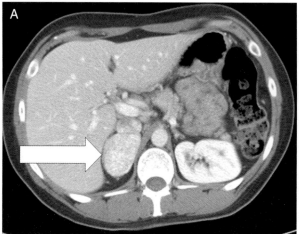

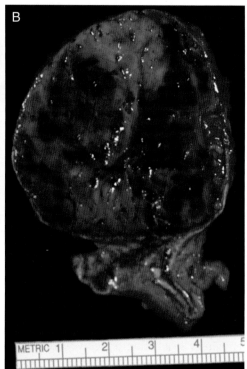

Fig. 96.1 The proband. (A) Axial image from a contrast-enhanced computed tomography scan showed a 5-cm mixed-density mass (*arrow*) in the right adrenal gland. (B) Gross pathology photograph of cut section of the right adrenal that weighed 40.1 g (normal, 4–5 g) containing a pheochromocytoma that measured 5.3 × 5.0 × 2.0 cm.

neoplasms. Her father had a history of hypertension and coronary artery disease but had not been screened for pheochromocytoma. Our patient had two brothers and one sister and none had been screened for pheochromocytoma.

Her medications included phenoxybenzamine, 10 mg twice daily, and carvedilol, 6.25 mg twice daily. On physical examination her body mass index was 24.1 kg/m², blood pressure 102/67 mmHg, and heart rate 100 beats per minute. The retinal examination was normal, and no Lisch nodules were evident on examination of the iris bilaterally. The thyroid gland was normal to palpation. Examination of the skin was normal, with absence of café au lait spots, axillary or inguinal freckling, and subcutaneous neurofibromas.

INVESTIGATIONS

Laboratory studies at Mayo Clinic reconfirmed a noradrenergic catecholamine-secreting tumor (Table 96.1). The echocardiogram was normal with no

regional wall motion abnormalities, and the ejection fraction was normal at 61%. The exercise sestamibi study was normal with no evidence of provokable ischemia.

TABLE 96.1	Laboratory Tests	
Biochemical Test	**Result**	**Reference Range**
Sodium, mmol/L	140	135–145
Potassium, mmol/L	4.3	3.6–5.2
Creatinine, mg/dL	0.9	0.7–1.2
Plasma metanephrine, nmol/L	<0.2	<0.5
Plasma normetanephrine, nmol/L	28.6	<0.9
24-Hour urine:		
Metanephrine, mcg	117	<400
Normetanephrine, mcg	8760	<900
Norepinephrine, mcg	781	<80
Epinephrine, mcg	2.4	<20
Dopamine, mcg	197	<400

TREATMENT

The patient underwent laparoscopic right adrenalectomy, and the pheochromocytoma was resected intact with great care to avoid tumor capsule rupture. The tumor measured 5.3 × 5.0 × 2.0 cm (see Fig. 96.1).

OUTCOME AND FOLLOW-UP

The patient recovered well from the operation and was discharged from the hospital on the second postoperative day. The plasma fractionated metanephrine levels obtained 2 days postoperatively were normal. The blood pressure was normal without medications. Germline genetic testing did not detect a pathogenic variant in any of the genes known to be associated with PPGL. She was followed with annual biochemical testing, which remained normal at last follow-up 15 years later.

THE GENETIC MYSTERY SOLVED

Given the known family history of pheochromocytoma but negative results from clinically available germline genetic testing that was available in 2005 (*VHL*, *RET*, *SDHB*, *SDHD*, *SDHC*), we advised that the patient's parents and siblings have biochemical testing for pheochromocytoma. Her 72-year-old father proved to have a 2.8-cm right adrenal gland pheochromocytoma (Fig. 96.2). Her 34-year-old brother had a 1.8-cm right adrenal gland pheochromocytoma (Fig. 96.3).

Subsequently, we discussed her family with Patricia Dahia, MD, PhD (Professor of Medicine at the University of Texas Health Science Center at San Antonio). Her career has been dedicated to research on the genetics of cancer, with emphasis on inherited endocrine tumors and discovery of cancer susceptibility genes. Dr. Dahia completed exome sequencing of our proband's germline DNA, and it revealed no missense or truncating mutations in known PPGL susceptibility genes. However, a heterozygous, synonymous variant was detected in exon 2 of the *VHL* gene (c.414A>G, p.Pro138Pro).

For the nongeneticist, this finding requires some background information. Most disease-causing pathogenic variants result in defective synthesis of a specific protein and are due to one of the following: (1) *missense mutation*, in which a change in a single nucleotide results in the substitution of one amino acid for another in the protein; (2) a *nonsense mutation*, in which a change in a single nucleotide results in a stop codon that signals the cell to stop building the protein prematurely; (3) an *insertion*, in which the number of DNA base pairs in a gene is increased by adding a piece of DNA; (4) a *deletion*, in which the number of DNA base pairs in a gene is reduced by removing a piece of DNA; (5) a *duplication*, in which a section of DNA is abnormally copied one or more times; (6) a *frameshift*

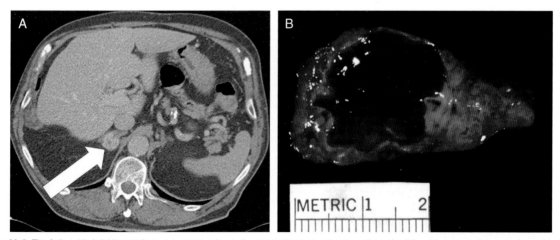

Fig. 96-2 The father. (A) Axial image from a contrast enhanced computed tomography scan showed a 2.3-cm hypervascular mass (*arrow*) in the right adrenal gland. (B) Gross pathology photograph of cut section of the right adrenal that weighed 16.4 g (normal, 4–5 g) containing a pheochromocytoma that measured 2.8 × 2.0 × 1.7 cm.

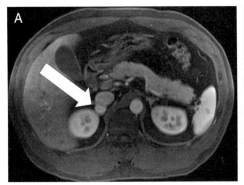
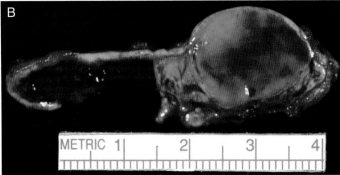

Fig. 96-3 The brother. (A) Axial image from magnetic resonance imaging of the abdomen after intravenous gadolinium showed a 1.8-cm hypervascular mass (*arrow*) in the right adrenal gland. (B) Gross pathology photograph of cut section of the right adrenal that weighed 10.4 g (normal, 4–5 g) containing a pheochromocytoma that measured 1.8 × 1.5 × 1.2 cm.

mutation, in which an addition or loss of DNA base pairs changes a gene's reading frame (the frameshift can be caused by insertions, deletions, or duplications); or (7) *repeat expansion*, in which a short DNA sequence is repeated.

A synonymous variant is similar to a missense mutation in that a single nucleotide is substituted for another, but because of the redundancy of the genetic code, the amino acid remains the same. The genetic code is composed of units known as codons, which are sequences of three nucleotides. Each codon corresponds to a specific amino acid of the 20, which are the building blocks of proteins. There are four DNA bases: adenine (A), guanine (G), cytosine (C), and thymine (T). The codon AGC, for example, codes the amino acid serine. As there are four bases in 3–base pair combinations, there are 64 possible codons; 61 specify amino acids and 3 specify stop signals. Thus most of the 20 amino acids are coded by more than one codon. For example, proline is coded by codons CCT, CCC, CCA, and CCG. In our patient's case, in codon 138, instead of CCA, adenine (A) was replaced by guanine (G), so the new codon became CCG. Both CCA and CCG code for proline, so the amino acid did not change. Synonymous variants are often assumed to be neutral or functionally silent, as there is no change in the product protein sequence. However, synonymous variants have the potential to disrupt splice sites, transcription, or mRNA transport or translation, which can potentially alter phenotype.

Sanger sequencing of germline DNA from 16 relatives showed that the c.414A>G *VHL* variant segregated with pheochromocytoma in this family.[1] Despite its location away from the canonical splice-site regions, the c.414A>G *VHL* variant was found to promote exon 2 skipping.[1] This same *VHL* pathogenic variant was identified in four additional families.[1] With the availability of germline genetic testing for this pathogenic variant, our patient's children were tested. Her son, who was born at the time of her pheochromocytoma discovery and who was now 14 years old, had inherited the pathogenic variant. The 24-hour urine excretion of normetanephrine (2392 mg; normal, <900 mcg) was diagnostic of a catecholamine-secreting tumor. Abdominal magnetic resonance imaging detected a left periadrenal 2.7-cm mass, which proved to be a paraganglioma (Fig. 96.4).

Key Points

- Pheochromocytoma in the setting of pregnancy is a high-risk scenario for both mother and fetus.[2]
- Myocardial infarction with nonobstructed coronary arteries is an atypical presentation of pheochromocytoma.[3,4]
- Medications and situations that may precipitate a PPGL crisis include metoclopramide (as seen in the aforementioned case), β-adrenergic blocker, high-dosage corticosteroid, anesthesia induction, glucagon, and angiography.
- All patients with PPGL should be counseled on the role for germline genetic testing.

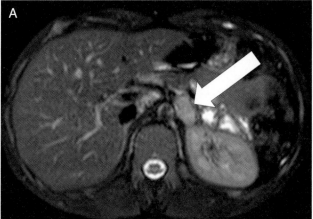

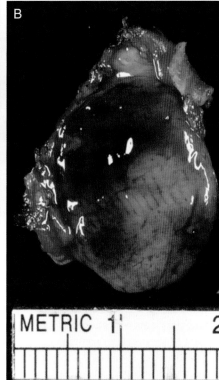

Fig. 96.4 The son. (A) Axial image from magnetic resonance imaging of the abdomen showed an ovoid 2.7 × 1.3 × 3.1–cm mass (*arrow*) adjacent to the left adrenal gland. (B) Gross pathology photograph of cut section of the paraganglioma that measured 3.2 × 2.5 × 2.2 cm.

- When a patient with a PPGL has a first-degree relative with a PPGL, there must be a germline pathogenic variant in a PPGL susceptibility gene.

REFERENCES

1. Flores SK, Cheng Z, Jasper AM, et al. A synonymous VHL variant in exon 2 confers susceptibility to familial pheochromocytoma and von Hippel-Lindau disease. *J Clin Endocrinol Metab*. 2019;104(9):3826–3834.

2. Bancos I, Atkinson E, Eng C, Young WF Jr, Neumann HPH, and International-Pheochromocytoma-and-Pregnancy-Study Group. Maternal and fetal outcomes in pheochromocytoma and pregnancy: a multi-center retrospective cohort study and systematic review of literature. *Lancet Diabetes Endocrinol*. 2021;9(1):13–21.

3. Melson E, Amir S, Shepherd L, Kauser S, Freestone B, Kempegowda P. Myocardial Infarction with non-obstructed coronaries – atypical presentation of pheochromocytoma. *Endocrinol Diabetes Metab Case Rep*.2019:EDM190089. doi: 10.1530/EDM-19-0089.

4. Boulkina LS, Newton CA, Drake AJ 3rd, Tanenberg RJ. Acute myocardial infarction attributable to adrenergic crises in a patient with pheochromocytoma and neurofibromatosis 1. *Endocr Pract*. 2007;13(3):269–273.

History of Pregnancy in a 41-Year-Old Woman With Undiagnosed Cushing Syndrome

Workup for corticotropin (ACTH)-independent hypercortisolism is required in any patient with an adrenal mass, regardless of symptoms of hormone excess. Unfortunately, only a minority of patients with adrenal incidentalomas undergo appropriate workup.[1] Although Cushing syndrome (CS) is associated with physical and metabolic changes, approximately half of patients with adrenal CS are diagnosed incidentally, suggesting poor recognition of CS in the clinical practice. Undiagnosed CS may present with abnormal menses and infertility.[2] During pregnancy, unrecognized and untreated CS may be associated with adverse maternal and fetal outcomes.[3,4]

Case Report

A 41-year-old woman presented for evaluation of an adrenal mass. After searching online for a reason for her symptoms, she came across a description of "Cushing syndrome" and requested further workup. She reported a 5-year history of progressive muscle weakness, weight gain, episodes of diaphoresis, and menstrual irregularity. Over the prior 2 years, she developed moon facies, dorsocervical and supraclavicular pads, erythema, insomnia, difficulty concentrating, and an increase in anxiety and depression. She was diagnosed with new onset hypertension and dyslipidemia 2 years ago. Overall, she gained 50 pounds over the prior 5 years, and 20 pounds in the prior 2 years.

Several years ago, after unsuccessfully attempting to conceive for 12 months, she pursued fertility therapy. During pregnancy, she developed gestational diabetes that necessitated insulin therapy.

Otherwise, her medical history was positive for nephrolithiasis. Two years prior, an abdominal computed tomography (CT) scan was performed that described a 3-cm right adrenal mass. No hormonal workup was performed at that time.

Her current medications included carvedilol, losartan, sertraline, and alprazolam. On physical examination, her blood pressure was 138/88 mmHg and body mass index was 46.64 kg/m^2. She had no striae or proximal myopathy but did have a dorsocervical pad, supraclavicular pads, and rounding and erythema of the face. She had minimal edema of the lower extremities.

INVESTIGATIONS

Contrast-enhanced CT of the abdomen that was performed recently was reviewed and compared to the CT performed 2 years prior. The most recent CT demonstrated a stable $3.3 \times 2.1 \times 3.1$–cm right adrenal mass (Fig. 97.1). The left adrenal gland was atrophic. Hormonal workup for hypercortisolism was performed, including morning measurement of ACTH and dehydroepiandrosterone sulfate (DHEA-S), 1-mg overnight dexamethasone suppression test (DST), and 24-hour urinary free cortisol excretion. The laboratory data were consistent with ACTH-independent hypercortisolism (Table 97.1). Laparoscopic adrenalectomy was recommended.

TREATMENT

The patient was treated with a laparoscopic right adrenalectomy at an institution other than ours, with pathologic analysis demonstrating an adrenocortical adenoma. She was educated on adrenal insufficiency and initiated on hydrocortisone therapy.

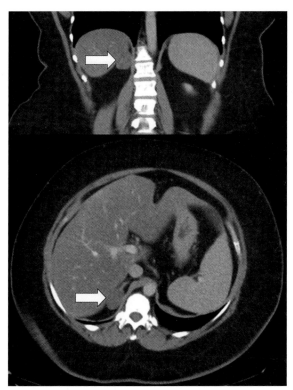

Fig. 97.1 Axial (*below*) and coronal (*above*) images from a contrast-enhanced computed tomography scan showed a 3.3 × 2.1 × 3.1–cm right adrenal mass (*arrows*).

TABLE 97.1 Laboratory Tests

Biochemical Test	Result	Reference Range
1-mg overnight DST, mcg/dL	12.4	<1.8
Morning cortisol, mcg/dL	13	7–25
ACTH, pg/mL	<5	7.2–63
DHEA-S, mcg/dL	14	27–240
Urine free cortisol, mcg/24 h	"Elevated," not repeated at our institution	3.5–45
Aldosterone, ng/dL	4.4	<21
Plasma renin activity, ng/mL per hour	2.1	2.9–10.8
Plasma metanephrine, nmol/L	<0.20	<0.5
Plasma normetanephrine, nmol/L	0.38	<0.9

ACTH, Corticotropin; *DHEA-S,* dehydroepiandrosterone-sulfate; *DST,* dexamethasone suppression test.

Discussion

The patient presented with unrecognized, progressive ACTH-independent CS of at least 5 years duration. An opportunity for an earlier diagnosis was lost when the incidental discovery of an adrenal mass several years prior was dismissed as not clinically significant, without any workup at that time. Assuming another diagnosis is not obvious (e.g., pheochromocytoma), a DST should be performed in all patients with an adrenal mass, regardless of symptoms of hormone excess. Our patient was diagnosed with overt CS, as she presented with clinical features of hypercortisolism on examination (Box C.1). Biochemical workup was consistent with ACTH-independent hypercortisolism with undetectable ACTH and DHEA-S, abnormal DST, and elevated 24-hour urine cortisol. With confirmation of ACTH-independent hypercortisolism, the unilateral adrenal mass was considered the culprit lesion, and adrenalectomy was recommended. Adrenal insufficiency and glucocorticoid withdrawal should be anticipated and properly treated in these cases (see Section C for more details).

In retrospect, the patient's irregular menses and infertility may have been caused or exacerbated by the undiagnosed and untreated CS.[2] A systematic review of the literature reported adrenal CS as the most common CS subtype diagnosed during pregnancy.[4] Patients with untreated CS during pregnancy had higher rates of pregnancy-related complications such as gestational diabetes mellitus (37%), gestational hypertension (41%), and preeclampsia (26%).[4] Preterm delivery and low birth weight were the most common adverse fetal outcomes.[4]

Depending on the severity of CS and gestation week, if diagnosed during pregnancy, conservative management of comorbidities, antepartum adrenalectomy, or medical therapy can be considered. Metyrapone is the most commonly used medication used for treatment of CS during pregnancy.[4,5] In-depth monitoring is required in these cases to document optimal therapy of hypercortisolism, prevent or appropriately treat adrenal insufficiency, observe for possible metyrapone-induced side effects of hypertension and hypokalemia, and adapt any ongoing management of hyperglycemia.

Key Points

- Workup for ACTH-independent hypercortisolism is recommended in all patients with an adrenal mass, regardless of symptoms.
- Untreated CS is associated with adverse maternal and fetal outcomes during pregnancy.
- Management of CS during pregnancy depends on its severity, etiology, and the gestational stage at diagnosis, and includes conservative management of comorbidities, surgery, or medical therapy.

REFERENCES

1. Ebbehoj A, Li D, Kaur RJ, et al. Epidemiology of adrenal tumours in Olmsted County, Minnesota, USA: a population-based cohort study. *Lancet Diabetes Endocrinol.* 2020;8(11):894–902.

2. Lado-Abeal J, Rodriguez-Arnao J, Newell-Price JD, et al. Menstrual abnormalities in women with Cushing's disease are correlated with hypercortisolemia rather than raised circulating androgen levels. *J Clin Endocrinol Metab.* 1998;83(9):3083–3088.

3. Lindsay JR, Jonklaas J, Oldfield EH, Nieman LK. Cushing's syndrome during pregnancy: personal experience and review of the literature. *J Clin Endocrinol Metab.* 2005;90(5):3077–3083.

4. Caimari F, Valassi E, Garbayo P, et al. Cushing's syndrome and pregnancy outcomes: a systematic review of published cases. *Endocrine.* 2017;55(2):555–563.

5. Azzola A, Eastabrook G, Matsui D, et al. Adrenal Cushing syndrome diagnosed during pregnancy: successful medical management with metyrapone. *J Endocr Soc.* 2021;5(1):bvaa167.

Pregnancy in a Patient With Primary Adrenal Insufficiency

Pregnancy is a state of physiologic hypercortisolism. Management of adrenal insufficiency during pregnancy includes adjustment of therapy to physiologic needs and avoidance of adrenal crisis through an in-depth education, availability, and comfort with stress-dose glucocorticoid use. Here we discuss the approach to glucocorticoid and mineralocorticoid therapy before and during pregnancy.

Case Report

The patient was a 36-year-old woman with history of Addison disease and celiac disease. Her medications included hydrocortisone 15 mg on waking, 5 mg in early afternoon and 2.5 mg at 5 pm, and fludrocortisone 0.05 mg every other day. She had an excellent compliance with medical therapy and never experienced an adrenal crisis. The patient had yearly monitoring for autoimmune disorders, including testing for pernicious anemia and thyroid dysfunction. She presented for her yearly evaluation with her endocrinologist 2 months early to discuss management of adrenal insufficiency during pregnancy. On physical examination, her body mass index was 26.1 kg/m^2, blood pressure 103/75 mmHg, and heart rate 78 beats per minute. She had no hyperpigmentation, no features suggestive of iatrogenic Cushing syndrome, and no lower extremity edema. She was not orthostatic. Pregnancy was confirmed 1 week earlier, at 9 weeks of gestation. She reported a high comfort level with adrenal insufficiency self-management, including the awareness of situations in which she should increase her dosage of hydrocortisone therapy. She never had to self-inject glucocorticoid, but she did receive education on self-injection, and felt comfortable to use it if necessary. She recently

refilled her prescription and had three vials of hydrocortisone solution available for use. She had a medical alert bracelet stating "adrenal insufficiency, needs cortisone." Her partner participated in the education session on adrenal insufficiency.

FOLLOW-UP AND MANAGEMENT

At 19 weeks of gestation, hydrocortisone was increased to 17.5 mg on waking, 5 mg early afternoon, and 2.5 mg at 5 PM. Sick day rules were carefully rereviewed. She was reevaluated again at 28 weeks and 34 weeks of gestation. She had no symptoms, physical examination was not suggestive for under- or overreplacement with glucocorticoid or mineralocorticoid therapy, and her electrolytes were within the normal range. Thus no changes in hydrocortisone and fludrocortisone were made.

Before the planned cesarean section, her medical team followed the plan agreed on between her endocrinologist and obstetrician to inject 100 mg of hydrocortisone solution, followed by 50 mg every 6 hours until able to have oral intake. At that point, she took oral hydrocortisone at slightly increased dose of 20 mg on waking, 10 mg at noon, and 5 mg at 5 PM for 1 week, and then reverted to her prepregnancy regimen.

Discussion

When appropriately managed, women with adrenal insufficiency experience excellent fetal and maternal outcomes.[1] Usually an adjustment in daily hydrocortisone dose is needed in the second or third trimester. [1–3] The need for adjustment depends on prepregnancy glucocorticoid dose and clinical assessment during pregnancy. Because progesterone has an antimineralocorticoid effect, fludrocortisone therapy may need to be modified during pregnancy. Assessment of

TABLE 98.1	Patient and Clinician-Related Measures to Ensure Appropriate Management of Adrenal Insufficiency and Prevention of Adrenal Crisis
Patient	**Clinician**
Chronic Management of Adrenal Insufficiency	
Consistency with taking hydrocortisone and fludrocortisone exactly as prescribed	Provide a written adrenal action plan that includes both standard glucocorticoid replacement and increased doses at times of illness (i.e., sick day guidelines).
Understanding symptoms of under- and overreplacement with glucocorticoids and mineralocorticoids to effectively communicate dosing issues to the health care team	Evaluate for appropriate glucocorticoid and mineralocorticoid replacement during each visit.
Ensuring an optimal supply of hydrocortisone and fludrocortisone tablets and injectable glucocorticoid (including during travel)	Provide an optimal supply of medications, including for the times of a need to increase.
Prevention and Treatment of Adrenal Crisis	
Participation in an education session on sick day guidelines	Educate patients on importance of wearing medical alert identification and maintaining a copy of adrenal action plan for cases of emergency.
Taking stress dose glucocorticoids when indicated	
Understanding the situations when stress dose glucocorticoids are required	Review indications for stress dose glucocorticoid at every visit and maintain an active prescription for injectable glucocorticoid.
Compliance with wearing medical alert identification (e.g., bracelet, necklace)	
Availability of injectable glucocorticoid and comfort with administration if needed	Provide education for emergency department staff regarding identification and prompt management of adrenal crisis.

Adapted from refs. 2, 4, and 5.

mineralocorticoid replacement therapy should rely on the physical examination (blood pressure measurement) and electrolyte assessment. Notably, plasma renin concentrations increase during pregnancy and should not be used in decision making. It is important to provide a detailed education on management during sickness and the importance of prevention of adrenal crisis (Table 98.1).[4,5] In addition, the patient's obstetrical team and the patient should be well aware of the glucocorticoid plans for during labor, delivery, and postpartum period.

Key Points

- Glucocorticoid and mineralocorticoid management during pregnancy may change in women with adrenal insufficiency and is based on clinical assessment.
- As plasma renin concentrations increase with pregnancy, measurement of renin is not helpful to guide mineralocorticoid replacement. Clinical

assessment and measurement of serum electrolytes should be used instead.
- All patients with adrenal insufficiency need an adequate plan for stress dose glucocorticoids during labor and delivery.

REFERENCES

1. Bothou C, Anand G, Li D, et al. Current management and outcome of pregnancies in women with adrenal insufficiency: experience from a multicenter survey. *J Clin Endocrinol Metab*. 2020;105(8).
2. Hahner S, Ross RJ, Arlt W, et al. Adrenal insufficiency. *Nat Rev Dis Primers*. 2021;7(1):19.
3. Lebbe M, Arlt W. What is the best diagnostic and therapeutic management strategy for an Addison patient during pregnancy? *Clin Endocrinol (Oxf)*. 2013;78(4):497–502.
4. Li D, Genere N, Behnken E, et al. Determinants of self-reported health outcomes in adrenal insufficiency: a multisite survey study. *J Clin Endocrinol Metab*. 2021;106(3):e1408–e1419.
5. Bancos I, Hahner S, Tomlinson J, Arlt W. Diagnosis and management of adrenal insufficiency. *Lancet Diabetes Endocrinol*. 2015;3(3):216–226.

Pregnancy in a Patient With 21-Hydroxylase Deficiency

The most common type of congenital adrenal hyperplasia (CAH) is 21-hydroxylase deficiency, which occurs in 1 in 10,000 live births.[1] The goals of therapy in CAH include (1) replacement therapy for glucocorticoid and mineralocorticoid deficiency and (2) controlling androgen excess. Women with 21-hydroxylase deficiency may present with impaired fertility; however, normal pregnancy rates can be achieved with optimal glucocorticoid replacement therapy.[2,3] Here we discuss the approach to glucocorticoid replacement therapy before and during pregnancy.

Case Report

The patient was a 27-year-old woman with history of 21-hydroxylase deficiency who presented for advice on management during future pregnancy. Her husband had genetic testing for 21-hydroxylase deficiency and was not a carrier.

PREVIOUS HISTORY

The patient was diagnosed with 21-hydroxylase deficiency at birth when she developed symptoms consistent with an adrenal crisis, and physical examination revealed ambiguous genitalia. Glucocorticoid and mineralocorticoid replacement therapy was initiated in the hospital. Over the years, her glucocorticoid therapy varied, initially consisting of hydrocortisone and later prednisone for 9 years, and, more recently, dexamethasone. At age 2 and 7 years, she was treated with clitoral repair operations. Menarche occurred at age 12 years, and menstrual cycles have been irregular.

She achieved her first pregnancy spontaneously at age 26. Before this, she and her husband had unprotected intercourse for 4 years without success.

CURRENT EVALUATION

The patient's medications included 0.75 mg dexamethasone daily and 150 mcg fludrocortisone daily, with an excellent compliance. On physical examination, her body mass index was 34.22 kg/m², blood pressure 103/72 mmHg, and heart rate 76 beats per minute. She had no hirsutism and no acne. Pale striae were noted under the axillary area and over the lower abdomen. The serum androstenedione concentration was low-normal at 53 ng/dL (normal range, 30–200), and the serum concentration of 17-hydroxyprogesterone was undetectable. She was advised that her dexamethasone dose was excessive and it was gradually decreased to 0.25 mg daily, at which point her serum androstenedione concentrations were mid-normal. She was also advised that as dexamethasone crosses the placenta, hydrocortisone would be a better choice for glucocorticoid replacement therapy when pregnancy is planned.

FOLLOW-UP

Dexamethasone was replaced by hydrocortisone, and she was able to conceive her second child at age 29 years (after one cycle of clomiphene therapy). She conceived her third child at age 35 years without any reproductive assistance therapy. During both pregnancies, she had significant morning nausea and vomiting. Because of an inability to take glucocorticoid therapy in the morning, she switched to prednisone at bedtime (5–7.5 mg at night). Her prednisone was titrated to mid-normal androstenedione concentrations. At the time of planned cesarean section, she received hydrocortisone 100 mg before surgery and then 50 mg every 6 hours during the first 24 hours. She was able to switch to oral glucocorticoids the second day after delivery.

After pregnancy, she was able to change her glucocorticoid regimen to hydrocortisone three times a day.

Discussion

Women with 21-hydroxylase deficiency may present with impaired fertility as a result of androgen excess, progesterone excess, and oligoanovulation.[3,4] Normal pregnancy rates can be achieved with adequate suppression of follicular phase progesterone through optimization of glucocorticoid therapy.[2] Hydrocortisone is the glucocorticoid of choice throughout the pregnancy, as it does not traverse the placenta.[5] Management of glucocorticoid and mineralocorticoid therapy during pregnancy should be reevaluated during the second and third trimesters. Assessment of symptoms, physical examination, and biochemical workup (electrolytes, androstenedione) aid decision making on individualization of therapy. As in adrenal insufficiency of any cause (see Case 98), all patients with 21-hydroxylase deficiency should have a clear and adequate plan for stress doses of glucocorticoids to be administered during labor and delivery.

Key Points

- Women with 21-hydroxylase deficiency may present with impaired fertility. Adequate suppression of follicular phase progesterone through optimization of glucocorticoid therapy improves fertility.

- Hydrocortisone is the glucocorticoid of choice throughout the pregnancy, as it does not traverse the placenta.

- Glucocorticoid and mineralocorticoid dosages need to be periodically reevaluated during pregnancy.

- All patients with 21-hydroxylase deficiency need an adequate plan for stress dose glucocorticoids during labor and delivery.

REFERENCES

1. Merke DP, Auchus RJ. Congenital adrenal hyperplasia due to 21-hydroxylase deficiency. *N Engl J Med.* 2020;383(13):1248–1261.

2. Casteras A, De Silva P, Rumsby G, Conway GS. Reassessing fecundity in women with classical congenital adrenal hyperplasia (CAH): normal pregnancy rate but reduced fertility rate. *Clin Endocrinol (Oxf).* 2009;70(6):833–837.

3. Hagenfeldt K, Janson PO, Holmdahl G, et al. Fertility and pregnancy outcome in women with congenital adrenal hyperplasia due to 21-hydroxylase deficiency. *Hum Reprod.* 2008;23(7):1607–1613.

4. Bidet M, Bellanne-Chantelot C, Galand-Portier MB, et al. Fertility in women with nonclassical congenital adrenal hyperplasia due to 21-hydroxylase deficiency. *J Clin Endocrinol Metab.* 2010;95(3):1182–1190.

5. Speiser PW, Arlt W, Auchus RJ, et al. Congenital adrenal hyperplasia due to steroid 21-hydroxylase deficiency: an Endocrine Society clinical practice guideline. *J Clin Endocrinol Metab.* 2018;103(11):4043–4088.

Primary Aldosteronism in Pregnancy

Primary aldosteronism (PA) is uncommon in pregnancy, with fewer than 64 cases reported in the medical literature; most of these reported patients had aldosterone-producing adenomas (APAs).[1] PA can lead to intrauterine growth retardation, preterm delivery, intrauterine fetal demise, and placental abruption. Case-detection testing for PA in a pregnant woman is the same as for nonpregnant patients: morning blood sample for the measurement of aldosterone and renin. The combination of suppressed renin and an aldosterone level >10 ng/dL is a positive case-detection test for PA. If spontaneous hypokalemia is present in the woman with high plasma aldosterone concentration (≥20 ng/dL) and suppressed renin, confirmatory testing is not needed. In a normokalemic woman with a positive case-detection test, confirmatory testing should be pursued. However, the captopril stimulation test is contraindicated in pregnancy, and the saline infusion test may not be well tolerated. One option is measurement of sodium and aldosterone in a 24-hour urine collection on an ambient sodium diet. Subtype testing with abdominal magnetic resonance imaging (MRI) without gadolinium is the test of choice. Computed tomography (CT) and adrenal venous sampling (AVS) should be avoided in pregnancy. In patients with vigorous PA who are less than 35 years old and have a clear-cut, unilateral adrenal adenoma on MRI, AVS is not needed. The type of treatment for PA in pregnancy depends on how difficult it is to manage the hypertension and hypokalemia. If the patient is in the subset of those who have a pregnancy-related remission in the degree of PA during pregnancy, then surgery or treatment with a mineralocorticoid receptor antagonist (MRA) can be avoided until after delivery. However, if PA accelerates during pregnancy and

hypertension and hypokalemia are marked, then surgical and/or targeted medical intervention with a MRA is indicated. Unilateral laparoscopic adrenalectomy during the second trimester can be considered in those women with confirmed PA and a clear-cut unilateral adrenal macroadenoma (>10 mm).

Case Report

A 22-year-old woman (gravida 2, para 1) was initially seen elsewhere at 12 weeks of gestation for increasing weakness and fatigue. She was hypertensive and hypokalemic. The plasma aldosterone concentration was >20 ng/dL and the plasma renin activity was suppressed. She was treated with potassium chloride and spironolactone. Because of worsening hypertension (160/105 mmHg), at 28 weeks of gestation she was referred to Mayo Clinic.

INVESTIGATIONS

Laboratory studies at Mayo Clinic were diagnostic for PA. The plasma aldosterone concentration was 230 ng/dL (normal, <21 ng/dL) and the plasma renin activity was suppressed. An abdominal magnetic resonance imaging (MRI) without gadolinium detected a 3.0 × 2.0 × 2.0–cm right adrenal mass with imaging characteristics consistent with an adenoma (Fig. 100.1).

TREATMENT

Treatment with spironolactone was discontinued. Despite additional antihypertensive medications, over the next 4 weeks she had worsening hypertension (165/115 mmHg) and proteinuria (24-hour urine protein was 4800 g). She subsequently underwent induction of labor at 32 weeks of gestation for superimposed preeclampsia. She delivered a 1705-g male

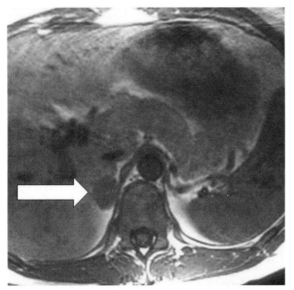

Fig. 100.1 Axial image from magnetic resonance imaging of the abdomen without gadolinium completed at 28 weeks of gestation showed a 3.0 × 2.0 × 2.0–cm right adrenal mass (*arrow*).

infant. Examination of the genitalia was normal. The infant required 15 days of neonatal intensive care for respiratory distress syndrome and nutritional support. At 2 months postpartum the mother underwent right adrenalectomy without complication. Pathology showed a 2-cm benign adrenocortical adenoma consistent with an APA.

OUTCOME AND FOLLOW-UP

At 1 month after operation the plasma aldosterone concentration was <1 ng/dL. At last follow-up, 1 year later, she was normotensive and normokalemic. She did not require potassium supplementation or antihypertensive medications.

Discussion

A unique feature of PA during pregnancy is that the degree of disease may be either improved or aggravated. In some women with PA, the high blood levels of pregnancy-related progesterone are antagonistic at the mineralocorticoid receptor and partially block the action of aldosterone; these patients have an improvement in the manifestations of PA during pregnancy.[2,3] In other pregnant women, increased expression of

luteinizing hormone choriogonadotropin receptor has been documented in APAs that harbor β-catenin mutations, and the degree of hyperaldosteronism is aggravated by the increased pregnancy-related blood levels of human chorionic gonadotropin.[4,5]

The optimal treatment for PA in pregnancy depends on how difficult it is to manage the hypertension and hypokalemia. If the patient is in the subset of patients who have a remission in the degree of PA, then surgery or treatment with a MRA can be avoided until after delivery. However, if hypertension and hypokalemia are marked, then surgical and/or medical intervention is indicated. Unilateral laparoscopic adrenalectomy during the second trimester can be considered in those women with confirmed PA and a clear-cut unilateral adrenal macroadenoma (>10 mm).

Spironolactone crosses the placenta and is a US Food and Drug Administration (FDA) pregnancy category C drug because feminization of newborn male rats has been documented. However, there is only one human case in the medical literature where treatment with spironolactone in pregnancy led to ambiguous genitalia in a male infant; this occurred in a woman treated with spironolactone for polycystic ovary syndrome prepregnancy and through the fifth week of gestation.[6] Eplerenone is an FDA pregnancy category B drug. Therefore, for those pregnant women who will be managed medically, the hypertension should be treated with standard antihypertensive drugs approved for use during pregnancy. Hypokalemia, if present, should be treated with oral potassium supplements. For those patients with refractory hypertension and/or hypokalemia, the addition of eplerenone may be cautiously considered.[7,8]

Key Points

- PA in the setting of pregnancy is a high-risk scenario for both mother and fetus. The most frequent complication is superimposed preeclampsia, which, in some cases, leads to preterm delivery (as occurred in the patient presented herein). The optimal way to prevent this difficult clinical scenario is a broader awareness of PA by clinicians and patients, which should lead to prepregnancy diagnosis and treatment. All woman with hypertension in their reproductive years should have case detection testing for PA—especially before starting a family.

- Case detection testing for PA in pregnancy is the same as in nonpregnant women. However, captopril, CT, and AVS should be avoided.
- Patients with PA in the setting of pregnancy can be managed successfully with standard antihypertensive medications and potassium supplementation. Another treatment option is laparoscopic adrenalectomy during the second trimester—assuming that a unilateral adrenal macroadenoma is identified on MRI. Treatment with spironolactone should be avoided.

REFERENCES

1. Zelinka T, Petrák O, Rosa J, Holaj R, Štrauch B, Widimský J Jr. Primary aldosteronism and pregnancy. *Kidney Blood Press Res*. 2020;45(2):275–285.
2. Campino C, Trejo P, Carvajal CA, et al. Pregnancy normalized familial hyperaldosteronism type I: a novel role for progesterone? *J Hum Hypertens*. 2015;29(2):138–139.
3. Ronconi V, Turchi F, Zennaro MC, Boscaro M, Giacchetti G. Progesterone increase counteracts aldosterone action in a pregnant woman with primary aldosteronism. *Clin Endocrinol (Oxf)*. 2011;74(2):278–279.
4. Albiger NM, Sartorato P, Mariniello B, et al. A case of primary aldosteronism in pregnancy: do LH and GNRH receptors have a potential role in regulating aldosterone secretion? *Eur J Endocrinol*. 2011;164(3):405–412.
5. Teo AE, Brown MJ. Pregnancy, primary aldosteronism, and somatic CTNNB1 mutations. *N Engl J Med*. 2016;374(15):1494.
6. Shah A. Ambiguous genitalia in a newborn with spironolactone exposure (abstract). *93rd Annual Meeting of the Endocrine Society*. 2011;4:227.
7. Riester A, Reincke M. Progress in primary aldosteronism: mineralocorticoid receptor antagonists and management of primary aldosteronism in pregnancy. *Eur J Endocrinol*. 2015;172(1):R23–R30.
8. Cabassi A, Rocco R, Berretta R, Regolisti G, Bacchi-Modena A. Eplerenone use in primary aldosteronism during pregnancy. *Hypertension*. 2012;59(2):e18–e19.

Index

Page numbers followed by *f* indicate figures, *t* indicate tables, and *b* indicate boxes.

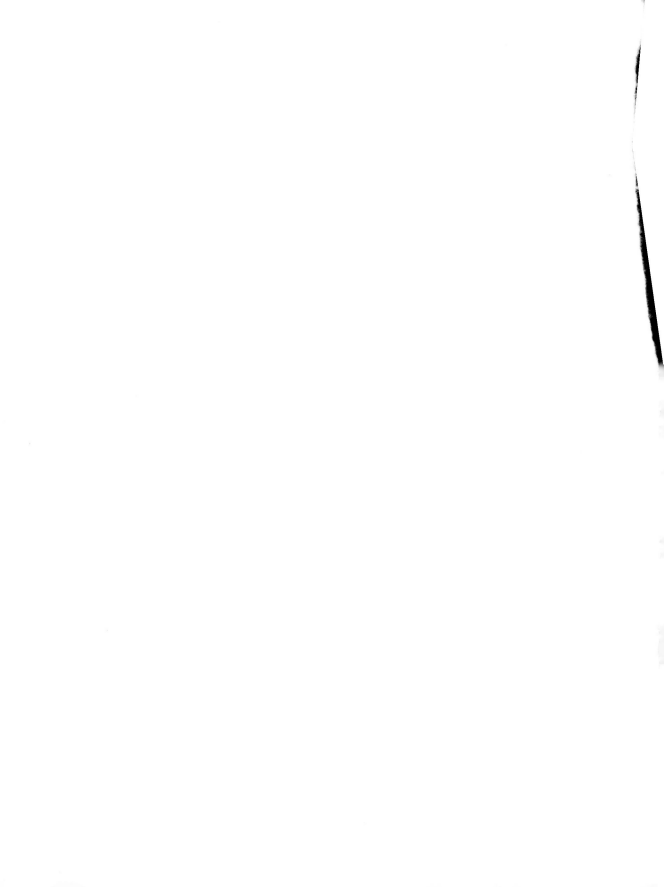